THE AMERICAN PSYCHIATRIC ASSOCIATION PUBLISHING
TEXTBOOK OF
SCHIZOPHRENIA

SECOND EDITION

The American Psychiatric Association Publishing

Textbook of
SCHIZOPHRENIA

SECOND EDITION

Edited by

Jeffrey A. Lieberman, M.D.
T. Scott Stroup, M.D., M.P.H.
Diana O. Perkins, M.D., M.P.H.
Lisa B. Dixon, M.D., M.P.H.

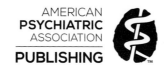

AMERICAN
PSYCHIATRIC
ASSOCIATION
PUBLISHING

If you wish to buy 50 or more copies of the same title, please go to www.appi.org/specialdiscounts for more information.

Copyright © 2020 American Psychiatric Association Publishing

ALL RIGHTS RESERVED

Second Edition

Manufactured in the United States of America on acid-free paper
24   23   22   21   20   5   4   3   2   1

American Psychiatric Association Publishing
800 Maine Avenue SW
Suite 900
Washington, DC 20024-2812
www.appi.org

Library of Congress Cataloging-in-Publication Data
Names: Lieberman, Jeffrey A., 1948- editor. | Stroup, T. Scott, 1960- editor. | Perkins, Diana O., 1958- editor. | Dixon, Lisa B., editor. | American Psychiatric Association, issuing body.
Title: The American Psychiatric Association Publishing textbook of schizophrenia / edited by Jeffrey A. Lieberman, T. Scott Stroup, Diana O. Perkins, Lisa B. Dixon.
Other titles: American Psychiatric Publishing textbook of schizophrenia | Textbook of schizophrenia
Description: Second edition. | Washington, D.C. : American Psychiatric Association Publishing, [2020] | Preceded by The American Psychiatric Publishing textbook of schizophrenia / edited by Jeffrey A. Lieberman, T. Scott Stroup, Diana O. Perkins. 1st ed. c2006. | Includes bibliographical references and index.
Identifiers: LCCN 2019045877 (print) | LCCN 2019045878 (ebook) | ISBN 9781615371723 (hardcover ; alk. paper) | ISBN 9781615372911 (epub)
Subjects: MESH: Schizophrenia
Classification: LCC RC514 (print) | LCC RC514 (ebook) | NLM WM 203 | DDC 616.89/8–dc23
LC record available at https://lccn.loc.gov/2019045877
LC ebook record available at https://lccn.loc.gov/2019045878

British Library Cataloguing in Publication Data
A CIP record is available from the British Library.

Contents

Contributors ix

Preface xiii

PART I

Presentation of Schizophrenia

1 Epidemiology 3

Bernardo Ng, M.D., DFAPA
Stephanie Martinez, M.D.
Steve Koh, M.D.
Mauricio Tohen, M.D., Dr.P.H., M.B.A.
James E. Gangwisch, Ph.D.

2 Natural History 13

Diana O. Perkins, M.D., M.P.H.
Jeffrey A. Lieberman, M.D.

3 Psychopathology 35

Ryan E. Lawrence, M.D.
Michael B. First, M.D.

4 Cultural Variations 53

Neil Krishan Aggarwal, M.D., M.B.A., M.A.
Roberto Lewis-Fernández, M.D., M.T.S.

PART II

Etiology and Pathophysiology

5 Causes 79

Matcheri S. Keshavan, M.D.
Paulo L. Lizano, M.D., Ph.D.
Seth W. Perry, Ph.D.
Konasale M. Prasad, M.D.
Julio Licinio, M.D., Ph.D.

6 Pathophysiological Theories 105

Donald C. Goff, M.D.

7 Neurobiology 127

L. Fredrik Jarskog, M.D.
T. Wilson Woo, M.D., Ph.D.

PART III

Treatment and Rehabilitative Therapies

8 Pharmacological and Somatic Therapies 149

T. Scott Stroup, M.D., M.P.H.
Diana O. Perkins, M.D., M.P.H.
Daniel C. Javitt, M.D.

9 Psychosocial and Rehabilitative Therapies 185

Alice Medalia, Ph.D.
Alice Saperstein, Ph.D.
Paul Grant, Ph.D.

10 Co-occurring Disorders and Conditions 205

Sarah Pratt, Ph.D.
Melanie Bennett, Ph.D.
Mary F. Brunette, M.D.

11 Evidence-Based Models of Service Delivery 251

Michael T. Compton, M.D., M.P.H.
Marc W. Manseau, M.D., M.P.H.

12 Person- and Family-Centered Care 273

Nev Jones, Ph.D.
Lisa B. Dixon, M.D., M.P.H.

Index 289

Contributors

Neil Krishan Aggarwal, M.D., M.B.A., M.A.
Assistant Professor of Clinical Psychiatry, Department of Psychiatry, Columbia University Medical Center; Research Psychiatrist, New York State Psychiatric Institute, New York, New York

Melanie Bennett, Ph.D.
Professor of Psychiatry, Department of Psychiatry, University of Maryland School of Medicine, Baltimore, Maryland

Mary F. Brunette, M.D.
Associate Professor of Psychiatry, Department of Psychiatry, Geisel School of Medicine at Dartmouth, Hanover, Dartmouth-Hitchcock Medical Center, Lebanon, New Hampshire

Michael T. Compton, M.D., M.P.H.
Professor of Psychiatry, Department of Psychiatry, Columbia University Vagelos College of Physicians and Surgeons; New York State Psychiatric Institute, New York, New York

Lisa B. Dixon, M.D., M.P.H.
Edna L. Edison Professor of Psychiatry, Columbia University Vagelos College of Physicians and Surgeons; Director, Division of Behavioral Health Services and Policy Research and Center for Practice Innovations, New York State Psychiatric Institute, New York, New York

Michael B. First, M.D.
Professor of Clinical Psychiatry, Department of Psychiatry, Columbia University Irving Medical Center, New York, New York

James E. Gangwisch, Ph.D.
Assistant Professor of Clinical Psychiatric Social Work (in Psychiatry), Columbia University Irving Medical Center, New York, New York

Donald C. Goff, M.D.
Marvin Stern Professor of Psychiatry and Vice Chair for Research, Department of Psychiatry, NYU School of Medicine, New York; Director, Nathan Kline Institute for Psychiatric Research, Orangeburg, New York

Paul Grant, Ph.D.
Research Assistant Professor of Psychology, Department of Psychiatry, Perelman School of Medicine, University of Pennsylvania, Philadelphia, Pennsylvania

L. Fredrik Jarskog, M.D.
Professor and Director, North Carolina Psychiatric Research Center, Department of Psychiatry, University of North Carolina at Chapel Hill, Chapel Hill, North Carolina

Daniel C. Javitt, M.D.
Professor of Psychiatry, Columbia University Vagelos College of Physicians and Surgeons, New York, New York; Director, Division of Experimental Therapeutics, New York State Psychiatric Institute; Director, Schizophrenia Research, Nathan Kline Institute for Psychiatric Research, Orangeburg, New York

Nev Jones, Ph.D.
Assistant Professor, Department of Psychiatry and Behavioral Neurosciences, Morsani College of Medicine, University of South Florida, Tampa, Florida

Matcheri S. Keshavan, M.D.
Stanley Cobb Professor and Vice-Chair for Public Psychiatry, Department of Psychiatry, Beth Israel Deaconess Medical Center and Massachusetts Mental Health Center, Harvard Medical School, Boston, Massachusetts

Steve Koh, M.D.
Associate Professor and Director, Outpatient Psychiatric Services, Hillcrest; Director, Community Psychiatry Program; Director, TeleMentalHealth Program, University of California, San Diego, California

Ryan E. Lawrence, M.D.
Assistant Professor, Department of Psychiatry, Columbia University Irving Medical Center, New York, New York

Roberto Lewis-Fernández, M.D., M.T.S.
Professor of Clinical Psychiatry, Department of Psychiatry, Columbia University Medical Center; Director, New York State Center of Excellence for Cultural Competence, New York, New York

Julio Licinio, M.D., Ph.D.
Professor of Psychiatry, Pharmacology, and Medicine; Dean, College of Medicine; and Senior Vice President and Executive Dean, SUNY Upstate Medical University, Syracuse, New York

Jeffrey A. Lieberman, M.D.
Lawrence C. Kolb Professor and Chairman of Psychiatry, Columbia University Vagelos College of Physicians and Surgeons; Director, New York State Psychiatric Institute; Psychiatrist-in-Chief, NewYork-Presbyterian Hospital-Columbia University Irving Medical Center, New York, New York

Paulo L. Lizano, M.D., Ph.D.
Instructor in Psychiatry, Department of Psychiatry, Beth Israel Deaconess Medical Center, Boston, Massachusetts

Marc W. Manseau, M.D., M.P.H.
Clinical Assistant Professor, Department of Psychiatry, New York University School of Medicine, New York, New York

Stephanie Martinez, M.D.
Resident Physician, Department of Psychiatry, University of California, San Diego, California

Alice Medalia, Ph.D.
Professor of Medical Psychology, Department of Psychiatry, Columbia University Vagelos College of Physicians and Surgeons, New York, New York

Bernardo Ng, M.D., DFAPA
Medical Director, Sun Valley Behavioral and Research Centers; Clinical Assistant Professor, Department of Psychiatry, University of California, San Diego, California

Diana O. Perkins, M.D., M.P.H.
Professor, Department of Psychiatry, University of North Carolina School of Medicine, Chapel Hill, North Carolina

Seth W. Perry, Ph.D.
Associate Professor of Psychiatry and of Neuroscience and Physiology, College of Medicine, SUNY Upstate Medical University, Syracuse, New York

Konasale M. Prasad, M.D.
Associate Professor, Departments of Psychiatry and Bioengineering, University of Pittsburgh; Investigator, Veterans Affairs Pittsburgh Health System, Pittsburgh, Pennsylvania

Sarah Pratt, Ph.D.
Assistant Professor of Psychiatry, Department of Psychiatry, Geisel School of Medicine at Dartmouth, Hanover, Dartmouth-Hitchcock Medical Center, Lebanon, New Hampshire

Alice Saperstein, Ph.D.
Assistant Professor of Medical Psychology, Department of Psychiatry, Columbia University Vagelos College of Physicians and Surgeons, New York, New York

T. Scott Stroup, M.D., M.P.H.
Professor of Psychiatry and Vice Chair for Academic Affairs and Faculty Development, Department of Psychiatry, Columbia University Vagelos College of Physicians and Surgeons, New York, New York

Mauricio Tohen, M.D., Dr.P.H., M.B.A.
Professor and Chairman, Department of Psychiatry and Behavioral Sciences, University of New Mexico Health Sciences Center, Albuquerque, New Mexico

T. Wilson Woo, M.D., Ph.D.
Director, Laboratory of Cellular Neuropathology, Department of Psychiatry, Harvard Medical School, Boston, Massachusetts

Disclosure of Competing Interests

The following contributors to this book have indicated a financial interest in or other affiliation with a commercial supporter, a manufacturer of a commercial product, a provider of a commercial service, a nongovernmental organization, and /or a government agency, as listed below:

Michael B. First, M.D.   *Faculty member*: Lundbeck International Neuroscience Foundation; *Author*: Chapter in the *Merck Manual*

L. Fredrik Jarskog, M.D.   *Research grant support*: In past 12 months from Teva/Auspex, Boehringer Ingelheim, Otsuka, and National Institutes of Health

Matcheri S. Keshavan, M.D.   *Consultant*: Alkermes Pharmaceuticals

Alice Medalia, Ph.D.   Oxford University Press, Boehringer Ingelheim, Otsuka America Pharmaceutical

Diana O. Perkins, M.D., M.P.H.   *Consultant*: Alkermes; *Funding support*: Boehringer Ingelheim for a sponsored research study

Alice Saperstein, Ph.D.   *Royalties*: Oxford University Press

T. Scott Stroup, M.D., M.P.H.   *Participant*: CME presentation for Medscape, sponsored by an independent educational grant from Intra-Cellular Therapies, Inc.

The following contributors to this book have indicated no competing interests to disclose during the year preceding manuscript submission:

Neil Krishan Aggarwal, M.D., M.B.A., M.A.; Melanie Bennett, Ph.D.; Mary F. Brunette, M.D.; Michael T. Compton, M.D., M.P.H.; Lisa B. Dixon, M.D., M.P.H.; James E. Gangwisch, Ph.D.; Donald C. Goff, M.D.; Paul Grant, Ph.D.; Steve Koh, M.D.; Ryan E. Lawrence, M.D.; Roberto Lewis-Fernández, M.D., M.T.S.; Julio Licinio, M.D., Ph.D.; Jeffrey A. Lieberman, M.D.; Paulo L. Lizano, M.D., Ph.D.; Marc W. Manseau, M.D., M.P.H.; Stephanie Martinez, M.D.; Bernardo Ng, M.D., D.F.A.P.A.; Seth W. Perry, Ph.D.; Konasale M. Prasad, M.D.; Sarah Pratt, Ph.D.; Mauricio Tohen, M.D., Dr.P.H., M.B.A.; T. Wilson Woo, M.D., Ph.D.

Preface

Schizophrenia remains the most challenging of mental disorders confronted by psychiatrists and other mental health providers. Its primary manifestations—psychotic symptoms and cognitive impairment—profoundly affect functioning. Because schizophrenia typically begins as people approach or enter adulthood and persists indefinitely, it is one of the leading causes of disability worldwide. Researchers have made substantial but uneven progress in understanding this brain disorder since the first edition of this textbook was published in 2006. Rapid progress in knowledge about genetics and neurobiology has not been accompanied by breakthroughs in pharmacotherapy. However, new models of service delivery and psychosocial treatments are making a difference in people's lives.

An updated textbook covering the current state of knowledge about schizophrenia, including its causes, nature, and treatment, is now warranted. We invited a roster of experts to join us in creating this work by writing chapters on specific topics. We are grateful to them for their outstanding scholarly contributions.

Part I, "Presentation of Schizophrenia," begins with a chapter on epidemiology that discusses risk factors and outcomes in addition to descriptive epidemiology. Chapter 2 focuses on stages of illness and the course of schizophrenia, including how antipsychotics and other factors affect prognosis. The symptoms of schizophrenia and its diagnosis are described in Chapter 3. Chapter 4 examines how culture influences the presentation of schizophrenia from the perspective of experts in cultural psychiatry who developed the DSM-5 Cultural Formulation Interview.

Part II, "Etiology and Pathophysiology," is largely based on research conducted since the first edition of this textbook was published in 2006. Chapter 5 describes genetic, environmental, and epigenetic causes of schizophrenia. Chapter 6 reviews pathophysiological theories of schizophrenia, including genetic, molecular, and circuit models. Chapter 7, on neurobiology, discusses schizophrenia's histopathology and neurochemistry.

Part III, "Treatment and Rehabilitative Therapies," explores clinical aspects of schizophrenia and interventions. Chapter 8 focuses on medications and somatic therapies; although there have been no breakthroughs with new pharmacotherapies, more is now known about how to use existing treatments, including adjunctive medications and combinations of antipsychotics. The promising field of neuromodulation is also discussed. Chapter 9 shifts attention to evidence-based psychosocial treatments and their deployment. Chapter 10 covers the evaluation and treatment of comorbidities, including substance use disorders and psychiatric conditions. Chapter 11 describes service delivery models with a focus on how to provide services to individuals with schizophrenia; included are assertive community treatment, critical time intervention, coordinated specialty care for early psychosis, and integrated dual diagnosis treatment. Finally, Chapter 12 presents the rationale and evidence for actively involving patients and family members in interventions and in decision making about treatments.

Jeffrey A. Lieberman, M.D.

T. Scott Stroup, M.D., M.P.H.

Diana O. Perkins, M.D., M.P.H.

Lisa B. Dixon, M.D., M.P.H.

PART I

Presentation of Schizophrenia

CHAPTER 1

Epidemiology

Bernardo Ng, M.D., DFAPA
Stephanie Martinez, M.D.
Steve Koh, M.D.
Mauricio Tohen, M.D., Dr.P.H., M.B.A.
James E. Gangwisch, Ph.D.

Epidemiological studies of schizophrenia have provided improved estimates of its incidence and prevalence, clues about etiology, and impetus for further research into potential risk and protective factors for the disorder. Schizophrenia is theorized to originate from a disruption in brain development from faulty interaction among genes and between genes and the environment (Owen et al. 2016), eventually crossing a threshold of clinical expression (Stilo and Murray 2010). The complex etiology of schizophrenia and its heterogeneous behavioral and cognitive symptoms make the interpretation of epidemiological findings challenging (Owen et al. 2016). According to the World Health Organization (2016, 2018), schizophrenia affects 12 million men and 9 million women around the world, but the prevalence varies widely by region. The lifetime prevalence of schizophrenia has been estimated to be between 0.3% and 0.7% of the general population, but this is affected by demographic, social, economic, health, cultural, and genetic factors (American Psychiatric Association 2013). Outcomes of schizophrenia vary by patient age, paternal age, gender, ethnic group, location (i.e., urban vs. rural), geographical site (i.e., country or region), climate, migratory status, month of birth, childhood and adult adversity, relocation, and socioeconomic level (American Psychiatric Association 2013; McGrath 2006; Owen et al. 2016). This chapter provides a review of prevalence and incidence estimates and their variation by demographic and other risk factors. Associated comorbidities and selected outcomes are also discussed.

Descriptive Epidemiology

The estimated incidence of schizophrenia per year is approximately 15 per 100,000 males and 10 per 100,000 females. The estimated point prevalence of schizophrenia is 4.6–5 per

1,000 people, and the lifetime risk is 0.7 per 100 (Messias et al. 2007; Owen et al. 2016). One systematic review included a total of 56 epidemiological studies from Europe ($n=29$), Asia ($n=13$), North America ($n=10$), Africa ($n=8$), and Oceania ($n=4$) published from 1990 through 2013 (Simeone et al. 2015). Lifetime prevalence of schizophrenia ranged from a low of 0.06% in Tanzania to a high of 1.46% in Canada and 1.54% in Finland. The review's authors concluded that among the general population, approximately 1 in 200 people will be diagnosed with schizophrenia at some point during their lifetime.

The typical age at onset of schizophrenia is late adolescence, with men generally experiencing an earlier onset than women. The concept of late-onset schizophrenia—the emergence of nonaffective, nonorganic psychotic symptoms after age 45—has been widely discussed. A 3-year longitudinal study from the Netherlands Mental Health Survey and Incidence Study divided 5,618 subjects into three groups based on age: young (18–34 years), middle (35–49 years), and older (50–64 years) (Köhler et al. 2007). The researchers found the cumulative incidence for psychosis onset to be surprisingly similar for each age group (1.3% for young, 1.1% for middle, and 0.8% for older), with a nonsignificant difference between groups ($P=0.097$). These findings highlight the possibility of a higher incidence than expected at older ages of new-onset psychotic symptoms attributable to schizophrenia. Women have an increased risk of developing schizophrenia around menopause, often referred to as the second peak of onset. This elevated risk may be due to the loss of antidopaminergic action of estrogens (Messias et al. 2007; Owen et al. 2016; Stilo and Murray 2010).

Schizophrenia is more common in men than in women. The degree to which schizophrenia prevalence among men surpasses that among women varies according to study type and region. Multiple meta-analyses have found that approximately 60% of those who develop schizophrenia are men (Aleman et al. 2003; Longenecker et al. 2010; McGrath et al. 2004, 2008). The consistency of these results helps rule out systematic bias in diagnostic systems and confirms that the disease is more prevalent among males. It appears, however, that nonepidemiological studies have historically exaggerated this disparity. In a review of 220 articles, investigators found that the proportion of men diagnosed with schizophrenia differed significantly between nonepidemiological and epidemiological studies, with nonepidemiological studies consistently reporting higher proportions of men (Longenecker et al. 2010). These results add to the evidence that men are diagnosed with schizophrenia more frequently than are women but that the gender difference is not as large as once thought.

Risk Factors for Development of Schizophrenia

The dominant paradigm for understanding the environmental contributions to schizophrenia etiology has been the neurodevelopmental hypothesis, which tries to explain the impact of the environment on the development of an individual's brain (Owen et al. 2016). This section provides a review of data on factors external to the individual that have an impact on the epidemiology of schizophrenia.

Ethnicity, Culture, and Immigration

The concept of *ethnicity* includes a wide range of features, including cultural, racial, national, tribal, religious, and linguistic origins and backgrounds. *Culture* is a collection of beliefs, attitudes, shared understandings, knowledge, customs, habits, and patterns of behavior that influence cognitions and social development of individuals. Culture plays a significant role in conceptions of both normality and deviance through which abnormality is defined and identified. The varying prevalence estimates for schizophrenia reported by country are affected by cultural differences. DSM-5 underscores the value of cultural studies to demonstrate the challenge of reliably diagnosing schizophrenia among different populations (American Psychiatric Association 2013). Similarities and differences in the expression of symptoms are closely linked to a patient's ethnicity, social context, cultural background, and degree of comfort and willingness to cooperate during a psychiatric assessment (Eack et al. 2012; McLean et al. 2014). Cultural differences are also likely to impact differences in reporting of disease by native and foreign-born residents.

Immigrants and their descendants have been found to be approximately 2.5 times more likely to have a psychotic disorder than the majority ethnic group in given settings (Cantor-Graae and Selten 2005). There are a number of plausible explanations for immigrants' increased risk for psychosis. Migrants can experience a grief reaction to the loss of language, social structures, and social support. Resettlement can bring difficulties in resuming education, finding work, and obtaining adequate housing and health care. Immigrants are less likely than native-born counterparts to be referred to or to seek out mental health treatment, and finding affordable and linguistically and culturally accessible services presents additional challenges (Shekunov 2016).

Paternal Age

The male germ line is a major source of new mutations in humans. Advanced age of the father at conception increases the mutation rate, likely due to an accumulation of replication errors in spermatogonial cell lines. In a large Israeli birth cohort, older paternal age was a strong and significant predictor of schizophrenia diagnosis. Compared with the risk in offspring of fathers younger than age 25 years, the relative risk (RR) of schizophrenia increased in each 5-year-older age group, doubling the risk in offspring of men ages 45–49 years and almost tripling the risk in children of men 50 years or older (Malaspina et al. 2001). Analyses of data from the Prenatal Determinants of Schizophrenia study also showed that advanced paternal age increased the risk of adult schizophrenia (Brown et al. 2002).

Prenatal Exposure to Infection and Inflammation

Numerous studies have found evidence that infection is a risk factor for schizophrenia. Microbial pathogens that cause disease such as influenza and toxoplasmosis have long been known to cause congenital brain abnormalities. The original studies on influenza and schizophrenia were limited because they were based on whether the individual was in gestation during an influenza epidemic, with no actual confirmation of maternal influenza infection. Consequently, a new approach was necessary to corroborate a connection between schizophrenia and prenatal exposure to infection. Advances were made through birth cohort studies, in which biological specimens were obtained during pregnancy and offspring were systematically assessed longitudinally. Maternal exposure during pregnancy to herpes simplex virus type 2, *Toxoplasma gondii*, and the influenza virus has been found to be associated with increased risk for schizophrenia in offspring (Brown and Derkits 2010). A more recent analysis of Finnish Prenatal Studies data including inflammatory factors revealed that serum C-reactive protein was higher in pregnant women whose offspring later developed schizophrenia (Canetta et al. 2014). One potential mechanism by which infection and inflammation during pregnancy could increase the risk for schizophrenia in offspring is the reduction of iron bioavailability to the developing fetus (Aguilar-Valles et al. 2010).

Infection and Inflammation During Childhood

Khandaker et al. (2012) conducted a systematic review and meta-analysis of seven large population-based cohort studies that included minors with central nervous system (CNS) infection (n=13,458) and control subjects (n=1,218,776). Participants in the studies were followed for the development of schizophrenia (n=1,035). The most commonly identified viral agents—cytomegalovirus, Coxsackie B5, and mumps—accounted for about half of the identified cases. CNS viral infections in childhood were shown to be associated with a greater than twofold increased risk of adult nonaffective psychosis (RR=2.12; 95% confidence interval [CI]=1.17–3.84). The authors proposed that a link between the CNS infection, an inflammatory process, and an immune system dysfunction might explain the increased risk of adult schizophrenia (Khandaker et al. 2012).

Latitude and Seasonality of Birth

Mounting evidence has identified increased distance from the equator and birth during winter or spring as risk factors for schizophrenia. A meta-analysis including 49 prevalence study samples from Africa, east and south Asia, Europe, North America, Argentina, and New Zealand revealed that the prevalence of schizophrenia across these samples varied widely, from 0.09% in Accra, Ghana, near the equator to 2.8% in Oxford Bay, Canada, near the Arctic Circle. The prevalence was greater among samples from geographical locations of higher latitude and colder climate. The correlations of schizophrenia prevalence with latitude (r=0.46, P<0.001) and mean temperature (r=−0.60, P<0.001) were both significant. These findings suggest that the risk of developing schizophrenia may increase with perinatal exposure to adverse environmental factors associated with higher latitudes and lower temperatures (Kinney et al. 2009). In addition, a widely replicated finding indicates that compared with births in the summer or fall, births in the winter or spring are associated with a higher risk of developing schizophrenia (Brown 2011). The seasonal risk has been seen to become even more elevated as the distance from the equator increases. Researchers hypothesize that higher latitude and lower temperature are associated with greater prenatal exposure to infections such as influenza and toxoplasmosis, which in turn may increase the incidence of schizophrenia (Kinney et al. 2009).

Urban Versus Rural Areas

Schizophrenia is overrepresented in the most deprived sectors of society. In 1939, it was reported that there were more schizophrenia-related hospital admissions in the poorer central areas of Chicago than in the suburbs. For a long time, this disparity was explained as the result of preschizophrenic individuals "drifting" into the deprived inner cities. However, studies from Sweden, the Netherlands, Denmark, the United Kingdom, and other countries have shown that the incidence of the disorder is higher among individuals born and raised in urban areas, especially in areas with less social cohesion (Stilo and Murray 2010). In results from analyses of data from the Environmental Risk (E-Risk) Longitudinal Twin Study, which tracks the development of a nationally representative birth cohort of 2,232 British twins, urbanicity was significantly associated with psychotic symptoms by age 12 years (odds ratio [OR]=1.76; 95% CI=1.15–2.69), with almost 25% of the effect explained by low social cohesion and crime victimization by age 5 years (Newbury et al. 2016). A prospective study in France found that the raw incidence of psychotic disorders in urban areas was 36.02 per 100,000 person-years versus 17.2 per 100,000 person-years in rural areas (Szöke et al. 2014). A systematic review of incidence rates of schizophrenia and other forms of psychosis in England from 1950 to 2009 found that the incidence of schizophrenia increased in larger cities (e.g., London) and decreased in smaller cities (e.g., Nottingham) during that time period. Changes in the clinical presentation of the disorder, as well as in diagnostic practice and the organization of mental health services, are thought to have led to these shifting patterns (Kirkbride et al. 2012).

Socioeconomic Status and Disparities

A socioeconomic gradient is observed worldwide for a number of health outcomes (e.g., cancer, coronary heart disease); decrements in social class are associated with increased morbidity and mortality rates. It has long been thought that socioeconomic status may also be causally related to schizophrenia. An Israeli population-based cohort study from 1964 to 1976, which included 88,829 births, followed offspring until schizophrenia diagnosis. The study found that the offspring of fathers in the lowest socioeconomic status category had a 40% increased risk of developing the disorder (RR=1.4; 95% CI =1.1–1.8) (Corcoran et al. 2009). Another Israeli study reported that children born to parents with lower educational attainment or of lower occupational class had an elevated risk for developing schizophrenia (Werner et al. 2007). A systematic review of 110 studies from 28 countries published from 1975 to 2011 explored the relationship between a country's incidence of schizophrenia and its *Gini coefficient*, a commonly used measure of income inequality in which a higher coefficient indicates a higher degree of income inequality. The investigators found that for each one-point increase in the Gini coefficient, there was a two-point increase in the incidence rate of schizophrenia after controlling for urbanization, migration, and unemployment (Burns et al. 2014).

Childhood Trauma and Resilience

Exposure to adverse events in childhood has been found to be associated with a twofold to fourfold increase in risk of psychosis (Morgan and Gayer-Anderson 2016). One cross-sectional study showed that patients with schizophrenia reported more severe childhood trauma (e.g., emotional, physical, sexual abuse), lower resilience, and worse physical health than did nonpsychiatric control subjects (Lee et al. 2018). Childhood traumatic experiences also tend to co-occur, with exposure to one type of adversity increasing the risk for exposure to others, resulting in a cumulative effect on psychosis (Shevlin et al. 2008).

Outcomes

Comorbidities

Individuals with schizophrenia are at greater risk for metabolic and other chronic diseases. A Swedish population-based study found that the most common comorbidities among 7,284 individuals diagnosed with schizophrenia were essential hypertension, diabetes, and obesity. Those ages 50–59 years were seen to have the highest prevalence of these comorbidities compared with other age groups (Brostedt et al. 2017). The higher risk for cardiometabolic disorders may be attributable to metabolic effects of antipsychotic medications, poor nutrition, and lack of physical activity. In spite of having high rates of these disorders, patients with schizophrenia have lower than expected rates of diagnosis and treatment for cardiovascular disorders (Smith et al. 2013).

Premature Mortality

Individuals with schizophrenia have a significant reduction in life expectancy. Mortality increase is due to both natural and unnatural causes, which result in an estimated 10- to 15-year decrease in life expectancy (Bushe et al. 2010; Healy et al. 2012). A review of eight studies identified suicide (0%–46%), cardiovascular disease (12%–49%), cancer (7%–21%), accidents (4%–10%), cerebrovascular disease (3%–8%), and respiratory disease (17%) as the most common causes of premature death in those with schizophrenia (Bushe et al. 2010). Individuals with schizophrenia are two to three times more likely to die at younger ages than the general population (World Health Organization 2016, 2018).

Suicide and Other Unnatural Deaths

Up to 40% of the excess risk for premature death among those with schizophrenia is attributable to suicide and other unnatural deaths (Bushe et al. 2010). For individuals with schizophrenia, the lifetime suicide risk is estimated at 4%–6% (Palmer et al. 2005; Popovic et al. 2014). A systematic review conducted by a task force of experts and clinicians (Popovic et al. 2014) found that suicide risk in individuals with schizophrenia is highly correlated with affective symptoms, a history of suicide attempts, and number of psychiatric admissions. Other risk factors identified for suicide include younger age, proximity to illness onset, older age at illness onset, male sex, substance use, and the period during or following psychiatric discharge. Other causes of unnatural death include homicide and accidents. In a study of Medicaid recipients in the United States, accidents were found to account for more than twice as many deaths as suicide among adults with schizophrenia (Olfson et al. 2015). Drug-induced deaths, whether accidental or intentional, were a common source of mortality.

Substance Use and Substance Use Disorders

Substance use and misuse are common among people with schizophrenia, and their presence increases the risk of suicide, nonpsychiatric comorbidities, and premature mortality (Fazel et al. 2009; Sharifi et al. 2015). A large Swedish study found a 7.9% 1-year prevalence of substance use disorder among individuals with schizophrenia and a 24.8% 12-year prevalence (Brostedt et al. 2017). A review of the association between cannabis use and psychosis found that cannabis use increased the risk for development of schizophrenia. After controlling for multiple factors, Radhakrishnan and colleagues (2014) found that more frequent consumption (50 times or more in lifetime) and earlier use (<15 years of age) were associated with psychotic symptoms. The legalization of medicinal and recreational use of cannabis in certain parts of the world has therefore raised questions about its impact on mental health and specifically on the incidence of schizophrenia. A statewide study conducted in Colorado, where recreational cannabis use has been legal since 2012, showed a fivefold higher prevalence of mental health diagnoses in cannabis-associated emergency department visits compared with visits not involving cannabis (Hall et al. 2018).

Violent Behavior

Individuals with schizophrenia and other psychoses are at increased risk for engaging in violent behavior. A systematic review and meta-analysis of 20 studies found that schizophrenia and other psychoses were associated with interpersonal violence and violent criminality, particularly homicide. For men, the ORs for violence committed by those with schizophrenia and other psychoses versus those of general population samples ranged from 1 to 7 with considerable heterogeneity; in women, the ORs ranged from 4 to 29 with substantial variation. Most excess risk was attributable to substance use (Fazel et al. 2009). In a systematic review and meta-regression analysis of 110 studies, nonadherence to treatment regimens, recent substance misuse, poor impulse control, and criminal history were found to be risk factors for violence in adults with schizophrenia and adults with other psychoses (Witt et al. 2013).

Conclusion

Examination of the epidemiology of schizophrenia provides vital information for health care planning and informs prevention and early intervention efforts. More translational research will be necessary to link epidemiological research with molecular, cellular, and behavioral neuroscience (Messias et al. 2007). Cross-disciplinary projects will help to explore this complex and heterogeneous disease (McGrath and Richards 2009).

References

Aguilar-Valles A, Flores C, Luheshi GN: Prenatal inflammation-induced hypoferremia alters dopamine function in the adult offspring in rat: relevance for schizophrenia. PLoS One 5(6):e10967, 2010 20532043

Aleman A, Kahn RS, Selten JP: Sex differences in the risk of schizophrenia: evidence from meta-analysis. Arch Gen Psychiatry 60(6):565–571, 2003 12796219

American Psychiatric Association: Diagnostic and Statistical Manual of Mental Disorders, 5th Edition. Arlington, VA, American Psychiatric Association, 2013

Brostedt EM, Msghina M, Persson M, et al: Health care use, drug treatment and comorbidity in patients with schizophrenia or non-affective psychosis in Sweden: a cross-sectional study. BMC Psychiatry 17(1):416, 2017 29284436

Brown AS: Prenatal infection as a risk factor for schizophrenia. Schizophr Bull 32(2):200–202, 2006 16469941

Brown AS: The environment and susceptibility to schizophrenia. Prog Neurobiol 93(1):23–58, 2011 20955757

Brown AS, Derkits EJ: Prenatal infection and schizophrenia: a review of epidemiologic and translational studies. Am J Psychiatry 167(3):261–280, 2010 20123911

Brown AS, Schaefer CA, Wyatt RJ, et al: Paternal age and risk of schizophrenia in adult offspring. Am J Psychiatry 159(9):1528–1533, 2002 12202273

Burns JK, Tomita A, Kapadia AS: Income inequality and schizophrenia: increased schizophrenia incidence in countries with high levels of income inequality. Int J Soc Psychiatry 60(2):185–196, 2014 23594564

Bushe CJ, Taylor M, Haukka J: Mortality in schizophrenia: a measurable clinical endpoint. J Psychopharmacol 24(4)(suppl):17–25, 2010 20923917

Canetta S, Sourander A, Surcel HM, et al: Elevated maternal C-reactive protein and increased risk of schizophrenia in a national birth cohort. Am J Psychiatry 171(9):960–968, 2014 24969261

Cantor-Graae E, Selten JP: Schizophrenia and migration: a meta-analysis and review. Am J Psychiatry 162(1):12–24, 2005 15625195

Corcoran C, Perrin M, Harlap S, et al: Effect of socioeconomic status and parents' education at birth on risk of schizophrenia in offspring. Soc Psychiatry Psychiatr Epidemiol 44(4):265–271, 2009 18836884

Eack SM, Bahorik AL, Newhill CE, et al: Interviewer-perceived honesty as a mediator of racial disparities in the diagnosis of schizophrenia. Psychiatr Serv 63(9):875–880, 2012 22751938

Fazel S, Gulati G, Linsell L, et al: Schizophrenia and violence: systematic review and meta-analysis. PLoS Med 6(8):e1000120, 2009 19668362

Hall KE, Monte AA, Chang T, et al: Mental health-related emergency department visits associated with cannabis in Colorado. Acad Emerg Med 25(5):526–537, 2018 29476688

Healy D, Le Noury J, Harris M, et al: Mortality in schizophrenia and related psychoses: data from two cohorts, 1875–1924 and 1994–2010. BMJ Open 2(5):e001810, 2012 23048063

Khandaker GM, Zimbron J, Dalman C, et al: Childhood infection and adult schizophrenia: a meta-analysis of population-based studies. Schizophr Res 139(1–3):161–168, 2012 22704639

Kinney DK, Teixeira P, Hsu D, et al: Relation of schizophrenia prevalence to latitude, climate, fish consumption, infant mortality, and skin color: a role for prenatal vitamin D deficiency and infections? Schizophr Bull 35(3):582–595, 2009 19357239

Kirkbride JB, Errazuriz A, Croudace TJ, et al: Incidence of schizophrenia and other psychoses in England, 1950–2009: a systematic review and meta-analyses. PLoS One 7(3):e31660, 2012 22457710

Köhler S, van Os J, de Graaf R, et al: Psychosis risk as a function of age at onset: a comparison between early- and late-onset psychosis in a general population sample. Soc Psychiatry Psychiatr Epidemiol 42(4):288–294, 2007 17370045

Lee EE, Martin AS, Tu X, et al: Childhood adversity and schizophrenia: the protective role of resilience in mental and physical health and metabolic markers. J Clin Psychiatry 79(3):17m11776, 2018 29701938

Longenecker J, Genderson J, Dickinson D, et al: Where have all the women gone? Participant gender in epidemiological and non-epidemiological research of schizophrenia. Schizophr Res 119(1–3):240–245, 2010 20399612

Malaspina D, Harlap S, Fennig S, et al: Advancing paternal age and the risk of schizophrenia. Arch Gen Psychiatry 58(4):361–367, 2001 11296097

McGrath JJ: Variations in the incidence of schizophrenia: data versus dogma. Schizophr Bull 32(1):195–197, 2006 16135560

McGrath JJ, Richards LJ: Why schizophrenia epidemiology needs neurobiology—and vice versa. Schizophr Bull 35(3):577–581, 2009 19273583

McGrath J, Saha S, Welham J, et al: A systematic review of the incidence of schizophrenia: the distribution of rates and the influence of sex, urbanicity, migrant status and methodology. BMC Med 2:13–35, 2004 15115547

McGrath J, Saha S, Chant D, et al: Schizophrenia: a concise overview of incidence, prevalence, and mortality. Epidemiol Rev 30(1):67–76, 2008 18480098

McLean D, Thara R, John S, et al: DSM-IV "Criterion A" schizophrenia symptoms across ethnically different populations: evidence for differing psychotic symptom content or structural organization? Cult Med Psychiatry 38(3):408–426, 2014 24981830

Messias EL, Chen CY, Eaton WW: Epidemiology of schizophrenia: review of findings and myths. Psychiatr Clin North Am 30(3):323–338, 2007 17720026

Morgan C, Gayer-Anderson C: Childhood adversities and psychosis: evidence, challenges, implications. World Psychiatry 15(2):93–102, 2016 27265690

Newbury J, Arseneault L, Caspi A, et al: Why are children in urban neighborhoods at increased risk for psychotic symptoms? Findings from a UK longitudinal cohort study. Schizophr Bull 42(6):1372–1383, 2016 27153864

Olfson M, Gerhard T, Huang C, et al: Premature mortality among adults with schizophrenia in the United States. JAMA Psychiatry 72(12):1172–1181, 2015 26509694

Owen MJ, Sawa A, Mortensen PB: Schizophrenia. Lancet 388(10039):86–97, 2016 26777917

Palmer BA, Pankratz VS, Bostwick JM: The lifetime risk of suicide in schizophrenia: a reexamination. Arch Gen Psychiatry 62(3):247–253, 2005 15753237

Popovic D, Benabarre A, Crespo JM, et al: Risk factors for suicide in schizophrenia: systematic review and clinical recommendations. Acta Psychiatr Scand 130(6):418–426, 2014 25230813

Radhakrishnan R, Wilkinson ST, D'Souza DC: Gone to pot—a review of the association between cannabis and psychosis. Front Psychiatry 5(54):54, 2014 24904437

Sharifi V, Eaton WW, Wu LT, et al: Psychotic experiences and risk of death in the general population: 24-27 year follow-up of the Epidemiologic Catchment Area study. Br J Psychiatry 207(1):30–36, 2015 25953893

Shekunov J: Immigration and risk of psychiatric disorders: a review of existing literature. The American Journal of Psychiatry Residents' Journal 11(2):3–5, 2016

Shevlin M, Houston JE, Dorahy MJ, Adamson G: Cumulative traumas and psychosis: an analysis of the National Comorbidity Survey and the British Psychiatric Morbidity Survey. Schizophr Bull 34(1):193–199, 2008 17586579

Simeone JC, Ward AJ, Rotella P, et al: An evaluation of variation in published estimates of schizophrenia prevalence from 1990–2013: a systematic literature review. BMC Psychiatry 15:193, 2015 26263900

Smith DJ, Langan J, McLean G, et al: Schizophrenia is associated with excess multiple physical-health comorbidities but low levels of recorded cardiovascular disease in primary care: cross-sectional study. BMJ Open 3(4):e002808, 2013 23599376

Stilo SA, Murray RM: The epidemiology of schizophrenia: replacing dogma with knowledge. Dialogues Clin Neurosci 12(3):305–315, 2010 20954427

Szöke A, Charpeaud T, Galliot AM, et al: Rural-urban variation in incidence of psychosis in France: a prospective epidemiologic study in two contrasted catchment areas. BMC Psychiatry 14:78, 2014 24636392

Werner S, Malaspina D, Rabinowitz J: Socioeconomic status at birth is associated with risk of schizophrenia: population-based multilevel study. Schizophr Bull 33(6):1373–1378, 2007 17443013

Witt K, van Dorn R, Fazel S: Risk factors for violence in psychosis: systematic review and meta-regression analysis of 110 studies. PLoS One 8(2):e55942, 2013 23418482

World Health Organization: Information sheet: Premature death among people with severe mental disorders, 2016. Available at: http://www.who.int/mental_health/management/info_sheet.pdf?ua=1. Accessed May 21, 2019.

World Health Organization: Schizophrenia, fact sheet, April 9, 2018. Available at: http://www.who.int/en/news-room/fact-sheets/detail/schizophrenia. Accessed May 21, 2019.

CHAPTER 2

Natural History

Diana O. Perkins, M.D., M.P.H.

Jeffrey A. Lieberman, M.D.

Schizophrenia typically emerges in late adolescence to early adulthood (Huber and Gross 1989; Mayer-Gross 1932). Most individuals who develop schizophrenia have a chronic course. However, the severity of positive, negative, cognitive, and mood symptoms is highly variable, as is the course of social and vocational disability. Long-term outcomes range from sustained, complete recovery to severe disability from chronic residual symptoms. In this chapter, we review the stages of illness and the variable course that characterize schizophrenia. We also examine long-term outcomes, as well as factors that impact prognosis, including pharmacological and psychotherapeutic treatments.

Stages of Illness

The natural history of schizophrenia may be conceptualized in stages that include premorbid, prodromal, first-episode, early-course, and chronic phases. The duration, course, and severity of symptoms in each phase are highly variable.

Premorbid Phase

Premorbid phase refers to the period before the emergence of psychotic symptoms. Childhood premorbid features include delayed motor milestones (Filatova et al. 2017), deficits in cognitive function (Mollon et al. 2018), and measured IQ that is on average 8 points lower than expected (Fuller et al. 2002; Khandaker et al. 2011). During adolescence, cognitive functions—especially information processing speed, attention, and verbal memory—further decline (Mollon and Reichenberg 2018; Mollon et al. 2018). Social understanding and social function are also impaired (Niemi et al. 2003). However, the distribution of cognitive and functional deficits overlaps considerably with that in the general population. Thus, in the premorbid period, most individuals who develop schizophrenia are not clearly distinguishable from their peers.

Prodromal Phase

About 75%–80% of individuals who go on to develop schizophrenia experience a pro-dromal phase, marked by attenuated, subsyndromal, psychotic-like symptoms prior to the onset of frank psychosis (Häfner and an der Heiden 1999). Attenuated psy-chotic symptoms involve disturbances in thought content, thought process, percep-tion, and abilities to organize thoughts and behaviors that are compelling, are disturbing, and impact function. The symptoms occur relatively frequently, at least several times a month. The main feature that distinguishes attenuated psychotic symptoms from fully psychotic symptoms is retention of insight. The person experi-encing attenuated psychotic symptoms understands that the experiences are not real and that his or her "mind is playing tricks."

Other symptoms characteristic of schizophrenia, including negative symptoms, typically emerge during the prodromal phase (Piskulic et al. 2012). By the time that prodromal symptoms emerge, cognitive impairments are at the severity level found in persons with first-episode schizophrenia (Bora and Murray 2014). Dysphoric moods, such as depression, anxiety, and irritability, are common; about 75% of persons with attenuated psychotic symptoms meet criteria for a mood or anxiety disorder (Addington et al. 2017). Attenuated psychotic, negative, cognitive, and mood symp-toms typically impair a person's ability to function at school, at work, or in social situ-ations, and the functional difficulties are often what brings the person to clinical attention. Much of the decline in social and occupational function associated with schizophrenia occurs during the prodromal phase, prior to the onset of frank psychosis (Velthorst et al. 2017, 2018).

It is critical to appreciate that attenuated psychotic symptoms indicate elevated risk but not a certainty of developing a schizophrenia spectrum disorder. Persons with attenuated psychosis meeting research criteria for a high-risk psychosis syndrome have approximately a 25% risk of developing a psychotic disorder within 2 years and about a 30%–35% risk within 5 years of follow-up (Fusar-Poli et al. 2012). Among non-converters, roughly half continue to experience attenuated symptoms and about half experience complete remission of the symptoms (Simon et al. 2013).

Interventions alter the likelihood of conversion to psychosis in a person experiencing attenuated psychosis symptoms (Davies et al. 2018). Meta-analyses of psychotherapy studies find moderate effects, with the risk of subsequent psychosis reduced by about half (Devoe et al. 2019; Hutton and Taylor 2014). The results of studies examining an-tipsychotics have been mixed (Deas et al. 2016). Importantly, antipsychotics are not considered first-line treatment, because the majority of persons with attenuated psy-chosis are not actually prodromal for schizophrenia and because psychotherapy ap-pears similarly effective without carrying the risks of antipsychotics. Pharmacological interventions targeting glutamate receptors are promising (Lieberman et al. 2018). There are conflicting results from trials that tested whether omega-3 fatty acids pre-vent conversion to psychosis (Amminger et al. 2010; Cadenhead et al. 2017).

Onset of Schizophrenia

Typically, schizophrenia spectrum disorders, including schizophrenia, schizoaffec-tive disorder, and schizophreniform disorder, emerge in late adolescence or early adulthood, with the period of highest risk in the decade between ages 20 and 30 (van der Werf et al. 2014). The risk of schizophrenia is higher in men than in women prior to age 30, but the risk is higher in women than in men after age 30. Overall, the risk of schizophrenia is slightly (about 15%) higher for men (van der Werf et al. 2014).

The emergence of symptoms varies on a spectrum ranging from abrupt, over days to weeks, to insidious, over months to years. For about half of individuals who develop psychotic symptoms, the emergence of psychosis is relatively acute, occurring over a period of a month or less (Harrison et al. 2001).

Course and End State After the First Episode

The course of illness after the first episode of psychosis is variable. Psychotic symptoms may remit or persist at varying levels of severity and may recur or worsen episodically. Associated symptoms, including negative symptoms, mood symptoms, and cognitive impairments, range from being nondetectable to severe. Social and vocational functioning ranges from premorbid levels to severe impairments. The severity of symptoms and level of disability often stabilize after 5–10 years, ranging from chronic severe symptoms and disability to complete recovery and return to premorbid level of function. Persons with schizophrenia have elevated mortality rates; important contributors to this are increased risks of death due to suicide, accidents, lung diseases, and cardiovascular diseases (Olfson et al. 2015).

Treatment with antipsychotic medications potentially affects the natural course of schizophrenia, increasing the likelihood of psychotic symptom remission, reducing the risk of relapse, and possibly improving the end state. Studies prior to the antipsychotic era shed light on the natural history of schizophrenia, independent of the influence of antipsychotics.

Course and End State Prior to Availability of Antipsychotic Medication

The clinical criteria used to diagnose schizophrenia are still evolving and are an important consideration because the clinical course varies depending on the diagnostic criteria. Diagnostic criteria used today were shaped by the observations of Emil Kraepelin (1919) and Eugen Bleuler (1934) early in the twentieth century, prior to the availability of antipsychotics. Kraepelin developed the concept of *dementia praecox*, a syndrome that required psychosis but often included negative symptoms and cognitive impairments. Kraepelin characterized the course of dementia praecox as either episodic or chronic and as typically progressing toward severe disabling symptoms. However, Kraepelin also observed heterogeneity in the end state and noted that a minority of individuals did not have a progressive course and that complete spontaneous recoveries, while rare, did occur. Kraepelin differentiated dementia praecox from manic-depressive insanity, based on prominent mood symptoms and a more benign course in the latter.

Eugen Bleuler coined the term *schizophrenia* to differentiate it from dementia praecox because "the disease needs not progress as far as dementia and does not always appear *praecociter*, i.e., during puberty or soon after" (Bleuler 1934, p. 373). Bleuler emphasized the cross-sectional presentation rather than the clinical course, with the primary feature of schizophrenia involving disturbances of thought process (delusions, disorganized ideas, poverty of thought) and disorganized speech. The severity of accessory features varied and included disturbances of perception (hallucinations, illusions), affect (mania, depression, anxiety), and cognition (attention, ambivalence, "dementia"), as well as negative symptoms (decreased motivation, blunting of emotions). Bleuler's formulation resulted in the diagnosis of schizophrenia in persons who would today, based on current criteria, be diagnosed with bipolar disorder or depression with psychosis; that is, he included people with disorders that have a better prognosis than does more narrowly defined schizophrenia (Harrison et al. 2001; Modestin et al. 2003).

Course

The contributions of Kraepelin and Blueler provide insights into the course of schizophrenia prior to the use of antipsychotic medications. Both Kraepelin and Bleuler noted schizophrenia's variable course. Kraepelin (1919) observed, "The general course of dementia praecox is very variable" (p. 181), and Bleuler (1934) noted, "This disease may clear up very much or altogether; but if it progresses, it leads to a dementia of a definite character" (p. 373).

Kraepelin (1919) described the course of illness in a cohort of 488 patients with whom he had been involved from the early stages of their illness. He found that 74% of patients had a chronic deteriorating course: "In the majority of cases with a distinctly marked commencement a certain terminal state with unmistakable symptoms of weak-mindedness is usually reached at latest in the course of about two to three years" (p. 181). Regarding the remaining patients, Kraepelin reported, "I myself found real improvement in 26% of my cases, when that of the duration of a few months was also taken into account" (p. 181). He gave an example of such an improved patient:

> We find the patient who up till then appeared to be quite confused in his aimless activity or his hopeless degradation, all at once quiet and reasonable in every way. He knows time and place and the people round about him, remembers all that has happened, even his own nonsensical actions, admits that he is ill, writes a connected and sensible letter to his relatives. (p. 188)

Kraepelin found that the severity of residual symptoms varied in the patients with improvements, with 16 of 488 (3%) "completely well" (p. 183). Kraepelin (1919) also found that most improved patients eventually relapsed. "The fact is of great significance that the course of the disease, as we have seen, is frequently interrupted by more or less complete remissions of the morbid phenomena; the duration of these may amount to a few days or weeks, but also to years and even decades, and then give way to a fresh exacerbation with terminal dementia" (p. 181).

Bleuler (1934) gave a similar description of the course of schizophrenia:

> In every course exacerbations may appear at any time, but after the disease has lasted from two to three decades they are pretty rare. Complete arrests of the diseases are not frequent in asylum patients. In the course of decades an increase of the dementia can usually be noted. Among the more mildly afflicted, who maintain themselves outside of asylums, some seem not to go beyond a certain stage of the disease.
>
> Improvements also may occur at every stage; but they relate primarily, to the accessory symptoms. Schizophrenic dementia itself no longer actually regresses. But to be

sure all acute syndromes show a tendency to disappear, and chronic hallucinations and delusions may also regress, though much more rarely. (p. 190)

Other investigators following Kraepelin's diagnostic conceptualization gave similar descriptions of the courses of "dementia praecox." For example, in a 4.5- to 10-year follow-up of a cohort of 571 hospitalized first-episode patients, 65% never improved, remaining chronically symptomatic and severely disabled (Hunt et al. 1938). Psychotic symptoms remitted for 18% and improved for an additional 17% of patients. Half of these patients relapsed and half did not relapse during the follow-up period, with relapses occurring on average 28 months after discharge. The majority (68%) of patients who relapsed became chronically psychotic. Another 5- to 10-year follow-up study of 519 patients similarly reported that 74% experienced a chronic, unremitting course, with most of these chronic patients continuously hospitalized during the follow-up period (Rupp and Fletcher 1940). Psychotic symptoms remitted for 8% and improved for an additional 18%. Relapses occurred during the follow-up period for 38% of the improved patients; 24% of the relapsed patients did not recover.

To summarize, the "natural" course of schizophrenia as described by studies early in the twentieth century was variable, with two-thirds to three-quarters of patients experiencing a chronic, deteriorating course. The rest experienced "spontaneous" improvements in the severity of psychosis, ranging from partial to complete symptom remission and generally an improvement in function. Most of the improved patients experienced recurrent episodes, sometimes with good recovery between episodes but more often with further functional deterioration, emergence of negative symptoms, cognitive impairments, and/or residual psychosis, resulting in chronic illness and disability. After a period that varied from a few years to a decade or more, patients who were chronically psychotic sometimes experienced a reduction or remission of psychosis; however, these patients typically remained functionally disabled by negative symptoms, cognitive impairments, and disorganization.

End State

The typical outcome for the majority of patients with schizophrenia prior to the availability of antipsychotic medication involved a progressive deterioration that led to severe impairments in capacity to interact with others and to function independently. Kraepelin (1919) described the terminal states with varying severity of negative symptoms, cognitive deficits, mood symptoms, and psychotic symptoms. Manfred Bleuler, the son of Eugen Bleuler, vividly depicted the range of pathology in his outcome rating scale (Bleuler 1978). He described patients with the most severe end state as those

> who never carry on coherent, understandable conversations. They are either mutistic, or they speak in such confusion that, in response to simple questions, an occasionally applicable remark interspersed with confusing nonsense is the best one can expect in the way of a reply, although usually no sensible answers at all can be expected. They either do no work at all, or at best do purely mechanical chores, such as hauling a cart, plucking horse hair, etc., under intensively supervised work-therapy methods. They appear to disregard and to remain indifferent to their surroundings. Any human contact with them is impossible. They require constant care, and usually cause trouble for those who care for them by acts of violence, vocal abuses, noisy behavior, uncleanliness, or their inability to properly and independently care for their bodily needs, etc. (pp. 190–191)

As Bleuler (1978) described, somewhat less severely ill patients "generally behaved as did the seriously idiotic, except that in one respect or another they consistently proved that their mental equipment was better preserved than outward appearance would indicate" (p. 191). Examples include patients who, on occasion, would "thaw out and establish contact"; "unequivocally and regularly reveal thought disturbances, even in conversation on impersonal topics, but who can still communicate in such a way as to convey their thoughts on a subject with reasonable clarity"; or "while remaining totally uncommunicative, still perform hard work or become actively involved in caring for others" (p. 191). Severely ill patients often lived out their lives in institutions. Patients with a mild or moderate end state were able to

> maintain a sensible conversation, at least about topics that do not concern their delusional or hallucinatory experiences, despite the fact that definite, schizophrenia symptoms do exist. Their overt behavior is generally normal, and their illness is not immediately obvious if one becomes involved in conversations. They perform useful work. They live either outside the institution or on quiet wards. (p. 191)

A patient described as recovered

> could be fully employed in gainful work, and...he could reassume his former role in society, particularly in the family as head of the family or, in women, as homemaker in the home. It was further required that his family accept him as "rational"; that is, that he was no longer considered by them as being mentally ill. Brief medical examinations should no longer reveal any psychotic symptoms. (p. 191)

However, a patient was still considered recovered even if a thorough examination revealed "some residues of delusional ideas, faulty perception relative to [his] former psychosis, eccentricity, or constriction in his fields of interest or activity" (p. 192).

In the first half of the twentieth century, several psychiatrists who ran inpatient services conducted long-term follow-up studies of the first-episode schizophrenia patients they had treated, motivated to document the long-term end state of schizophrenia without the benefits of "somatic" treatments, in particular, "shock therapy" (seizures induced by drugs or insulin) (Achté and Apo 1967; Cheney and Drewry 1938; Hastings 1958; Hunt et al. 1938; Rupp and Fletcher 1940). Similar to the descriptions provided by Kraepelin (1919) and Bleuler (1934), these studies provide a sense of the prognosis of schizophrenia without interventions such as shock therapy or antipsychotics. At that time, Kraepelin's conceptualization of schizophrenia dominated in the United States and strongly influenced the schizophrenia diagnostic criteria in use at that time, as set forth in the *Statistical Manual for the Use of Institutions for the Insane* (Kendler 2016; National Committee for Mental Hygiene 1934). Three studies of first-episode schizophrenia (Cheney and Drewry 1938; Hunt et al. 1938; Rupp and Fletcher 1940) used these criteria, which required the presence of hallucinations, delusions, and/or disorganization symptoms but, importantly, did not specify the course or end state. A fourth study (Guttmann et al. 1939) did not specify the diagnostic criteria, but the diagnostic approach described in the paper followed the Kraepelinian conceptualization. The studies listed in Figure 2–1 also used a similar set of criteria to define the clinical state at follow-up, criteria that were in line with the clinical descriptions painted by Manfred Bleuler (see above). "Recovered" included persons who resumed premorbid levels of social function and work function and who were without

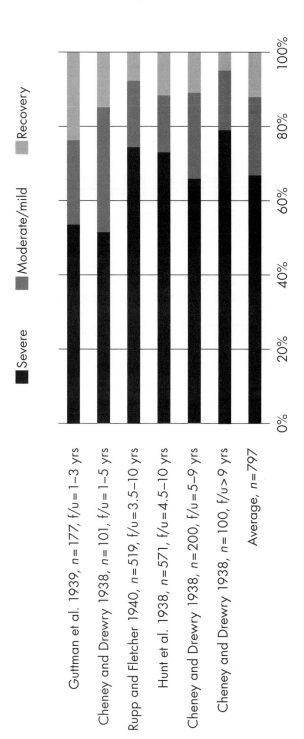

FIGURE 2–1. Long-term outcomes for persons with first-episode schizophrenia never treated with antipsychotics.
f/u=follow-up.

obvious residual psychosis or significant negative symptoms. "Moderately severe/ severe" included those without abatement in severity of psychosis and those who progressed to a "dementia" and required close supervision, either in or outside a psychiatric hospital. "Mild/moderate" included those with improvements in psychotic symptoms, an ability to interact socially with others, and an ability to perform some sort of work (as either an inpatient or outpatient).

As shown in Figure 2–1, the long-term outcomes were similar to those described by Bleuler (1934) and Kraepelin (1919); on average, 67% were severely ill, 21% had mild to moderate symptoms and varying ability to function socially and vocationally, and 12% were categorized as completely recovered. Consistent with the fact that most patients with spontaneous improvements from a first episode relapsed and the fact that patients might not fully recover from relapses, studies with longer duration of follow-up reported greater proportions of patients with severe outcomes.

Studies of hospital admission cohorts may include patients who, during a previous hospitalization, recovered sufficiently to be discharged and thus are potentially biased to patients with better prognoses. Nevertheless, follow-up studies of admission schizophrenia cohorts identified at various stages, diagnosed within Kraepelin's (Bond and Braceland 1937; Hastings 1958; Rennie and Fowler 1939; Romano and Ebaugh 1938; Wooton et al. 1935) or Eugen Bleuler's (Malamud and Render 1939) framework, have yielded similar results.

The capricious nature of schizophrenia challenged the characterization of long-term outcomes. Kraepelin, Eugen Bleuler, and others described cases of spontaneous and unexplained improvements at any point, even after decades of illness. However, the majority of persons who developed schizophrenia prior to the availability of antipsychotic medications in Europe and the United States had an illness that ultimately was socially and vocationally incapacitating. Improvements in psychosis and in function were reported in some patients as they aged, but disability remained severe. A small percentage—up to 5%—experienced just a single episode of psychosis with full recovery.

Course and End State in the Antipsychotic Era

The pharmacological treatment era for schizophrenia began in the early 1950s with chlorpromazine, a drug first used as a preanesthetic by Henri Laborit in 1951. As described by the historian Judith Swazey (1974), Laborit noted the drug's propensity to induce disinterest and so promoted its use to psychiatric colleagues. Pierre Deniker heard about chlorpromazine's effects from his brother-in-law, a surgeon, and with Jean Delay tried chlorpromazine in a series of patients with schizophrenia. Impressed with the results, Deniker and Delay investigated and promoted the use of chlorpromazine, advocating relatively low doses (thus avoiding neurological side effects). By the end of the 1950s, the "antipsychotic era" began, as use of chlorpromazine and other antipsychotics became common practice in the treatment of schizophrenia.

Course

In the mid to late twentieth century, after the introduction of antipsychotics, various investigators developed systems to delineate the course of schizophrenia. These systems characterized the onset (acute vs. insidious), course (episodic or chronic, as well as the level of recovery between episodes), and end state (Carpenter and Kirkpatrick 1988).

Studies generally reported that about 20%–30% of patients experienced a chronic, symptomatic course, with most of the remainder having an episodic course (Bleuler 1978; Harrison et al. 2001; Henry et al. 2010; Kaleda 2008; Revier et al. 2015; Shibre et al. 2015). These studies also reported that most patients received antipsychotic medication. Thus, it is conceivable that the lower proportion of patients with a chronic course in the antipsychotic era (20%–30%) compared with the proportion in the era prior to antipsychotic availability (~60%–75%) was related to antipsychotic medication use, given the clear efficacy of antipsychotics in ameliorating psychotic symptoms.

End State

Since the introduction of antipsychotics, the criteria used by research studies to define a "poor" outcome have shifted to include persons who would have been considered to have mild or moderate outcomes in the preantipsychotic era. For example, modern studies (Crumlish et al. 2009; Harrison et al. 2001; Möller et al. 2011) often defined poor outcome as a score of less than 60 on the Global Assessment of Functioning (GAF) Scale (Hall 1995). However, GAF scores of 31 and 60 are consistent with moderate symptoms as described by Bleuler (1978) (see above). Thus, many of the participants classified as having a poor outcome in modern studies would have been rated as having moderate outcome using criteria from the preantipsychotic era studies. Severe illness outcomes as described by studies from the preantipsychotic era and by Bleuler's scale (1978) are consistent with a GAF score of less than 31: "Behavior is considerably influenced by delusions or hallucinations OR serious impairment in communication or judgment...OR inability to function in almost all areas."

Several studies of first-episode schizophrenia cohorts diagnosed after the mid-1950s provided GAF ratings and/or used Bleuler's (1978) characterization of end state, which allowed classification of long-term outcome by criteria comparable to those used in the preantipsychotic era (Bertelsen et al. 2009; Bland and Orn 1978; DeLisi et al. 1998; Harrison et al. 2001; Henry et al. 2010; Holmboe et al. 1968; Kaleda 2008; Morgan et al. 2014). For Figure 2-2, rating of "recovered" required psychotic and negative symptom remission and good social and vocational function outcomes. A "moderately severe/severe" rating required chronic, severe symptoms and lack of meaningful social or vocational function (GAF<31 *and/or* Bleuler's [1978] scale rating of "poor" outcome). Persons not meeting recovered or severe criteria were considered to have a mild/moderate outcome. As shown in Figure 2–2, over half (54%) of participants were rated as having mild to moderate long-term outcomes, and 21% were considered recovered. A minority, 25%, had a severe outcome. In addition, there is no clear pattern of end-state outcomes worsening with a longer follow-up period.

Compared with the proportion of participants who experienced a full recovery, somewhat higher proportions of participants experienced either symptom remission or functional recovery. For example, results of the World Health Organization's schizophrenia incidence cohort study showed that at 15-year follow-up, 34% of participants had been asymptomatic over the past 2 years; 9% had no psychotic symptoms but some residual negative symptoms; 17% had episodes of psychosis lasting less than 6 months, with recovery between episodes; and 34% were chronically psychotic (Harrison et al. 2001). In addition, 57% of participants had been working full time for most of the previous 2 years, 37% for pay and 20% maintaining a household. Another example comes from the first specialty treatment program for early psycho-

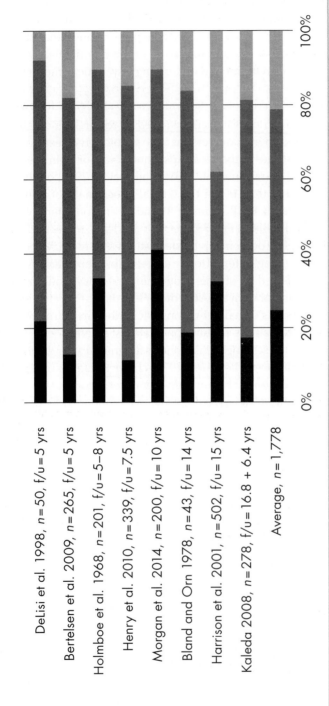

FIGURE 2–2. Long-term outcomes for persons with first-episode schizophrenia diagnosed after the availability of antipsychotics.

f/u=follow-up.

sis, the Early Psychosis Prevention and Intervention Centre (EPPIC) schizophrenia cohort (Henry et al. 2010). At long-term follow-up, 29% of participants were in symptomatic remission for both psychotic and negative symptoms, and an additional 21% were without psychosis but still experienced negative symptoms. At follow-up, 22% were rated as socially and vocationally recovered, and 53% were working.

Although outcome information from the Suffolk County Mental Health Project study of 175 first-episode schizophrenia patients recruited between 1990 and 1995 was insufficient to be included in Figure 2–2, it is worth mentioning that the 20-year outcomes were remarkably poor (Kotov et al. 2017). The average severity of symptoms and functional level as rated by the GAF Scale was 46 at 10-year follow-up and declined to 34 at 20-year follow-up—ratings that are consistent with a severe outcome. Only 4% of participants were rated as recovered (with a GAF score >60). This cohort may have included a high proportion of persons with poor prognostic features and a poor response to treatment, as most participants had a chronic (74%) rather than an episodic (25%) course, even though most patients were prescribed antipsychotic medications. In addition, on average, premorbid functioning was rated as highly impaired, consistent with an especially poor prognosis cohort (Velthorst et al. 2017, 2018).

In the studies included in Figure 2–2, almost none of the participants were hospitalized for the duration of the follow-up period, including those participants rated as "severe" in outcome. In contrast, in the twentieth century prior to the advent of antipsychotics, almost all of the patients considered severely ill were hospitalized for the duration of the follow-up period. Although changing psychiatric practice may explain this difference, it could also be that among those with poor outcomes the most debilitating of outcomes have become relatively rare. Manfred Bleuler's (1978) studies spanned the 1940s to 1960s, and his observations suggest that the latter may be true:

> A comparison between today's statistics and those of about half a century ago forces acceptance of the following conclusion: Among those schizophrenic psychoses that proceed to long-term, stable conditions, the most severe, chronic conditions of illness have become more rare, and milder ones more frequent in the past decades. (p. 209)

Bleuler also wrote the following:

> The numerical shift in frequency discovered from severe to mild chronic conditions ("end states") corresponds to the experience from the practice of most clinicians. If comparisons were made from memory, between wards of schizophrenics as we saw them decades ago in most localities, and the schizophrenic wards of today, one is impressed by the obvious progress. On the wards for chronic schizophrenics there are more patients who are quiet, communicative, working, content, and not requiring restraint, than there were years ago.... While decades ago nearly all the wards for the most severely ill were almost always overcrowded, these wards today often contain empty beds, and space is scarce much more often in the wards for mild schizophrenics cases. (p. 206)

Symptomatic and Functional Recovery

Full Recovery

As discussed above, the "natural" (without somatic intervention) course of schizophrenia includes a small proportion of people who have a single episode of psychosis followed by symptomatic and functional recovery. However, as pointed out by Krae-pelin (1919), "the degree of recovery must be taken into account" (p. 186). One issue relates to whether there are residual impairments in other symptom domains, espe-cially as "all the more striking morbid phenomena may disappear, while less import-ant changes of the psychic personality remain, which for the discharging of the duties of life have no importance, but are perceptible to the careful observer, who need not always be a relative" (p. 186), Kraepelin (1919) referred to such patients as "recovery with defect" (p. 186).

The proportion of patients with a single psychosis episode followed by full recovery is small. After a decade of follow-up, Kraepelin (1919) reported a single patient (out of 488) who was completely well; other studies have reported the proportion as 5% (Cheney and Drewry 1938) and 6% (Rupp and Fletcher 1940). Studies from the anti-psychotic era with 10 or more years of follow-up similarly found that 2%–8% of pa-tients had a single episode with full recovery, without any relapses (Mason et al. 1996; Möller et al. 2010; Thara 2004).

In contrast to research conducted at the turn of the twentieth century, studies in the antipsychotic era reported higher recovery rates at the time of follow-up (Figure 2–2), averaging 22%. Long-term studies not included in Figure 2–2 similarly reported re-covery rates that ranged from 14% to 31% at follow-up (Crumlish et al. 2009; Harrow et al. 2005; Hegelstad et al. 2012; Robinson et al. 1999). One observational study re-ported that 40% of patients met recovery criteria at some point during the course of their illness, although recovery was not sustained long term for most (Harrow et al. 2005). The recovery rates reported in Figure 2–2 include both persons who were tak-ing antipsychotic medications and those who were not. For example, Harrison and colleagues (2001) reported that slightly less than half of the recovered participants from the World Health Organization's schizophrenia incidence cohort study were pre-scribed antipsychotics in the 2 years prior to the 15-year follow-up, and half were not.

Morbidity and Mortality

The risk of death for persons with schizophrenia, beginning with the first episode, is substantially higher than that found in the general population. For example, in one U.S. study, the standardized mortality ratio (observed deaths divided by age- and sex-matched expected deaths) in the year after diagnosis with a first episode was 24 and varied from 8 to 73 depending on sex and age at treatment (Schoenbaum et al. 2017). A Finnish population-based registry study found that the overall all-cause standardized mortality ratio was twice as high for persons with schizophrenia as for the general population (Tanskanen et al. 2018). A meta-analysis of studies published before 2017 found a standardized mortality ratio of 3, but there was substantial het-erogeneity among studies (Oakley et al. 2018).

The increased risk of death for persons with schizophrenia is due to suicide, acci-dents, cardiovascular diseases, smoking-related cancers and lung diseases, and a vari-ety of other health problems (Oakley et al. 2018; Tanskanen et al. 2018). In addition, evidence suggests that the elevated mortality rate is related in part to psychotic relapse. For example, a Finnish study reported that the risk of death for first-episode patients who discontinued antipsychotics was roughly double that for those who continued antipsychotic medications over a 16-year follow-up period (Tanskanen et al. 2018).

Potential Factors Affecting the "Natural" History of Schizophrenia

Treatment

The second half of the twentieth century marked a turning point for persons with schizophrenia, coincident with the introduction of antipsychotic medications. Antipsychotic medications are unquestionably efficacious in treating hallucinations, delusions, and disorganization symptoms in persons with schizophrenia, and they dramatically decrease the time to symptom remission compared with placebo (Leucht et al. 2018). Maintenance treatment with antipsychotic medications has reduced the risk of subsequent episodes of psychosis (Leucht et al. 2012; Taipale et al. 2018; Tiihonen et al. 2017, 2018); repeated episodes of psychosis are tied to the emergence of more severe residual psychotic and negative symptoms (Robinson et al. 1999; Wiersma et al. 1998). Furthermore, shorter duration of untreated psychosis is associated with better short-term and long-term outcomes (Perkins et al. 2005). These observations support the conclusion that antipsychotics improve short-term outcomes in persons with schizophrenia and alter the course of schizophrenia by reducing the frequency of relapses.

However, the relationship between antipsychotics and better long-term outcomes has been questioned (Harrow et al. 2014; Whitaker 2016). Reasons for this questioning include the increase in hospital discharge rates in Europe and the United States that began in the 1940s, before the introduction of antipsychotics. One likely explanation for the increase in discharge rates during the 1940s was the widespread use of shock therapy (induction of seizures via hypoglycemia or metrazol), which was expected to produce short-term improvements in psychosis severity and thus shorten hospital stays. However, relapse rates were high in shock-treated patients, and follow-up studies found no difference in short-term outcomes for patients treated with shock therapy (Ackner and Oldham 1962).

Long-term observational studies have found that the proportion of persons not taking antipsychotics who have good outcomes is greater than the proportion of persons taking antipsychotic medications who have good outcomes. For example, the World Health Organization–sponsored international study of 502 persons with incident (first-episode) schizophrenia found that at 15-year follow-up, 31% of participants had been symptomatically and functionally recovered for the prior 2 years. Although almost all participants had been prescribed antipsychotics at some point during follow-up, 128 had not received antipsychotics during the prior 2 years. Eighty-one (63%) of these subjects were rated as recovered, compared with 109 of the 374 participants (29%) who had received antipsychotics during the 2-year period. Other studies have similarly reported higher rates of recovery at long-term follow-up for participants who were not prescribed compared with those who were prescribed antipsychotic medications, although, again, most of these participants had been prescribed antipsychotic medications at some point during their illness (Harrow and Jobe 2005, 2018; Harrow et al. 2005; Morgan et al. 2014; Wils et al. 2017).

Interpretation of the finding that at long-term follow-up, persons not taking antipsychotics have higher recovery rates than persons currently taking antipsychotics is not straightforward. One possibility is that long-term maintenance treatment, despite reducing relapse risk, also has negative consequences that impact recovery (Harrow and Jobe 2018). Alternatively, the direction of causality could be the reverse: persons who fully recover could be more likely to stop taking antipsychotics than persons who partially recover (Correll et al. 2018b). Patients might agree to take antipsychotics while actively psychotic but could be reluctant to take antipsychotics to prevent future relapse and might therefore discontinue medication during a period of recovery. Relapse may occur days to months to years after stopping antipsychotics; studies report that the proportion of remitted patients who relapsed after stopping antipsychotics ranged from 20% to 40% at 1 year, 50% to 60% at 2 years, and 80% to 90% at 5 years (Chen et al. 2010; Gitlin et al. 2001; Robinson et al. 1999; Winton-Brown et al. 2017; Wunderink et al. 2007). Thus, it is impossible to disentangle the direction of cause and effect from the results of long-term observational studies, and in fact these two alternative explanations are not mutually exclusive.

Nonpharmacological treatment interventions may also alter the course and long-term outcomes of schizophrenia. This idea is the basis for early-psychosis coordinated specialty care (CSC) programs, which include a multidisciplinary team offering, in addition to pharmacotherapy, a range of services such as individual and family therapy and vocational support services. CSC programs appear to improve short-term outcomes (Bertelsen et al. 2009; Correll et al. 2018a; Henry et al. 2010; Kane et al. 2016; McGorry et al. 1996). Furthermore, a variety of psychosocial interventions have been shown to improve functional and symptomatic outcomes in persons with schizophrenia (Dixon et al. 2010).

Finally, it is possible that the improvements in the course and long-term outcome of schizophrenia since the 1950s are a result of changes in the pathology of schizophrenia—for example, related to changes in environmental risk factors (e.g., emergence of schizophrenia related to marijuana use) (Manrique-Garcia et al. 2012) or changes in human vulnerability to the most severe type of schizophrenia. This possibility is not without precedent, as the natural histories of various disorders, including infectious diseases, are known to change over time (Karlsson et al. 2014). With infectious disease, the change is due to selection pressures from the interactions between host vulnerability and pathogen virulence; often, a disease course becomes milder as hosts that survive are better able to defend against the pathogen, and less pathogenic strains are selectively transmitted if their hosts live longer. Thus, factors other than antipsychotic use may contribute to the less severe outcomes in schizophrenia that emerged in the second half of the twentieth century.

Other Prognostic Factors

The cause of the extreme heterogeneity in long-term outcome—from complete recovery to incapacitating symptoms and disability—is unknown but of obvious interest. Some individuals may have a worse prognosis due to their genetics and/or exposure to early environmental events that affect brain development. Features associated with a worse prognosis include poor premorbid social and vocational function, prominent negative symptoms, more severe cognitive impairments, insidious onset, and male sex (Austin et al. 2013; Harrison et al. 2001; Rund et al. 2004; White et al. 2009). These features are intercorrelated, suggesting that together they characterize a poor-prognosis illness. However, the finding that greater impairments in function at baseline predict greater impairments at long-term follow-up is somewhat tautological. Thus, these predictors, although perhaps useful in predicting prognosis, do not shed light on factors contributing to poor prognosis.

Substance use is estimated to be four times more common among persons with schizophrenia than among the general population (Hartz et al. 2014). Use of alcohol or other drugs has been associated with greater severity of positive psychotic symptoms, more depressive symptoms, greater risk of suicide, and more frequent hospitalizations (Addington and Addington 2007; Koola et al. 2012). Substance use may influence prognosis, at least in part, by increasing the likelihood of treatment nonadherence (Coldham et al. 2002). In addition, substance use disorders are themselves associated with increased risk of suicide and functional impairments and thus may exacerbate the symptomatic and functional consequences of the psychotic disorder.

Marijuana use, especially a pattern of use that begins during early adolescence, or heavy use in late adolescence or early adulthood, has emerged as an environmental risk factor for the development of psychosis, increasing risk about fourfold (Arseneault et al. 2002; Davis et al. 2013; Hickman et al. 2007; Manrique-Garcia et al. 2012; van Os et al. 2002). Interestingly, at the first episode of psychosis, the "kind" of schizophrenia associated with heavy marijuana use is characterized by less severe negative symptoms and cognitive impairments (Burns et al. 2010; Segev and Lev-Ran 2012) as well as earlier age at onset (Donoghue et al. 2014). Possible reasons include the following: marijuana exerts some therapeutic benefit, the type of schizophrenia for which marijuana is a risk factor is more benign than the type of schizophrenia that develops for other reasons, obtaining marijuana requires intact social skills, and/or some other confounding factor. However, once schizophrenia develops, continued use of marijuana is associated with relapse, rehospitalization, and worse functional outcomes (D'Souza et al. 2009; Faber et al. 2012).

Summary

Premorbidly, persons with schizophrenia score lower than average on tests of intellectual ability and have more social and academic difficulties but not to the extent that the persons who later develop schizophrenia are clearly distinguishable from their peers. As schizophrenia emerges, most persons experience a prodromal phase, characterized by attenuated, subclinical psychotic symptoms, negative symptoms, and mood symptoms. However, only about one-third of persons who report prodromal-severity symptoms develop schizophrenia. Full-blown psychosis emerges abruptly, over a period of weeks, for about half of persons with schizophrenia. The remainder have an insidious onset, with psychosis emerging over months to years.

Once schizophrenia develops, its course is highly heterogeneous, with outcomes ranging from complete recovery to chronic incapacity. At the turn of the twentieth century, treatment institutions offered patients with schizophrenia various combinations of therapies, including individual psychotherapy, milieu therapy, physiotherapy (e.g., massage), recreational therapy, and occupational therapy (Cheney and Drewry 1938; Rupp and Fletcher 1940). Such interventions did not prevent the progressive worsening of psychotic, negative, and cognitive symptoms or the development of severe impairments in most patients. After a first psychotic episode, about one-third of patients showed spontaneous improvements in severity of psychosis, typically improving over a period of 6–18 months. About 10% of patients were completely well and returned to their premorbid level of function. However, most of the patients with meaningful clinical improvements subsequently relapsed, and in the end a small percentage—at most 5%—remained asymptomatic a decade or more later. The "natural" course of schizophrenia was described by Kraepelin, Eugen Bleuler, and others as typically, but not always, progressing to a state in which the person has extremely limited capacity to communicate with others or to engage in meaningful activities.

The evidence base clearly indicates that antipsychotics impact the course of schizophrenia, effectively reducing or eliminating psychotic symptoms in most patients. Maintenance treatment with antipsychotics reduces the risk of relapse and improves short-term outcomes. Evaluating the impact of antipsychotics on long-term outcomes is complicated due to nonadherence and the time lag between stopping antipsychotics and psychosis relapse. At present, schizophrenia still remains a disorder characterized by high risk of relapse, emergence of chronic symptoms, and functional disability. However, the proportion of patients who develop the most severe end state is much lower than it was at the turn of the twentieth century.

Conclusion

Researchers investigate and clinicians offer pharmacotherapy and psychosocial treatments with the intent of altering the natural course of schizophrenia and improving outcomes. When a patient is first diagnosed with schizophrenia, patients and their families are often interested in the expected course and prognosis. Providing patients and family members with information about the natural history of schizophrenia and the potential impact of treatment on its course and prognosis is an essential part of medical management of first-episode schizophrenia.

All patients with schizophrenia should be offered antipsychotic medications and the following information: Antipsychotics dramatically improve the short-term course of schizophrenia; spontaneous improvement of psychosis without antipsychotic treatment is highly unlikely; and without the use of antipsychotics, the long-term outcomes are extremely poor. The longer psychosis goes untreated, the worse the prognosis is; therefore, treatment with antipsychotics and other interventions should occur as close to psychosis onset as possible. Clinicians should also inform patients about the importance of antipsychotic medication adherence, because even brief gaps in treatment are associated with delayed response and symptom exacerbation (Winton-Brown et al. 2017). In developing their personalized treatment plan, patients and their family members should also be informed of other available interventions, especially psychosocial interventions, that may improve residual symptoms and thereby potentially impact the course of illness and improve long-term outcomes.

Although not every patient requires maintenance antipsychotic treatment to prevent relapse, it is not possible at this point in time to discern reliably the minority of individuals destined for a benign course from the majority who will have a more severe course of schizophrenia. In determining the duration of maintenance antipsychotic treatment, clinicians and patients need to weigh the risks of discontinuation, especially the high risk of relapse, versus the long-term known (and as yet unclear) risks of antipsychotics. As part of this discussion, clinicians should inform patients that prevention of recurrent episodes is likely to be critical in preventing disease progression (Lieberman 1999), that for most patients recovery from a relapse is often less complete and takes longer than recovery from the first psychotic episode, and that the severity of residual symptoms increases with each successive relapse. Clinicians and patients should also discuss the impact that relapse could have on social and vocational gains made while taking antipsychotic medications. Patients who use marijuana, alcohol, and other drugs should be informed that substance use may negatively impact course and long-term outcome.

To summarize, effective management of schizophrenia requires the clinician to know and to explain to patients and family members the natural history of schizophrenia and the potential impact of available treatments on the course and prognosis. This includes an appreciation that without intervention the outcomes are dismal and that only a small proportion of patients spontaneously improve.

References

Achté KA, Apo M: Schizophrenic patients in 1950–1952 and 1957–1959: a comparative study. Psychiatr Q 41(3):422–441, 1967 4294876

Ackner B, Oldham AJ: Insulin treatment of schizophrenia: a three-year follow-up of a controlled study. Lancet 1(7228):504–506, 1962 13859190

Addington J, Addington D: Patterns, predictors and impact of substance use in early psychosis: a longitudinal study. Acta Psychiatr Scand 115(4):304–309, 2007 17355521

Addington J, Piskulic D, Liu L, et al: Comorbid diagnoses for youth at clinical high risk of psychosis. Schizophr Res 190:90–95, 2017 28372906

Amminger GP, Schäfer MR, Papageorgiou K, et al: Long-chain omega-3 fatty acids for indicated prevention of psychotic disorders: a randomized, placebo-controlled trial. Arch Gen Psychiatry 67(2):146–154, 2010 20124114

Arseneault L, Cannon M, Poulton R, et al: Cannabis use in adolescence and risk for adult psychosis: longitudinal prospective study. BMJ 325(7374):1212–1213, 2002 12446537

Austin SF, Mors O, Secher RG, et al: Predictors of recovery in first episode psychosis: the OPUS cohort at 10 year follow-up. Schizophr Res 150(1):163–168, 2013 23932664

Bertelsen M, Jeppesen P, Petersen L, et al: Course of illness in a sample of 265 patients with first-episode psychosis—five-year follow-up of the Danish OPUS trial. Schizophr Res 107(2–3):173–178, 2009 18945593

Bland RC, Orn H: 14-year outcome in early schizophrenia. Acta Psychiatr Scand 58(4):327–338, 1978 717003

Bleuler E: Textbook of Psychiatry. New York, Macmillan, 1934

Bleuler M: The Schizophrenic Disorders: Long-Term Patient and Family Studies. New Haven, CT, Yale University Press, 1978

Bond ED, Braceland FJ: Prognosis in mental disease. Am J Psychiatry 94(9):263–274, 1937

Bora E, Murray RM: Meta-analysis of cognitive deficits in ultra-high risk to psychosis and first-episode psychosis: do the cognitive deficits progress over, or after, the onset of psychosis? Schizophr Bull 40(4):744–755, 2014 23770934

Burns JK, Jhazbhay K, Emsley R: Cannabis use predicts shorter duration of untreated psychosis and lower levels of negative symptoms in first-episode psychosis: a South African study. Afr J Psychiatry (Johannesbg) 13(5):395–399, 2010 21390411

Cadenhead K, Addington J, Cannon T, et al: Omega-3 fatty acid versus placebo in a clinical high-risk sample from the North American Prodrome Longitudinal Studies (NAPLS) Consortium. Schizophr Bull 43:S16, 2017

Carpenter WT Jr, Kirkpatrick B: The heterogeneity of the long-term course of schizophrenia. Schizophr Bull 14(4):645–652, 1988 3064288

Chen EY, Hui CL, Lam MM, et al: Maintenance treatment with quetiapine versus discontinuation after one year of treatment in patients with remitted first episode psychosis: randomised controlled trial. BMJ 341:c4024, 2010 20724402

Cheney CO, Drewry PH Jr: Results of non-specific treatment in dementia præcox. Am J Psychiatry 95:203–217, 1938

Coldham EL, Addington J, Addington D: Medication adherence of individuals with a first episode of psychosis. Acta Psychiatr Scand 106(4):286–290, 2002 12225495

Correll CU, Galling B, Pawar A, et al: Comparison of early intervention services vs treatment as usual for early phase psychosis: a systematic review, meta-analysis, and meta-regression. JAMA Psychiatry 75(6):555–565, 2018a 29800949

Correll CU, Rubio JM, Kane JM: What is the risk-benefit ratio of long-term antipsychotic treatment in people with schizophrenia? World Psychiatry 17(2):149–160, 2018b 29856543

Crumlish N, Whitty P, Clarke M, et al: Beyond the critical period: longitudinal study of 8-year outcome in first-episode non-affective psychosis. Br J Psychiatry 194(1):18–24, 2009 19118320

Davies C, Cipriani A, Ioannidis JPA, et al: Lack of evidence to favor specific preventive interventions in psychosis: a network meta-analysis. World Psychiatry 17(2):196–209, 2018 29856551

Davis GP, Compton MT, Wang S, et al: Association between cannabis use, psychosis, and schizotypal personality disorder: findings from the National Epidemiologic Survey on Alcohol and Related Conditions. Schizophr Res 151(1–3):197–202, 2013 24200416

Deas G, Kelly C, Hadjinicolaou AV, et al: An update on: meta-analysis of medical and non-medical treatments of the prodromal phase of psychotic illness in at risk mental states. Psychiatr Danub 28 (Suppl 1):31–38, 2016 27663802

DeLisi LE, Sakuma M, Ge S, Kushner M: Association of brain structural change with the heterogeneous course of schizophrenia from early childhood through five years subsequent to a first hospitalization. Psychiatry Res 84(2–3):75–88, 1998 10710165

Devoe JD, Farris MS, Townes P, Addington J: Attenuated psychotic symptom interventions in youth at risk of psychosis: A systematic review and meta-analysis. Early Interv Psychiatry 13(1):3–17, 2019 29749710

Dixon LB, Dickerson F, Bellack AS, et al; Schizophrenia Patient Outcomes Research Team (PORT): The 2009 schizophrenia PORT psychosocial treatment recommendations and summary statements. Schizophr Bull 36(1):48–70, 2010 19955389

Donoghue K, Doody GA, Murray RM, et al: Cannabis use, gender and age of onset of schizophrenia: data from the ÆSOP study. Psychiatry Res 215(3):528–532, 2014 24461684

D'Souza DC, Sewell RA, Ranganathan M: Cannabis and psychosis/schizophrenia: human studies. Eur Arch Psychiatry Clin Neurosci 259(7):413–431, 2009 19609589

Faber G, Smid HG, Van Gool AR, et al: Continued cannabis use and outcome in first-episode psychosis: data from a randomized, open-label, controlled trial. J Clin Psychiatry 73(5):632–638, 2012 22394457

Filatova S, Koivumaa-Honkanen H, Hirvonen N, et al: Early motor developmental milestones and schizophrenia: a systematic review and meta-analysis. Schizophr Res 188:13–20, 2017 28131598

Fuller R, Nopoulos P, Arndt S, et al: Longitudinal assessment of premorbid cognitive functioning in patients with schizophrenia through examination of standardized scholastic test performance. Am J Psychiatry 159(7):1183–1189, 2002 12091197

Fusar-Poli P, Bonoldi I, Yung AR, et al: Predicting psychosis: meta-analysis of transition outcomes in individuals at high clinical risk. Arch Gen Psychiatry 69(3):220–229, 2012 22393215

Gitlin M, Nuechterlein K, Subotnik KL, et al: Clinical outcome following neuroleptic discontinuation in patients with remitted recent-onset schizophrenia. Am J Psychiatry 158(11):1835–1842, 2001 11691689

Guttmann E, Mayer-Gross W, Slater ETO: Short-distance prognosis of schizophrenia. J Neurol Psychiatry 2(1):25–34, 1939 21610940

Häfner H, an der Heiden W: The course of schizophrenia in the light of modern follow-up studies: the ABC and WHO studies. Eur Arch Psychiatry Clin Neurosci 249 (suppl 4):14–26, 1999 10654105

Hall RC: Global Assessment of Functioning: a modified scale. Psychosomatics 36(3):267–275, 1995 7638314

Harrison G, Hopper K, Craig T, et al: Recovery from psychotic illness: a 15- and 25-year international follow-up study. Br J Psychiatry 178:506–517, 2001 11388966

Harrow M, Jobe TH: Longitudinal studies of outcome and recovery in schizophrenia and early intervention: can they make a difference? Can J Psychiatry 50(14):879–880, 2005 16494256

Harrow M, Jobe TH: Long-term antipsychotic treatment of schizophrenia: does it help or hurt over a 20-year period? World Psychiatry 17(2):162–163, 2018 29856562

Harrow M, Grossman LS, Jobe TH, et al: Do patients with schizophrenia ever show periods of recovery? A 15-year multi-follow-up study. Schizophr Bull 31(3):723–734, 2005 16020553

Harrow M, Jobe TH, Faull RN: Does treatment of schizophrenia with antipsychotic medications eliminate or reduce psychosis? A 20-year multi-follow-up study. Psychol Med 44(14):3007–3016, 2014 25066792

Hartz SM, Pato CN, Medeiros H, et al; Genomic Psychiatry Cohort Consortium: Comorbidity of severe psychotic disorders with measures of substance use. JAMA Psychiatry 71(3):248–254, 2014 24382686

Hastings DW: Follow-up results in psychiatric illness. Am J Psychiatry 114(12):1057–1066, 1958 13533644

Hegelstad WT, Larsen TK, Auestad B, et al: Long-term follow-up of the TIPS early detection in psychosis study: effects on 10-year outcome. Am J Psychiatry 169(4):374–380, 2012 22407080

Henry LP, Amminger GP, Harris MG, et al: The EPPIC follow-up study of first-episode psychosis: longer-term clinical and functional outcome 7 years after index admission. J Clin Psychiatry 71(6):716–728, 2010 20573330

Hickman M, Vickerman P, Macleod J, et al: Cannabis and schizophrenia: model projections of the impact of the rise in cannabis use on historical and future trends in schizophrenia in England and Wales. Addiction 102(4):597–606, 2007 17362293

Holmboe R, Noreik K, Astrup C: Follow-up of functional psychoses at two Norwegian mental hospitals. Acta Psychiatr Scand 44(3):298–310, 1968 5722606

Huber G, Gross G: The concept of basic symptoms in schizophrenic and schizoaffective psychoses. Recenti Prog Med 80(12):646–652, 1989 2697899

Hunt RC, Feldman H, Fiero RP: "Spontaneous" remissions in dementia praecox. Psychiatr Q 12(3):414–425, 1938

Hutton P, Taylor PJ: Cognitive behavioural therapy for psychosis prevention: a systematic review and meta-analysis. Psychol Med 44(3):449–468, 2014 23521867

Kaleda VG: Endogenous psychoses with a first episode at the juvenile age: course and outcome (follow-up study) [in Russian]. Zh Nevrol Psikhiatr Im S S Korsakova 108(9):11–23, 2008 18833167

Kane JM, Robinson DG, Schooler NR, et al: Comprehensive versus usual community care for first-episode psychosis: 2-year outcomes from the NIMH RAISE early treatment program. Am J Psychiatry 173(4):449–468, 2016 26481174

Karlsson EK, Kwiatkowski DP, Sabeti PC: Natural selection and infectious disease in human populations. Nat Rev Genet 15(6):379–393, 2014 24776769

Kendler KS: The transformation of American psychiatric nosology at the dawn of the twentieth century. Mol Psychiatry 21(2):152–158, 2016 26692416

Khandaker GM, Barnett JH, White IR, et al: A quantitative meta-analysis of population-based studies of premorbid intelligence and schizophrenia. Schizophr Res 132(2–3):220–227, 2011 21764562

Koola MM, McMahon RP, Wehring HJ, et al: Alcohol and cannabis use and mortality in people with schizophrenia and related psychotic disorders. J Psychiatr Res 46(8):987–993, 2012 22595870

Kotov R, Fochtmann L, Li K, et al: Declining clinical course of psychotic disorders over the two decades following first hospitalization: evidence from the Suffolk County Mental Health Project. Am J Psychiatry 174(11):1064–1074, 2017 28774193

Kraepelin E: Dementia Praecox and Paraphrenia. Chicago, IL, Chicago Medical Book Company, 1919

Leucht S, Tardy M, Komossa K, et al: Antipsychotic drugs versus placebo for relapse prevention in schizophrenia: a systematic review and meta-analysis. Lancet 379(9831):2063–2071, 2012 22560607

Leucht S, Chaimani A, Leucht C, et al: 60 years of placebo-controlled antipsychotic drug trials in acute schizophrenia: meta-regression of predictors of placebo response. Schizophr Res 201:315–323, 2018 29804928

Lieberman JA: Is schizophrenia a neurodegenerative disorder? A clinical and neurobiological perspective. Biol Psychiatry 46(6):729–739, 1999 10494440

Lieberman JA, Girgis RR, Brucato G, et al: Hippocampal dysfunction in the pathophysiology of schizophrenia: a selective review and hypothesis for early detection and intervention. Mol Psychiatry 23(8):1764–1772, 2018 29311665

López-Muñoz F, Alamo C, Cuenca E, et al: History of the discovery and clinical introduction of chlorpromazine. Ann Clin Psychiatry 17(3):113–135, 2005 16433053

Malamud W, Render N: Course and prognosis in schizophrenia. Am J Psychiatry 95(5):1039–1057, 1939

Manrique-Garcia E, Zammit S, Dalman C, et al: Cannabis, schizophrenia and other non-affective psychoses: 35 years of follow-up of a population-based cohort. Psychol Med 42(6):1321–1328, 2012 21999906

Mason P, Harrison G, Glazebrook C, et al: The course of schizophrenia over 13 years: a report from the International Study on Schizophrenia (ISoS) coordinated by the World Health Organization. Br J Psychiatry 169(5):580–586, 1996 8932886

Mayer-Gross W: Die Klinik der Schizophrenie, in Handbuch der Geisteskrankheiten, Vol 9. Edited by Bunke O. Berlin, Germany, Springer, 1932, pp 293–578

McGorry PD, Edwards J, Mihalopoulos C, et al: EPPIC: an evolving system of early detection and optimal management. Schizophr Bull 22(2):305–326, 1996 8782288

Modestin J, Huber A, Satirli E, et al: Long-term course of schizophrenic illness: Bleuler's study reconsidered. Am J Psychiatry 160(12):2202–2208, 2003 14638591

Möller HJ, Jäger M, Riedel M, et al: The Munich 15-year follow-up study (MUFUSSAD) on first-hospitalized patients with schizophrenic or affective disorders: comparison of psychopathological and psychosocial course and outcome and prediction of chronicity. Eur Arch Psychiatry Clin Neurosci 260(5):367–384, 2010 20495979

Möller HJ, Jäger M, Riedel M, et al: The Munich 15-year follow-up study (MUFUSSAD) on first-hospitalized patients with schizophrenic or affective disorders: assessing courses, types and time stability of diagnostic classification. Eur Psychiatry 26(4):231–243, 2011 20621452

Mollon J, Reichenberg A: Cognitive development prior to onset of psychosis. Psychol Med 48(3):392–403, 2018 28735586

Mollon J, David AS, Zammit S, et al: Course of cognitive development from infancy to early adulthood in the psychosis spectrum. JAMA Psychiatry 75(3):270–279, 2018 29387877

Morgan C, Lappin J, Heslin M, et al: Reappraising the long-term course and outcome of psychotic disorders: the AESOP-10 study. Psychol Med 44(13):2713–2726, 2014 25066181

National Committee for Mental Hygiene: Statistical Manual for the Use of Institutions for the Insane. New York, National Committee for Mental Hygiene, 1934

Niemi LT, Suvisaari JM, Tuulio-Henriksson A, et al: Childhood developmental abnormalities in schizophrenia: evidence from high-risk studies. Schizophr Res 60(2–3):239–258, 2003 12591587

Oakley P, Kisely S, Baxter A, et al: Increased mortality among people with schizophrenia and other non-affective psychotic disorders in the community: a systematic review and meta-analysis. J Psychiatr Res 102:245–253, 2018 29723811

Olfson M, Gerhard T, Huang C, et al: Premature mortality among adults with schizophrenia in the United States. JAMA Psychiatry 72(12):1172–1181, 2015 26509694

Perkins DO, Gu H, Boteva K, et al: Relationship between duration of untreated psychosis and outcome in first-episode schizophrenia: a critical review and meta-analysis. Am J Psychiatry 162(10):1785–1804, 2005 16199825

Piskulic D, Addington J, Cadenhead KS, et al: Negative symptoms in individuals at clinical high risk of psychosis. Psychiatry Res 196(2–3):220–224, 2012 22445704

Rennie TAC, Fowler JB: Follow-up study of five hundred patients with schizophrenia admitted to the hospital from 1913 to 1923. Arch Neurol Psychiatry 42(5):877–891, 1939

Revier CJ, Reininghaus U, Dutta R, et al: Ten-year outcomes of first-episode psychoses in the MRC ÆSOP-10 Study. J Nerv Ment Dis 203(5):379–386, 2015 25900547

Robinson D, Woerner MG, Alvir JM, et al: Predictors of relapse following response from a first episode of schizophrenia or schizoaffective disorder. Arch Gen Psychiatry 56(3):241–247, 1999 10078501

Romano J, Ebaugh FG: Prognosis in schizophrenia. Am J Psychiatry 95:563–596, 1938

Rund BR, Melle I, Friis S, et al: Neurocognitive dysfunction in first-episode psychosis: correlates with symptoms, premorbid adjustment, and duration of untreated psychosis. Am J Psychiatry 161(3):466–472, 2004 14992972

Rupp C, Fletcher EK: A five- to ten-year follow-up study of 641 schizophrenic cases. Am J Psychiatry 96:877–888, 1940

Schoenbaum M, Sutherland JM, Chappel A, et al: Twelve-month health care use and mortality in commercially insured young people with incident psychosis in the United States. Schizophr Bull 43(6):1262–1272, 2017 28398566

Segev A, Lev-Ran S: Neurocognitive functioning and cannabis use in schizophrenia. Curr Pharm Des 18(32):4999–5007, 2012 22716156

Shibre T, Medhin G, Alem A, et al: Long-term clinical course and outcome of schizophrenia in rural Ethiopia: 10-year follow-up of a population-based cohort. Schizophr Res 161(2–3):414–420, 2015 25468171

Simon AE, Borgwardt S, Riecher-Rössler A, et al: Moving beyond transition outcomes: meta-analysis of remission rates in individuals at high clinical risk for psychosis. Psychiatry Res 209(3):266–272, 2013 23871169

Swazey JP: Chlorpromazine in Psychiatry: A Study of Therapeutic Innovation. Cambridge, MA, The MIT Press, 1974

Taipale H, Mehtala J, Tanskanen A, et al: Comparative effectiveness of antipsychotic drugs for rehospitalization in schizophrenia—a nationwide study with 20-year follow-up. Schizophr Bull 44(6):1381–1387, 2018 29272458

Tanskanen A, Tiihonen J, Taipale H: Mortality in schizophrenia: 30-year nationwide follow-up study. Acta Psychiatr Scand 138(6):492–499, 2018 29900527

Thara R: Twenty-year course of schizophrenia: the Madras Longitudinal Study. Can J Psychiatry 49(8):564–569, 2004 15453106

Tiihonen J, Mittendorfer-Rutz E, Majak M, et al: Real-world effectiveness of antipsychotic treatments in a nationwide cohort of 29,823 patients with schizophrenia. JAMA Psychiatry 74(7):686–693, 2017 28593216

Tiihonen J, Tanskanen A, Taipale H: 20-year nationwide follow-up study on discontinuation of antipsychotic treatment in first-episode schizophrenia. Am J Psychiatry 175(8):765–773, 2018 29621900

van der Werf M, Hanssen M, Köhler S, et al; RISE Investigators: Systematic review and collaborative recalculation of 133,693 incident cases of schizophrenia. Psychol Med 44(1):9–16, 2014 23244442

van Os J, Bak M, Hanssen M, et al: Cannabis use and psychosis: a longitudinal population-based study. Am J Epidemiol 156(4):319–327, 2002 12181101

Velthorst E, Fett AJ, Reichenberg A, et al: The 20-year longitudinal trajectories of social functioning in individuals with psychotic disorders. Am J Psychiatry 174(11):1075–1085, 2017 27978770

Velthorst E, Zinberg J, Addington J, et al: Potentially important periods of change in the development of social and role functioning in youth at clinical high risk for psychosis. Dev Psychopathol 30(1):39–47, 2018 28420458

Whitaker R: The Case Against Antipsychotics: A Review of Their Long-Term Side Effects. Cambridge, MA, Mad in America Foundation, 2016

White C, Stirling J, Hopkins R, et al: Predictors of 10-year outcome of first-episode psychosis. Psychol Med 39(9):1447–1456, 2009 19187566

Wiersma D, Nienhuis FJ, Slooff CJ, et al: Natural course of schizophrenic disorders: a 15-year followup of a Dutch incidence cohort. Schizophr Bull 24(1):75–85, 1998 9502547

Wils RS, Gotfredsen DR, Hjorthøj C, et al: Antipsychotic medication and remission of psychotic symptoms 10 years after a first-episode psychosis. Schizophr Res 182:42–48, 2017 28277310

Winton-Brown TT, Elanjithara T, Power P, et al: Five-fold increased risk of relapse following breaks in antipsychotic treatment of first episode psychosis. Schizophr Res 179:50–56, 2017 27745754

Wooton LH, Armstrong RW, Lilley D: An investigation into the after histories of discharged patients. J Ment Sci 81(332):168–172, 1935

Wunderink L, Nienhuis FJ, Sytema S, et al: Guided discontinuation versus maintenance treatment in remitted first-episode psychosis: relapse rates and functional outcome. J Clin Psychiatry 68(5):654–661, 2007 17503973

CHAPTER 3

Psychopathology

Ryan E. Lawrence, M.D.
Michael B. First, M.D.

Schizophrenia is characterized by psychosis, which may be divided into positive symptoms (hallucinations and delusions), negative symptoms (the absence of several normal traits), and disorganization (abnormal thought processes or behaviors). A variety of cognitive symptoms have also been observed in schizophrenia. Diagnosing schizophrenia requires close attention not only to these symptom domains but also to how they evolve over time. Importantly, schizophrenia is also associated with several potential complications, including mood symptoms, anxiety, substance use disorders, suicide, and violence. Box 3–1 provides the DSM-5 criteria for schizophrenia (American Psychiatric Association 2013).

Box 3–1. Diagnostic Criteria for Schizophrenia

A. Two (or more) of the following, each present for a significant portion of time during a 1-month period (or less if successfully treated). At least one of these must be (1), (2), or (3):

1. Delusions.
2. Hallucinations.
3. Disorganized speech (e.g., frequent derailment or incoherence).
4. Grossly disorganized or catatonic behavior.
5. Negative symptoms (i.e., diminished emotional expression or avolition).

B. For a significant portion of the time since the onset of the disturbance, level of functioning in one or more major areas, such as work, interpersonal relations, or self-care, is markedly below the level achieved prior to the onset (or when the onset is in childhood or adolescence, there is failure to achieve expected level of interpersonal, academic, or occupational functioning).

C. Continuous signs of the disturbance persist for at least 6 months. This 6-month period must include at least 1 month of symptoms (or less if successfully treated) that meet Criterion A (i.e., active-phase symptoms) and may include periods of prodromal or residual symptoms. During these prodromal or residual periods, the signs of the disturbance may be manifested by only negative symptoms or by two or more symptoms listed in Criterion A present in an attenuated form (e.g., odd beliefs, unusual perceptual experiences).

D. Schizoaffective disorder and depressive or bipolar disorder with psychotic features have been ruled out because either 1) no major depressive or manic episodes have occurred concurrently with the active-phase symptoms, or 2) if mood episodes have occurred during active-phase symptoms, they have been present for a minority of the total duration of the active and residual periods of the illness.

E. The disturbance is not attributable to the physiological effects of a substance (e.g., a drug of abuse, a medication) or another medical condition.

F. If there is a history of autism spectrum disorder or a communication disorder of child-hood onset, the additional diagnosis of schizophrenia is made only if prominent delu-sions or hallucinations, in addition to the other required symptoms of schizophrenia, are also present for at least 1 month (or less if successfully treated).

Specify if:

The following course specifiers are only to be used after a 1-year duration of the disorder and if they are not in contradiction to the diagnostic course criteria.

First episode, currently in acute episode: First manifestation of the disorder meet-ing the defining diagnostic symptom and time criteria. An *acute episode* is a time pe-riod in which the symptom criteria are fulfilled.

First episode, currently in partial remission: *Partial remission* is a period of time during which an improvement after a previous episode is maintained and in which the defining criteria of the disorder are only partially fulfilled.

First episode, currently in full remission: *Full remission* is a period of time after a previous episode during which no disorder-specific symptoms are present.

Multiple episodes, currently in acute episode: Multiple episodes may be deter-mined after a minimum of two episodes (i.e., after a first episode, a remission and a minimum of one relapse).

Multiple episodes, currently in partial remission

Multiple episodes, currently in full remission

Continuous: Symptoms fulfilling the diagnostic symptom criteria of the disorder are remaining for the majority of the illness course, with subthreshold symptom periods be-ing very brief relative to the overall course.

Unspecified

Specify if:

With catatonia (refer to the criteria for catatonia associated with another mental disorder, [DMS-5] pp. 119–120, for definition).

Coding note: Use additional code 293.89 (F06.1) catatonia associated with schizophrenia to indicate the presence of the comorbid catatonia.

Specify current severity:

Severity is rated by a quantitative assessment of the primary symptoms of psychosis, including delusions, hallucinations, disorganized speech, abnormal psychomotor be-havior, and negative symptoms. Each of these symptoms may be rated for its current severity (most severe in the last 7 days) on a 5-point scale ranging from 0 (not present) to 4 (present and severe). (See Clinician-Rated Dimensions of Psychosis Symptom Severity in the [DSM-5] chapter "Assessment Measures.")

Note: Diagnosis of schizophrenia can be made without using this severity specifier.

Core Symptoms of Schizophrenia

Positive Symptoms

Schneider and First-Rank Symptoms

In 1939, Kurt Schneider famously generated a list of "first-rank symptoms" that he considered pathognomonic of schizophrenia (Cutting 2015). These are audible thoughts (voices are speaking the subject's thoughts aloud), voices arguing (two or more voices are discussing the subject in the third person), voices commenting on one's action (voices are describing the subject's activities as they occur), influence playing on the body—somatic passivity (the subject experiences bodily sensations as if they are imposed by an external agent), thought withdrawal (the subject's thoughts cease and the subject simultaneously experiences them as removed by an external force), thought insertion (thoughts have a quality of not being one's own thoughts or are ascribed to an external agent), thought broadcasting (the subject feels his or her thoughts escape into the outside world, where they are experienced by others), made feelings (feelings do not seem to be the subject's own or are attributed to an external force), made impulses (the subject's drives or impulses seem to be alien and external), made volitional acts (actions and movements are experienced by the subject as under outside control), and delusional perception (a normal perception has a private and illogical meaning; common or insignificant events are experienced as having special significance).

According to current diagnostic criteria, first-rank symptoms are neither necessary nor sufficient to diagnose schizophrenia. They also are not specific to schizophrenia. Approximately half of patients with schizophrenia exhibit these symptoms. In one study of 196 patients experiencing their first psychiatric hospitalization, 70% of patients with schizophrenia had first-rank symptoms, but so did 29% of patients with "psychotic bipolar disorder" and 18% of patients with "psychotic depression," making first-rank symptoms 73.3% sensitive and 72.5% specific for schizophrenia (Tanenberg-Karant et al. 1995).

Epidemiology of Positive Symptoms

Hallucinations are common among persons with schizophrenia. Approximately 60%–80% of these patients endorse auditory hallucinations, which can be treatment refractory in a quarter of patients (Moseley et al. 2013). Visual hallucinations affect about 27% of patients with schizophrenia (Zmigrod et al. 2016). Olfactory, somatic, and gustatory hallucinations are much less common but have also been reported (Zmigrod et al. 2016).

Delusions are also common, affecting 71% of patients with schizophrenia experiencing an acute psychiatric hospitalization in one study (among 194 persons hospitalized with schizophrenia, 138 had delusions) (Appelbaum et al. 1999). In this study, among schizophrenia patients with delusions, 84.1% had persecutory delusions, 75.4% had body/mind control delusions, 48.6% had grandiose delusions, 52.2% had thought broadcasting, 35.5% had religious delusions, 10.1% had delusions of guilt, 10.9% had somatic delusions, and 34.1% had some other type of delusion. Patients often had more than one type of delusion.

Importantly, psychotic experiences are also reported among the general population in nonclinical samples. In self-report questionnaires, between 30% and 70% of college students reported that they had heard voices at least once in their lives (Stip and Letourneau 2009). In a study of more than 7,000 adults in the general population, 4.2% had experienced hallucinations or delusional symptoms attested to by a psychiatrist, and 17.5% reported at least one experience resembling psychosis (Stip and Letourneau 2009). Among patients in a general practice waiting room (not diagnosed with psychosis), 25% felt they were being persecuted in some way, 18% felt that people were looking at them strangely, and 21% felt particularly close to God (Stip and Letourneau 2009). Whereas these experiences tend to be frequent, intrusive, and distressing in psychiatric populations, these symptoms are likely to be temporary, nonthreatening, or positive in nonclinical samples (Stip and Letourneau 2009).

Differential Diagnosis for Positive Symptoms

Hallucinations can occur in a variety of medical and psychiatric conditions in addition to schizophrenia. For example, substance intoxication or withdrawal, major depressive disorder, bipolar disorder, borderline personality disorder, posttraumatic stress disorder (PTSD), and dissociative disorder (especially in cases of early childhood trauma) all can include auditory hallucinations (Larøi et al. 2012). Neurological conditions associated with hallucinations include Parkinson's disease, epilepsy, brain tumors, and traumatic brain injury (Waters and Fernyhough 2017). Although hallucinations have been reported in multi-infarct dementia and Alzheimer's disease, they are not common. Other medical conditions associated with hallucinations include hearing impairment (associated with auditory hallucinations) and diseases of the eye or afferent visual pathways (associated with visual hallucinations). Vitamin deficiencies (D and B_{12}), chromosomal disorders (e.g., Prader-Willi syndrome), autoimmune diseases, HIV/AIDS, and sleep disorders (e.g., narcolepsy) can have associated hallucinations. Transient hallucinations can happen during extreme physiological or psychological stress (e.g., severe fatigue, sensory deprivation, bereavement).

Delusions also appear in a variety of conditions. As with the occurrence of hallucinations, medical and neurological conditions need to be considered and ruled out (e.g., electrolyte abnormalities, multi-infarct dementia) when patients have delusions. Psychiatric disorders in which delusions are common include major depression and bipolar disorder (delusions can be mood congruent or incongruent), substance-related disorders, borderline personality disorder, obsessive-compulsive disorder, body dysmorphic disorder, illness anxiety disorder, and other psychotic disorders (e.g., delusional disorder, schizoaffective disorder, brief psychotic disorder, other specified schizophrenia spectrum and other psychotic disorder) (Bebbington and Freeman 2017).

Evidence does not support the notion that specific types of hallucinations or delusions can reliably and specifically predict a patient's diagnosis (Bebbington and Freeman 2017; Waters and Fernyhough 2017). When hallucinations or delusions occur, the clinician must consider the full differential diagnosis and conduct a thorough evaluation.

Proposed Etiologies for Hallucinations

A variety of theories have been proposed to explain the etiology of hallucinations, and it is possible that more than one mechanism is involved. One theory is that persons with schizophrenia who experience hallucinations may have difficulty distinguishing between internally generated stimuli (e.g., inner images or speech, voices, memories, vivid daydreams, bodily sensations) and externally generated stimuli. Evidence for this comes from multiple studies involving self-monitoring, source monitoring, or reality monitoring, which have been summarized by Moseley et al. (2013). Electromyography has recorded subvocalizations (tiny movements of the vocal musculature that occur during inner speech) while patients are experiencing auditory verbal hallucinations, suggesting that the hallucination is inner speech that was misattributed to an external source. In joystick tasks in which participants had to monitor errors without feedback, patients with schizophrenia were worse at self-monitoring. When listening to speech through headphones and asked to discriminate whether the voice was their own or someone else's, schizophrenia patients with auditory verbal hallucinations were worse at judging correctly. There is some evidence that schizophrenia patients with auditory hallucinations do not show a different response when a tickle sensation is evoked by themselves or others. Accordingly, it has been proposed that schizophrenia patients with auditory hallucinations have deficits in the *efference copy system* (i.e., the brain plans a motor action, sends an efferent copy of the plan to sensory areas to warn them the action is about to occur, then receives sensory information when the planned action occurs and labels the action as self-generated). A result is that patients with schizophrenia demonstrate externalizing bias—a higher likelihood of attributing stimuli to an external source.

Schizophrenia patients with hallucinations are prone to memory errors (source memory) that might play a role in hallucinatory experiences (Moseley et al. 2013). When tasked with distinguishing between self-generated words, experimenter-generated words, and words that had not previously appeared in the task, hallucinating patients and hallucination-prone patients were more likely to misattribute words to the experimenter. Other evidence suggests that schizophrenia patients with auditory verbal hallucinations are more likely than nonhallucinating patients and healthy control subjects to recall an imagined word as spoken or an imagined action as performed.

Other theories underlying hallucinatory experiences include unbidden thoughts (unintentional memory retrieval and failure to suppress irrelevant thoughts or memories) (Moseley et al. 2013). Studies have also implicated inappropriate emotional responses to hallucinated words (attributing excessive emotional salience to usually neutral stimuli) (Stip and Letourneau 2009).

Of note, neuroimaging studies indicate very different activation patterns during auditory verbal hallucinations and visual hallucinations, suggesting that different brain regions are involved in different hallucinatory experiences (Zmigrod et al. 2016).

Proposed Etiologies for Delusions

People with delusions have been found to make decisions on the basis of less evidence than do healthy individuals or people with nonpsychotic mental health problems (Dudley et al. 2016). This "jumping-to-conclusions" bias is also seen among persons at risk of developing psychosis and first-degree relatives of psychotic persons. The beads task measures this tendency: Participants are shown two jars with beads in equal but opposite ratios (85 red and 15 blue in one jar, vice versa in the other jar), the jars are hidden, participants are told that individual beads will be drawn from one jar, and participants have to guess from which jar the beads are being drawn. People with delusions make decisions after fewer beads are drawn and have higher rates of extreme responding (making decisions after two or fewer beads are drawn). A jumping-to-conclusions bias may lead to premature acceptance of implausible ideas or may prevent realistic alternatives from being considered.

Other psychological mechanisms that occur at higher rates among schizophrenia patients with delusions are biases against disconfirming evidence and liberal acceptance (overrating the plausibility of absurd interpretations) (Bebbington and Freeman 2017).

Learning mechanisms and prediction error may be involved in delusion formation (Knobel et al. 2008). Dopamine plays an important role in modulating how environmental stimuli are encoded in the brain. Proper encoding helps the brain to distinguish between relevant and irrelevant stimuli and to pair stimuli with rewards. Animal studies that pair stimuli with anticipated rewards show that dopaminergic neurons fire during these events. In psychosis, an increase in dopamine release could generate an abnormal signal-to-noise ratio, disrupting the brain's ability to filter stimuli, causing some stimuli to appear disproportionately important, and ultimately causing the person to draw incorrect conclusions. This process could form the basis of delusions.

Attentional bias has also been implicated. The brain does not give equal attention to every stimulus it processes. People direct attentional bias toward emotionally salient stimuli, and people with delusions (especially delusions of reference or persecutory delusions) might have attentional bias toward threatening stimuli. Supporting this theory, a functional magnetic resonance imaging (fMRI) study showed that while processing fearful versus neutral faces, persons with persecutory delusions had a greater stress response than control subjects (Knobel et al. 2008).

Negative Symptoms

Descriptions

In schizophrenia, *negative symptoms* refer to the absence of a psychological or cognitive function or attribute that is normally present. Several lists of negative symptoms have been proposed over the years. The list of negative symptoms in the DSM-5 definition of schizophrenia includes *diminished emotional expression* (affective flattening), *alogia* (decreased verbal output or verbal expressiveness), and *avolition* (the inability to initiate and persist in goal-directed activities) (American Psychiatric Association 2013). DSM-5 adds that *anhedonia* (loss of the ability to find or derive pleasure from activities or relationships) and *asociality* (lack of involvement in various kinds of social relationships) can exist as associated symptoms. The National Institute of Mental Health Measurement and Treatment Research to Improve Cognition in Schizophrenia (NIMH MATRICS) consensus panel lists blunted affect, alogia, asociality, avolition, and anhedonia as negative symptoms (Foussias et al. 2014). In other literature, factor analysis has suggested that attentional impairment, inappropriate affect, and poverty of speech content are more closely related to disorganization than to negative symptoms (Mitra et al. 2016).

Conceptually, negative symptoms can be divided into primary and secondary negative symptoms. Primary negative symptoms are directly caused by schizophrenia. Frequently, they are chronic and difficult to treat, persist during periods of clinical stability, and remain stable over many years. Primary enduring negative symptoms are sometimes labeled "deficit syndrome" (Foussias et al. 2014). Secondary negative symptoms, however, are not directly caused by schizophrenia. They might be iatrogenic, as when antipsychotics cause parkinsonism or other extrapyramidal side effects such as rigidity and bradykinesia that mimic negative symptoms. They might be environmental, as when chronic institutionalization, a low-stimulation environment, or poor social support leads to apathy, inactivity, or emotional unresponsiveness. Depression is also commonly associated with decreased interests, affective flattening, and psychomotor retardation. Positive symptoms, such as paranoia, can lead to suspicious withdrawal or other behaviors that resemble negative symptoms. Distinguishing between primary and secondary negative symptoms can be difficult. Nevertheless, clinicians should look for reversible or treatable etiologies and try to remedy them before concluding that a patient has primary negative symptoms (Foussias et al. 2014).

Anhedonia warrants special mention because research suggests that the term *anhedonia* is misleading. Evidence indicates that hedonic capacity is actually preserved in schizophrenia. Studies using emotion-eliciting stimuli (films, pictures, sounds, tastes) and assessing participants' emotions in the moment have shown that patients with schizophrenia experience pleasant and unpleasant emotions with the same intensity as healthy control subjects (Foussias et al. 2014). First-episode and chronic schizophrenia patients both seem to have intact experiences of emotions (Foussias et al. 2014). This evidence suggests that rather than labeling the experience "anhedonia," a more accurate description might be "reduced pleasure-seeking behavior" or "beliefs of low pleasure" (Foussias et al. 2014).

Research into amotivation suggests that this deficit might center around problems with learning, anticipating, and planning (Foussias et al. 2014). Patients with schizophrenia show impaired reward learning, impaired coupling of behaviors with the motivational properties of stimuli, difficulty integrating information about rewards and punishments, deficits in anticipating rewards, difficulty maintaining and updating internal value representations, and problems using this information to guide goal-directed behavior. In laboratory settings, they tend (more than control subjects) to prefer smaller, more immediate rewards and to discount the value of larger future rewards. Defeatist beliefs about performance have also been observed. What appears to be a lack of motivation might actually be caused by an impaired ability to learn how rewards are structured and to convert those experiences into action.

Epidemiology of Negative Symptoms

Negative symptoms are sometimes seen early in the course of schizophrenia and may appear before the onset of frank psychosis. Negative symptoms are common among both first-episode schizophrenia patients (15%) and chronic schizophrenia patients (25%–30%) (Kirkpatrick et al. 2001).

Negative symptoms are not specific to schizophrenia and can also be seen among patients with depression, Parkinson's disease, Alzheimer's disease, Huntington's disease, frontotemporal dementia, progressive supranuclear palsy, temporal lobe epilepsy, multiple sclerosis, and traumatic brain injury (Foussias et al. 2014). In these other conditions, the symptoms are sometimes labeled "apathy." Literature is mixed regarding whether negative symptoms are more frequent or more severe among schizophrenia patients versus nonschizophrenia mental health patients. There is some evidence that enduring primary negative symptoms are more common in schizophrenia than in major depression or other nonschizophrenia illnesses, suggesting that enduring primary negative symptoms are more specific to schizophrenia (Foussias et al. 2014). There is also evidence that negative symptoms (especially poverty of speech and affective flattening) tend to be more severe in schizophrenia than in schizoaffective disorder (Foussias et al. 2014).

Etiology

A variety of neuroimaging studies have looked for associations between brain structure and function and negative symptoms of schizophrenia. For example, studies focusing on brain networks have noted relationships between more severe negative symptoms and the following: a decrease in prefrontal white matter volume (especially in orbitofrontal regions); volume loss in the anterior cingulate, insular cortex, and left temporal cortex; and ventricular enlargement (Mitra et al. 2016). Severity of negative symptoms has also been associated with reduced cerebral blood perfusion in frontal, prefrontal, posterior cingulate, thalamus, some parietal, and striatal regions (Mitra et al. 2016). In regard to particular symptom domains, alogia and affective flattening have been associated with frontotemporal network dysfunction, motivational deficits correlate with ventral striatal dysfunction, and apathy has been related to reduced frontal lobe volumes and reduced ventral striatal responsiveness during reward anticipation (Foussias et al. 2014).

Biochemical pathways have also been implicated (Mitra et al. 2016). Consistent with theories that low cortical dopamine transmission in the mesocortical pathways contributes to negative symptoms, researchers have found that low plasma homovanillic acid levels predict more severe negative symptoms. The involvement of noradrenergic pathways has been suggested, based on observations that more severe negative symptoms are associated with decreased noradrenaline levels in cerebrospinal fluid, decreased urinary 3-methoxy-4-hydroxy-phenylglycol (a noradrenaline metabolite), and the (limited) benefits associated with noradrenergic drugs such as imipramine. Antipsychotics with serotonin receptor activity have sometimes been helpful to patients with negative symptoms, indicating that serotonin transmission may also play a role.

Additional causes of the negative symptoms of schizophrenia with some supporting evidence include neuroinflammation, hypofunction of the N-methyl-D-aspartate (NMDA) system, and genetic factors (Mitra et al. 2016).

Functional Outcomes

More severe negative symptoms are associated with worse functional outcomes, including poorer occupational functioning, economic status, household integration, social functioning (social interactions, interpersonal relationships), engagement in recreational activities, and quality of life (Foussias et al. 2014). Negative symptoms can directly affect functional outcomes and can also play an indirect role by exacerbating the relationship between cognitive problems and poor outcomes (Foussias et al. 2014). Motivational deficits are a particularly important predictor of impaired functioning (Foussias et al. 2014).

Disorganization

Description

Factor analysis studies indicate that disorganization is a distinct symptom domain, separate from positive and negative symptoms (Malla et al. 1993). Disorganization was once thought to be specific to schizophrenia, but it can also occur in individuals with affective psychoses or nonpsychotic illnesses and in individuals without psychiatric illness (Roche et al. 2015).

Disorganization is a heterogeneous entity, and its core clinical phenotype has not been definitively established (Roche et al. 2015). It may reflect a cluster of related cognitive, linguistic, behavioral, and affective disturbances (Roche et al. 2015). DSM-5 distinguishes between disorganized thinking, which is sometimes called formal thought disorder and is typically inferred from the individual's speech, and grossly disorganized or abnormal motor behavior, which includes childlike silliness, unpredictable agitation, and catatonic behavior. Disorganized behaviors might include eccentricity, mannerisms, paradoxical acts, aggression, agitation, rituals, stereotyped actions (Nestsiarovich et al. 2017), inappropriate affect or behavior, and inattention (Roche et al. 2015). Thought disorder can appear as distorted or inconsistent thinking, disrupted speech, ungrammatical construction of phrases, or tangentiality (Nestsiarovich et al. 2017). Patients may also respond to questions in an oblique manner, switch topics disjointedly, or use neologisms (made-up words) (Kerns and Berenbaum 2002). A distinction is sometimes made between positive thought disorder (incoherence, use of peculiar words, distractibility), which is part of the disorganization factor, and negative thought disorder (reduction in the amount and content of speech), which is part of the negative symptom factors (Kircher et al. 2001). Some studies have found pressured speech to be a symptom of disorganization (Roche et al. 2015).

Etiology

Research into disorganization has been limited, and much remains unknown about these symptoms (Nestsiarovich et al. 2017). Various studies have pointed toward contributions from genetics, NMDA receptor dysfunction, and environmental stressors, but many of these findings have not been replicated, and there is no consensus on the underlying pathological processes (Nestsiarovich et al. 2017). There is evidence that thought disorder is associated with impaired executive function and impaired processing of semantic information and that it has a small association with impaired language production (Kerns and Berenbaum 2002).

Neuroimaging studies on thought disorder in schizophrenia have resulted in diverse findings, and research in this area is ongoing. In structural studies, thought disorder correlated with bilateral gray matter deficits in the language network, including the bilateral inferior frontal gyrus, left frontal operculum, bilateral superior temporal gyrus, left superior temporal sulcus, and left angular gyrus (Cavelti et al. 2018). Thought disorder was also associated with diminished asymmetry of the planum temporale, indicating a decrease of the normal hemispheric lateralization of the language network (Cavelti et al. 2018). Most resting state fMRI studies suggest that thought disorder is related to hyperactivity in the bilateral language network, especially in the inferior frontal gyrus, superior temporal gyrus, middle temporal gyrus, and inferior parietal lobe (Cavelti et al. 2018). In short, thought disorder in schizophrenia is likely associated with aberrations in gray matter structure and neural activity of cortical regions involved with language processing. There is also evidence for altered gray matter structure (mostly volume loss) and neural activity (both hypoactivity and hyperactivity) in brain regions associated with aspects of speech production, namely, the middle and superior frontal gyri, the insular cortex, the cingulate gyrus, the precentral gyrus, the cuneus/lingual gyrus, the fusiform gyrus, the parahippocampal gyrus, and the cerebellum (Cavelti et al. 2018).

Epidemiology

The prevalence of thought disorder among patients with schizophrenia has been difficult to measure because rating scale validation studies have been limited in the general population, studies rarely use more than one thought disorder assessment scale for comparative purposes, and scales do not have well-defined cutoffs separating thought disorder from normal ranges. Existing data suggest a high prevalence of thought disorder among patients with schizophrenia, especially among inpatient samples. The largest study (N=1,665) reported that 50.39% of patients with schizophrenia have thought disorder (Breier and Berg 1999). Another study (N=660 inpatients with schizophrenia and other psychotic illnesses) reported a prevalence of 72.7% for the entire sample (Cuesta and Peralta 2011). The prevalence among inpatients was markedly lower (27.4%) when stricter criteria were used to define thought disorder (Howard et al. 1993). By comparison, an estimated 6% of individuals without psychiatric illness have thought disorder (Roche et al. 2015).

When patients are followed longitudinally, thought disorder seems to wax and wane for some diagnoses, but it tends to persist for patients with schizophrenia. In a 6-month study, thought disorder remitted more for patients with mania and schizoaffective disorder than for patients with schizophrenia (Andreasen and Grove 1986). In an 8-year longitudinal study, persistent thought disorder was rare in nonpsychotic disorders (4%) and was more common in schizophrenia (24%) (Roche et al. 2015). At follow-up, thought disorder was best predicted by diagnosis (premorbid social and academic functioning also predicted thought disorder), and severe thought disorder was usually associated with chronic unremitting schizophrenia rather than with acute relapse (Roche et al. 2015). Another study included 10- and 20-year follow-ups and reported that thought disorder was significantly more severe in patients with schizophrenia than in patients with other diagnoses (Wilcox et al. 2012). Thought disorder likely increases in the 6 years following a first episode of psychosis (Roche et al. 2015).

Few predictors of thought disorder have been identified, and it is not correlated with most common demographic variables. It may be more prevalent in early-onset schizophrenia (54.5%) than in late-onset schizophrenia (5.6%) (Roche et al. 2015). Cannabis abuse prior to the onset of schizophrenia is associated with more severe thought disorder (Roche et al. 2015).

Functional Outcomes

Disorganized behaviors can interfere with social functioning when they lead to illegal acts and make it difficult to communicate effectively with clinicians and/or social supports (Nestsiarovich et al. 2017).

Thought disorder is associated with worse social functioning, including poor conversation skills. Hospital admissions are more likely to occur, are more likely to be involuntary, and are more likely to be longer (Roche et al. 2015). In longitudinal studies, it is the clinical course (rather than baseline measures of thought disorder) that has the most influence on overall outcome, work functioning, rehospitalization, and clinical symptoms: a more persistent course predicts a worse outcome (Roche et al. 2015).

Diagnosis of Schizophrenia

The symptom pattern that defines DSM-5 schizophrenia comprises at least one active-phase syndrome (defined in Criterion A) plus periods of prodromal and/or residual symptoms so that the total continuous duration of symptoms is at least 6 months (Criterion C). The active-phase syndrome consists of at least two active-phase symptoms, each present for a significant portion of time during a 1-month period (although this period can be shorter than 1 month if the symptoms have been successfully treated). The active-phase symptoms included in DSM-5 are 1) delusions, 2) hallucinations, 3) disorganized speech, 4) grossly disorganized or catatonic behavior, and 5) negative symptoms. Moreover, although only two active-phase symptoms are required, at least one of them must be delusions, hallucinations, or disorganized speech in order for the patient to meet Criterion A of schizophrenia. The prodromal period (which precedes the first period of active-phase symptoms) and the residual periods (which occur between the active-phase periods) are manifested by either negative symptoms (without any positive symptoms) or two or more active-phase symptoms in an attenuated form (e.g., odd beliefs, unusual perceptual experiences). Although most cases of schizophrenia consist of a mixture of active-phase periods and prodromal/residual periods, some cases are characterized by continuous active-phase symptoms.

In addition to these symptomatic requirements, a diagnosis of schizophrenia requires that the patient's level of functioning since the onset of the disturbance (in areas such as work, interpersonal relations, or self-care) be markedly below the level achieved prior to the onset (Criterion B).

The remaining DSM-5 criteria require that certain other mental disorders be considered and ruled out before a diagnosis of schizophrenia can be made. In situations in which there is a mixture of both mood and psychotic symptoms, the competing diagnoses of schizoaffective disorder and mood disorder with psychotic features can be ruled out based on the temporal course of the mood and psychotic symptoms. If psychotic symptoms occur exclusively during mood episodes, a diagnosis of major depressive disorder or bipolar disorder with psychotic features would apply instead of schizophrenia. In cases in which there are periods with a mixture of mood and psychotic symptoms as well as other periods in which there are psychotic symptoms occurring in the absence of a major mood episode, the diagnosis of schizoaffective disorder would apply if mood episodes have been present for a majority of the total duration of the active and residual phases of the illness (Criterion D). If the psychotic symptoms are due to the direct physiological effects of a substance or a medical condition, the diagnosis is substance-induced psychotic disorder or psychotic disorder due to another medical condition (Criterion E).

Additional Symptoms Associated With Schizophrenia

Cognitive Symptoms

Description

Cognitive symptoms are estimated to affect 85% of patients with schizophrenia (Isaac and Januel 2016). Cognitive impairment is distinct from other schizophrenia symptoms and often remains after acute symptoms are stabilized.

The NIMH MATRICS group identified six cognitive domains affected in schizophrenia: speed of processing (e.g., the speed with which digit/symbol pairings can be completed); attention or vigilance (e.g., tasks requiring sustained attention); working memory (e.g., remembering and repeating a span of digits); verbal learning memory (e.g., immediate and delayed recall of word lists); visual learning memory (e.g., recognizing faces); and reasoning and problem solving (e.g., sorting cards by an abstract principle that changes over time) (Nuechterlein et al. 2004).

Longitudinal studies have identified mild neuropsychological deficits among children who later go on to develop schizophrenia. In the premorbid phase, persons who later develop schizophrenia have an 8-point IQ deficit relative to healthy control subjects (Woodberry et al. 2008). First-episode and chronic schizophrenia patients demonstrated a 14- to 21-point IQ deficit (Meier et al. 2014). One cohort study that followed approximately 1,000 participants from early childhood found that those who developed schizophrenia had an average IQ of 93.63 in childhood, which declined to 87.92 in adulthood (Meier et al. 2014). IQ was stable from ages 7 to 13 and then decreased significantly for the schizophrenia group between ages 13 and 38. The schizophrenia group showed decline in a variety of neurocognitive tests: Digit Symbol Coding (processing speed), Rey Total Recall (learning), Trails A (processing speed), Trails B (executive functioning), and Grooved Pegboard (motor functioning) (Meier et al. 2014).

Functional Outcomes

Among persons with schizophrenia, neurocognitive deficits predict 40%–50% of the variance in adaptive and community functioning (Velligan et al. 2000). One study of adults with schizophrenia recently discharged from a state hospital observed several associations between cognitive functions and social outcomes (Velligan et al. 2000). Verbal memory (Hopkins Verbal Learning Test and Digit Span) correlated with social and occupational functioning (Social and Occupational Functioning Assessment Scale), activities of daily living (Multnomah Community Ability Scale), and social competence (Multnomah Community Ability Scale). Executive function (reverse reaction time and Wisconsin Card Sorting Test) correlated with social and occupational functioning, activities of daily living, work and productivity, and social competence. Vigilance (Continuous Performance Test—Identical Pairs version) correlated with social and occupational functioning and social competence. Visual memory and organization (Rey-Osterrieth Complex Figure Test) correlated with activities of daily living.

Mood and Anxiety Symptoms

Although depression and anxiety are not among the defining symptoms, they are common among individuals with schizophrenia.

Depression

Schizophrenia and depression were historically treated as separate entities. However, both conditions can occur at the same time. An estimated 25% of patients with schizophrenia experience depression (estimates vary from 7% to 75% depending on the study criteria) (Siris 2000).

Diagnostically, it can be challenging to distinguish between schizophrenia with comorbid depression, bipolar depression with psychotic features, unipolar depression with psychotic features, and schizoaffective disorder. Accurate diagnosis requires thorough knowledge of the longitudinal course of both the mood and the psychotic symptoms. Bipolar depression and unipolar depression are likely if the psychosis resolves between mood episodes. In schizoaffective disorder as defined by DSM-5 criteria, the symptoms of a major mood episode must be present for the majority of the duration of the illness (American Psychiatric Association 2013). If the psychotic symptoms are persistent over time and if the depressive symptoms appear intermittently (not for a majority of the time), then schizophrenia and depression can both be diagnosed.

Comorbid depression is associated with a worse prognosis for patients with schizophrenia. For example, depressed patients with schizophrenia experience more impaired functioning, more personal suffering, higher rates of relapse and rehospitalization, and greater risk of suicide (Siris 2000). When depressive symptoms appear, it is important to consider the differential diagnosis. Depression-like symptoms can be caused by active medical problems, including cardiovascular disorders, pulmonary infections, autoimmune diseases, anemia, cancer, metabolic disorders, neurological problems, and endocrine disorders. Depression can occur as a medication side effect. The following have been implicated in depression: β-blockers, other antihypertensives, hypnotics, antineoplastics, barbiturates, nonsteroidal anti-inflammatory drugs, sulfonamides, and indomethacin. Depressive symptoms can also occur when some medications are stopped, especially corticosteroids and psychostimulants (including nicotine and caffeine, which are frequently stopped abruptly when patients are hospitalized) (Siris 2000).

Depression and negative symptoms of schizophrenia can look similar, especially reduced interest in activities, few experiences of pleasure, low energy, low motivation, psychomotor slowing, and impaired concentration. Classically, blunted affect is considered more suggestive of negative symptoms, whereas sad mood, guilty feelings, or suicidal thoughts are more suggestive of depression (Siris 2000).

Depressive symptoms can sometimes emerge as part of a prodrome that appears days or a few weeks before a psychotic relapse (Siris 2000). Depressive symptoms and dysphoria might be accompanied by anxiety, withdrawal, guilt, and shame. When patients are also hypervigilant, experience perceptual disturbances, or overinterpret perceptions or events, a psychotic relapse might be emerging.

The relationship between depressive symptoms and antipsychotics has long been the subject of debate. Dopamine blockade likely interacts with the brain's reward circuitry, so there is a theoretical possibility that antipsychotics could contribute to anhedonia and depression. However, the evidence suggests that depressive symptoms are often present before antipsychotics are given and that depressive symptoms frequently subside with antipsychotic treatment (Siris 2000). Moreover, patients with schizophrenia who receive antipsychotics do not have higher rates of depression than patients who do not receive antipsychotics (Siris 2000).

Anxiety Symptoms

A variety of anxiety disorders are especially common among patients with schizophrenia. Panic attacks have a prevalence of approximately 25%, and panic disorder has a prevalence of approximately 15% (Buckley et al. 2009). In contrast, the lifetime prevalence of panic disorder in the general population is between 2% and 5.1%. Panic symptoms have been associated with poorer initial outcomes, more severe psychopathology, and more positive symptoms of psychosis after 24 months. Panic symptoms may also increase the risk of suicidal ideation and behavior and increase vulnerability to substance abuse.

PTSD affects approximately 29% of persons with schizophrenia versus 7.8% of the general population (Buckley et al. 2009). Among patients with schizophrenia, the presence of PTSD has been associated with more severe psychopathology, cognitive impairment, more suicidal ideation and behavior, more frequent outpatient medical visits, and more hospitalizations. The increased prevalence of PTSD is not thought to be part of the schizophrenia illness, but rather to be caused by more environmental risk factors (e.g., increased rates of traumatic experiences related to substance use, homelessness, or incarceration).

Obsessive-compulsive disorder (OCD) may affect up to 23% of patients with schizophrenia (Buckley et al. 2009). True prevalence estimates are difficult to generate because of challenges involved in distinguishing obsessions and compulsions from delusions and disorganized behavior. Some evidence suggests that comorbid OCD is associated with earlier age at onset, more OCD-spectrum disorders (including tic disorder and body dysmorphic disorder), more paranoia and first-rank psychotic symptoms, more executive dysfunction, and more depression.

Complications of Schizophrenia

Suicide

Suicide risk is markedly increased among persons with schizophrenia. The lifetime suicide mortality rate is estimated at 4%–6%, and 2%–12% of all suicides in the general population are attributable to schizophrenia (Popovic et al. 2014). Many of the suicides happen early in the illness; an estimated 2.4% of patients with schizophrenia die by suicide in the first 5 years of their illness.

Several factors are known to increase the suicide risk in schizophrenia. A prior suicide attempt is one of the strongest risk factors (Hawton et al. 2005). Risk remains especially high for 2 years following a suicide attempt. Current depression, a prior depressive episode, and a family history of depression all increase risk (Hawton et al. 2005). It is estimated that half of patients with schizophrenia who commit suicide have depression (Popovic et al. 2014). Hopelessness is a risk factor for suicide, even in the absence of depression (Popovic et al. 2014). Having more psychiatric hospitalizations is associated with more suicide risk (Popovic et al. 2014). Suicide risk is high during and after hospitalizations; one-third of suicides happen in the hospital or in the week following discharge, and the risk remains elevated throughout the year after discharge (Popovic et al. 2014). Although suicide risk remains elevated throughout the life span, it is especially high among younger patients, among patients who are older when the illness develops, and during the first few years after illness onset (Popovic et al. 2014). Additional risk factors include living alone or not living with family, having a recent loss event, and being poorly adherent to treatment (Hawton et al. 2005). Those patients with a higher number of positive symptoms, paranoia or suspiciousness, or agitation or motor restlessness and those who fear mental disintegration are also at increased suicide risk (Hawton et al. 2005).

Data are more ambiguous for other factors sometimes associated with suicide in the general population. Suicides are more common among males than females, but the gender difference among those with schizophrenia is not as marked as among the general population (Popovic et al. 2014). Use of alcohol or stimulants (cocaine, amphetamines) likely increases suicide attempts, but the data are less clear about completed suicides (Popovic et al. 2014). Command hallucinations may not increase risk. Delusions have been associated with a decreased risk of suicide in some literature (Hawton et al. 2005). Negative symptoms and insight into the illness were not associated with increased risk (Hawton et al. 2005). Some putative biomarkers (cerebrospinal fluid monoamine metabolites, tryptophan hydroxylase 1 genetic locus) have not been shown to be associated with suicidal behavior in patients with schizophrenia (Popovic et al. 2014).

Substance Use

Substance use disorders (not including nicotine) affect 47% of patients with schizophrenia, which is triple the background rate in the general population (Green 2006). Alcohol use disorder is present among 34% of patients (three times the general population rate), and 28% have other substance use disorders (six times the general population rate). Nicotine use affects up to 75%–90% of patients with schizophrenia versus 21% of the general population. Substance use is an early comorbidity in schizophrenia: 37% of first-episode patients have a history of substance use disorders, especially involving cannabis (28%) and alcohol (21%).

One theory about these high rates of substance use disorders is that schizophrenia causes dysregulation of the dopamine-mediated mesocorticolimbic network, which disrupts the brain's reward circuitry. The use of substances might briefly allow patients with schizophrenia to experience normal rewards from daily life. There is also some evidence that substance use can lessen negative symptoms, but this has limited explanatory power because schizophrenia patients with negative symptoms are less likely to use substances compared with other schizophrenia patients (Green 2006).

There is probably not a simple cause-effect relationship between substance use and the development of schizophrenia; however, there is evidence linking substance use with an earlier age at schizophrenia onset. In one study, individuals who abused drugs showed the first signs of schizophrenia at age 17.7 years, whereas persons who did not engage in substance abuse showed the first signs at age 25.7 years (Hambrecht and Häfner 1996). In another study, male cannabis users had their first psychotic episode 6.9 years earlier than male nonusers (Veen et al. 2004).

Among patients with chronic schizophrenia, substance use disorders are associated with poorer outcomes, including higher relapse rates, more treatment nonadherence, poorer response to medications, more hospitalizations, more violence risk, and higher medical costs (Green 2006).

Violence

The vast majority of persons with schizophrenia are not violent. Nevertheless, researchers have frequently observed a link between schizophrenia and violent behavior. In a study examining several large registries in Sweden (the Hospital Discharge Registry, the Crime Register, the National Censuses, the Multi-Generation Register, the causes of death register, and the total population register), 12%–13% of patients with schizophrenia had a conviction for a violent crime, versus 5%–8% of control subjects (Fazel et al. 2009). These percentages correspond to an increased risk of violent crime among patients with schizophrenia compared with general population control subjects (adjusted odds ratio [OR]=2.0) and unaffected siblings (adjusted OR=1.6). Importantly, violent crimes were far more prevalent among schizophrenia patients with comorbid substance abuse (27.6%, OR=4.4) than among those not engaged in substance abuse (8.5%, OR=1.2). The study authors concluded that associations between schizophrenia and violent crimes are minimal in the absence of comorbid substance use.

Analyses from the Clinical Antipsychotic Trials of Intervention Effectiveness (CATIE) schizophrenia trial found that prospective predictors of violence include economic deprivation, living with family (vs. living alone), living with nonrelatives (vs. living alone), a history of childhood conduct problems, substance use, substance misuse/ dependence, and a history of violent victimization (Swanson et al. 2008). Negative psychotic symptoms decreased the risk of violence.

Patients with schizophrenia are also at very high risk of being the victims of violence. In a study of adults with schizophrenia living in the community (N=172) who were followed for 3 years, 65 individuals (38%) reported being the victim of a crime during the study period, of whom 59 individuals (34%) were the victims of violent crimes (robbery, rape, assault). Individuals experienced 118 separate incidents, of which 107 (91%) were violent crimes (Brekke et al. 2001). Another study compared adults with severe mental illness with the National Crime Victimization Survey and found that more than a quarter of adults with severe mental illness had been victims of a violent crime in the past year, which is 11 times higher than the general population rates (Teplin et al. 2005).

Conclusion

Persons with schizophrenia may experience a wide variety of symptoms affecting their lives in many domains. Patients, family members, and treaters must remain mindful that the illness can affect a person's life in many ways. Ideally, a comprehensive plan of care will create opportunities to identify symptoms quickly and provide appropriate support so that patients can continue pursuing their life goals.

References

American Psychiatric Association: Diagnostic and Statistical Manual of Mental Disorders, 5th Edition. Arlington, VA, American Psychiatric Association, 2013

Andreasen NC, Grove WM: Thought, language, and communication in schizophrenia: diagnosis and prognosis. Schizophr Bull 12(3):348–359, 1986 3764356

Appelbaum PS, Robbins PC, Roth LH: Dimensional approach to delusions: comparison across types and diagnoses. Am J Psychiatry 156(12):1938–1943, 1999 10588408

Bebbington P, Freeman D: Transdiagnostic extension of delusions: schizophrenia and beyond. Schizophr Bull 43(2):273–282, 2017 28399309

Breier A, Berg PH: The psychosis of schizophrenia: prevalence, response to atypical antipsychotics, and prediction of outcome. Biol Psychiatry 46(3):361–364, 1999 10435201

Brekke JS, Prindle C, Bae SW, et al: Risks for individuals with schizophrenia who are living in the community. Psychiatr Serv 52(10):1358–1366, 2001 11585953

Buckley PF, Miller BJ, Lehrer DS, et al: Psychiatric comorbidities and schizophrenia. Schizophr Bull 35(2):383–402, 2009 19011234

Cavelti M, Kircher T, Nagels A, et al: Is formal thought disorder in schizophrenia related to structural and functional aberrations in the language network? A systematic review of neuroimaging findings. Schizophr Res 199:2–16, 2018 29510928

Cuesta MJ, Peralta V: Testing the hypothesis that formal thought disorders are severe mood disorders. Schizophr Bull 37(6):1136–1146, 2011 21857008

Cutting J: First rank symptoms of schizophrenia: their nature and origin. Hist Psychiatry 26(2):131–146, 2015 26022465

Dudley R, Taylor P, Wickham S, et al: Psychosis, delusions and the "jumping to conclusions" reasoning bias: a systematic review and meta-analysis. Schizophr Bull 42(3):652–665, 2016 26519952

Fazel S, Långström N, Hjern A, et al: Schizophrenia, substance abuse, and violent crime. JAMA 301(19):2016–2023, 2009 19454640

Foussias G, Agid O, Fervaha G, et al: Negative symptoms of schizophrenia: clinical features, relevance to real world functioning and specificity versus other CNS disorders. Eur Neuropsychopharmacol 24(5):693–709, 2014 24275699

Green AI: Treatment of schizophrenia and comorbid substance abuse: pharmacologic approaches. J Clin Psychiatry 67 (suppl 7):31–35, quiz 36–37, 2006 16961422

Hambrecht M, Häfner H: Substance abuse and the onset of schizophrenia. Biol Psychiatry 40(11):1155–1163, 1996 8931919

Hawton K, Sutton L, Haw C, et al: Schizophrenia and suicide: systematic review of risk factors. Br J Psychiatry 187(1):9–20, 2005 15994566

Howard R, Castle D, Wessely S, et al: A comparative study of 470 cases of early-onset and late-onset schizophrenia. Br J Psychiatry 163:352–357, 1993 8401965

Isaac C, Januel D: Neural correlates of cognitive improvements following cognitive remediation in schizophrenia: a systematic review of randomized trials. Socioaffect Neurosci Psychol 6(6):30054, 2016 26993787

Kerns JG, Berenbaum H: Cognitive impairments associated with formal thought disorder in people with schizophrenia. J Abnorm Psychol 111(2):211–224, 2002 12003444

Kircher TT, Liddle PF, Brammer MJ, et al: Neural correlates of formal thought disorder in schizophrenia: preliminary findings from a functional magnetic resonance imaging study. Arch Gen Psychiatry 58(8):769–774, 2001 11483143

Kirkpatrick B, Buchanan RW, Ross DE, et al: A separate disease within the syndrome of schizophrenia. Arch Gen Psychiatry 58(2):165–171, 2001 11177118

Knobel A, Heinz A, Voss M: Imaging the deluded brain. Eur Arch Psychiatry Clin Neurosci 258 (suppl 5):76–80, 2008 18985300

Larøi F, Sommer IE, Blom JD, et al: The characteristic features of auditory verbal hallucinations in clinical and nonclinical groups: state-of-the-art overview and future directions. Schizophr Bull 38(4):724–733, 2012 22499783

Malla AK, Norman RM, Williamson P, et al: Three syndrome concept of schizophrenia: a factor analytic study. Schizophr Res 10(2):143–150, 1993 8398946

Meier MH, Caspi A, Reichenberg A, et al: Neuropsychological decline in schizophrenia from the premorbid to the postonset period: evidence from a population-representative longitudinal study. Am J Psychiatry 171(1):91–101, 2014 24030246

Mitra S, Mahintamani T, Kavoor AR, et al: Negative symptoms in schizophrenia. Ind Psychiatry J 25(2):135–144, 2016 28659691

Moseley P, Fernyhough C, Ellison A: Auditory verbal hallucinations as atypical inner speech monitoring, and the potential of neurostimulation as a treatment option. Neurosci Biobehav Rev 37(10 Pt 2):2794–2805, 2013 24125858

Nestsiarovich A, Obyedkov V, Kandratsenka H, et al: Disorganization at the stage of schizophrenia clinical outcome: clinical-biological study. Eur Psychiatry 42:44–48, 2017 28192769

Nuechterlein KH, Barch DM, Gold JM, et al: Identification of separable cognitive factors in schizophrenia. Schizophr Res 72(1):29–39, 2004 15531405

Popovic D, Benabarre A, Crespo JM, et al: Risk factors for suicide in schizophrenia: systematic review and clinical recommendations. Acta Psychiatr Scand 130(6):418–426, 2014 25230813

Roche E, Creed L, MacMahon D, et al: The epidemiology and associated phenomenology of formal thought disorder: a systematic review. Schizophr Bull 41(4):951–962, 2015 25180313

Siris SG: Depression in schizophrenia: perspective in the era of "atypical" antipsychotic agents. Am J Psychiatry 157(9):1379–1389, 2000 10964850

Stip E, Letourneau G: Psychotic symptoms as a continuum between normality and pathology. Can J Psychiatry 54(3):140–151, 2009 19321018

Swanson JW, Swartz MS, Van Dorn RA, et al; CATIE investigators: Comparison of antipsychotic medication effects on reducing violence in people with schizophrenia. Br J Psychiatry 193(1):37–43, 2008 18700216

Tanenberg-Karant M, Fennig S, Ram R, et al: Bizarre delusions and first-rank symptoms in a first-admission sample: a preliminary analysis of prevalence and correlates. Compr Psychiatry 36(6):428–434, 1995 8565447

Teplin LA, McClelland GM, Abram KM, et al: Crime victimization in adults with severe mental illness: comparison with the National Crime Victimization Survey. Arch Gen Psychiatry 62(8):911–921, 2005 16061769

Veen ND, Selten JP, van der Tweel I, et al: Cannabis use and age at onset of schizophrenia. Am J Psychiatry 161(3):501–506, 2004 14992976

Velligan DI, Bow-Thomas CC, Mahurin RK, et al: Do specific neurocognitive deficits predict specific domains of community function in schizophrenia? J Nerv Ment Dis 188(8):518–524, 2000 10972571

Waters F, Fernyhough C: Hallucinations: a systematic review of points of similarity and difference across diagnostic classes. Schizophr Bull 43(1):32–43, 2017 27872259

Wilcox J, Winokur G, Tsuang M: Predictive value of thought disorder in new-onset psychosis. Compr Psychiatry 53(6):674–678, 2012 22341649

Woodberry KA, Giuliano AJ, Seidman LJ: Premorbid IQ in schizophrenia: a meta-analytic review. Am J Psychiatry 165(5):579–587, 2008 18413704

Zmigrod L, Garrison JR, Carr J, Simons JS: The neural mechanisms of hallucinations: a quantitative meta-analysis of neuroimaging studies. Neurosci Biobehav Rev 69:113–123, 2016 27473935

CHAPTER 4

Cultural Variations

Neil Krishan Aggarwal, M.D., M.B.A., M.A.
Roberto Lewis-Fernández, M.D., M.T.S.

In this chapter, we discuss cultural variations in the presentation of schizophrenia. DSM-5 characterizes culture as "systems of knowledge, concepts, rules, and practices that are learned and transmitted across generations. Culture includes language, religion and spirituality, family structures, life-cycle stages, ceremonial rituals, and customs, as well as moral and legal systems" (American Psychiatric Association 2013, p. 749). DSM-5 further explains that all people construct unique, hybrid senses of selfhood because they are exposed to different cultural influences, which is why clinicians should not take a patient's cultural identity for granted:

> Cultures are open, dynamic systems that undergo continuous change over time; in the contemporary world, most individuals and groups are exposed to multiple cultures, which they use to fashion their own identities and make sense of experience. These features of culture make it crucial not to overgeneralize cultural information or stereotype groups in terms of fixed cultural traits. (p. 749)

We return to these characterizations of culture throughout the chapter.

Readers of a textbook on schizophrenia may wonder what is to be gained by assessing patients for cultural factors related to illness and treatment when the understanding of this disorder has been enriched through thousands of studies in genetics and neuroimaging since the 1970s (Kapur et al. 2012). However, research has also consistently found disparities in the identification and treatment of schizophrenia across social groups, notably among immigrants and racial and ethnic minorities. The past decade has witnessed the growth of professional guidelines and legal mandates specifying the need for clinicians at all levels of education to conduct thorough cultural assessments to address these disparities and to personalize care based on patients' and families' illness interpretations and treatment expectations. Medical students (Association of American Medical Colleges 2015), residents (American Board of Psychiatry and Neurology 2011), fellows and faculty at academic institutions (Accreditation

Council for Graduate Medical Education 2014), and clinicians in general (National Quality Forum 2012) are all expected to exhibit proficiencies in assessment, case formulation, patient communication, treatment planning, and clinical intervention that prioritize cultural competence, especially with the goal of eliminating disparities in quality of care across social groups. A firm grounding in cultural factors related to the diagnosis and treatment of schizophrenia is essential for all behavioral health clinicians.

With these goals and expectations in mind, this chapter is laid out in four sections. The first section reviews the legacy of Emil Kraepelin, who is widely regarded as a pioneer in studying the cross-cultural manifestations of mental illnesses, especially of psychotic disorders. The second and third sections provide an overview of studies on cultural variations in the incidence or prevalence, phenomenology, course, and treatment of schizophrenia, focusing particularly on differences by immigration status and by racial and ethnic background. Our intent is not to describe every instance of variation but rather to sensitize clinicians to consistent findings. The final section describes use of the DSM-5 Cultural Formulation Interview (CFI) as a cultural assessment tool that can elicit variations in symptom presentations and treatment preferences.

Emil Kraepelin and the Cross-Cultural Study of Mental Illnesses

The first known article to describe cultural variations in the manifestations of psychotic disorders comes from the German psychiatrist Emil Kraepelin (1856–1926). Today, Kraepelin is remembered for redefining psychiatric classification through clinical observations that distinguished mood from psychotic disorders and endogenous from exogenous disorders (Boroffka 1990). After a trip to Java in 1904, Kraepelin published his seminal article *"Vergleichende Psychiatrie"* ("Comparative Psychiatry"). Reading this article in our contemporary context demonstrates how certain scientific interests in cultural psychiatry have remained the same and others have evolved in conjunction with the social sciences. For example, Kraepelin lamented the lack of systematic research on the cross-cultural variations of mental illnesses: "The data hitherto available respecting mental illness in the races (*Rassen*) of other lands have been of very limited value even though the differences to be anticipated should make such a comparison fruitful and convincing" (Kraepelin 1904/1974, p. 108). Nine decades later, specialists in culture and mental health continued to express frustration at the dearth of studies that could meaningfully inform revisions to the diagnostic criteria that would constitute DSM-IV (American Psychiatric Association 1994): "The requirement that large-scale epidemiology and clinical validation studies be conducted on culture-related diagnoses poses a challenge that the largely ethnographic record of cultural psychiatry can, in most instances, not yet meet" (Kirmayer 1998, p. 340). Indeed, Kraepelin's voyage heralded a research agenda in cultural psychiatry that persists into the present—the extent to which illnesses manifest similarly or differently across societies (Kirmayer 2007).

Kraepelin attributed cross-cultural differences in illness manifestations to race, a link that cultural psychiatrists have questioned in modern times. One passage he wrote provides a particularly vivid illustration: "The early stages of a depression were rarely seen and violent excitement was also uncommon, but at the same time the very severe forms of dementia, so common in our own mental hospitals and found among the Europeans in Java as well, seem rarely to develop among the indigenous population" (Kraepelin 1904/1974, p. 111). Kraepelin's differentiation between "Europeans" and the "indigenous population" reflects the tendency of twentieth-century imperial medicine to describe symptom differences through the broad political categories of colonizer and colonized that psychiatrists now reject (Littlewood 1996). The terms *Europeans* and *indigenous populations* stereotype groups by making assumptions about fixed cultural traits; one needs only to go to Europe or Java to behold the diverse linguistic, religious, ethnic, and social diversity in these regions.

Kraepelin also drew connections between race, religion, nationhood, politics, and history that today's cultural psychiatrist would consider imprecise. Kraepelin (1904/1974) writes, "If the character of a nation is reflected in its religion and its customs, in its political actions and its historical development, then it will also find expression in the frequency and nature of its mental disorders, particularly those that are endogenous in origin" (p. 111). Kraepelin is clearly writing in the "culture and personality school" of psychology, which attempted to infer a nation's group psychology through the characteristics of a few studied individuals (Kirmayer 2007). However, empirical research that has compared national character ratings to average personality scores of people from those cultures shows that national character ratings did not converge with personality traits, leading to concerns that national character studies are unfounded stereotypes (Terracciano et al. 2005). Rather than start with categories such as "nation," "religion," "customs," "political actions," or "historical development," whose very meanings may differ among people, cultural psychiatrists recommend that today's psychiatrists adopt patient-centered approaches to cultural assessment that ask patients directly about their identities and how these identities relate to their manifesting illnesses (Aggarwal 2011). This approach departs from older models of cultural competence in which clinicians assumed that race, ethnicity, religion, nationality, or other categories influenced the manifestations of mental illnesses without probing how individuals fashion unique identities to make sense of their experiences with mental illness (Aggarwal 2012).

Our analysis of Kraepelin's work is not intended to judge him critically by today's standards but to delineate scientific areas of convergence and divergence. Definitions of culture and cultural assessment methods evolve in tandem with the social sciences such as anthropology, psychology, and sociology (Jayasuriya 2008). Therefore, clinicians can update their cultural knowledge as they would for other fields, such as neuroscience or pharmacology, by reading professional journals such as *Transcultural Psychiatry* or *Culture, Medicine, and Psychiatry* and by attending continuing education sessions addressing cultural assessment or health disparities (Aggarwal et al. 2016c).

Cross-Cultural Detection and Outcome of Schizophrenia

Distinguishing schizophrenia from other psychotic disorders and from experiences that appear psychotic but may not be ("psychotic-like symptoms") can be difficult, not only under cross-cultural circumstances but also when clinicians and participants share similar cultural backgrounds. Moreover, the outcome of schizophrenia appears to vary across cultural settings, suggesting that culture can affect illness course, including by impacting treatment options and utilization patterns. In this section, we discuss 1) difficulties that arise clinically in distinguishing psychotic disorders from psychotic-like symptoms; 2) methodological issues involved in the epidemiological assessment of schizophrenia; and 3) available cross-national findings on incidence, prevalence, and outcomes of schizophrenia.

Evaluating Psychotic-Like Symptoms

Across cultures, many individuals report symptoms that appear to be signs of psychosis but whose clinical status is uncertain. These symptoms usually consist of patient descriptions that sound like hallucinations and delusions that are not as functionally impairing but that lie on a continuum with more severe syndromes that meet criteria for a psychotic disorder. In a meta-analysis of 35 studies in the general population of numerous countries using self-report symptom scales, this "psychosis continuum" has a median prevalence of 5.3%, with an interquartile range of 1.9%–14.4%, a 7.6-fold difference. Although for some people these symptoms constitute a prodrome to clinical psychosis, most individuals reporting them never develop a diagnosable psychotic disorder (van Os et al. 2009).

The role of culture-related factors in the etiology, phenomenology, propensity to report, and distress associated with psychotic-like symptoms remains unclear, but the role of these factors is suggested by variations in their prevalence across countries, within racial and ethnic groups, and of endorsement of psychotic-like symptoms to acculturation, *acculturative stress* (defined as cognitive and/or behavioral difficulties during the acculturation process), and other culture-related factors. Systematic reviews of studies from multiple countries indicate that compared with majority populations, ethnic minorities have 1.35 higher odds of reporting psychotic-like experiences such as hallucinations or delusions that are clinically subthreshold and do not meet full criteria for a psychotic disorder (Linscott and van Os 2013). Acculturative stress was a key correlate of symptom endorsement in a subsample from the National Latino and Asian American Study (NLAAS) of first-generation immigrants to the United States ($N=2{,}434$). Greater acculturative stress showed a significant linear-trend relationship with visual and auditory hallucinations among Asians and with hearing voices among Latinos; younger age at immigration, indicating greater acculturation, was also associated with higher endorsement of any psychotic-like experiences among Latino immigrants (Devylder et al. 2013). This latter finding confirms research with the full Latino sample of the NLAAS (immigrants to and individuals born in the United States), which also showed that greater acculturation to U.S. society and reliance on religious/spiritual sources of help were associated with psychotic-like symptoms (Lewis-Fernández et al. 2009). Taken together, this research suggests that culture-related stressors and coping methods associated with the adverse aspects of immigration (e.g., family separation, discrimination) may be related to the emergence of psychotic-like experiences (Devylder et al. 2013; Lewis-Fernández et al. 2009; Vega et al. 2006).

Within the United States, chart reviews of Latino psychiatric outpatients demonstrate that 46%–95% have reported experiencing simple hallucinations (e.g., hearing steps, hearing voices calling their name, visual hallucinations of relatives or religious figures) that do not meet criteria for a psychotic disorder (Geltman and Chang 2004; Mischoulon et al. 2005). National epidemiological surveys using the DSM-IV Composite International Diagnostic Interview (CIDI) (N=16,423) confirm a higher prevalence of psychotic-like symptoms among U.S. Latinos than among other racial and ethnic groups, after adjusting for clinical covariates such as substance use disorder and PTSD (Cohen and Marino 2013). Only 7% of individuals endorsing these symptoms met criteria for a psychotic disorder on clinical reappraisal of a nationally representative Latino sample (N=2,554) using the Structured Clinical Interview for DSM-IV (SCID), confirming the nonpsychotic nature of most of these symptoms (Cohen and Marino 2013). Yet, compared with nonendorsers, individuals reporting psychotic-like symptoms had more physical and emotional distress, including significantly higher odds of suicidal ideation (OR=2.30), disability due to mental health problems (OR=1.81), and use of outpatient mental health services (OR=1.67) after adjustments for sociodemographic and clinical covariates (Lewis-Fernández et al. 2009). These associations were also found among Latinos accessing primary care services in New York City (Olfson et al. 2002). Careful clinical and cultural assessment is needed to distinguish between prodromal psychotic symptoms that can progress to severe conditions such as schizophrenia and psychotic-like experiences that constitute a marker of general psychiatric vulnerability (McGrath et al. 2016; Vega et al. 2006).

Methodological Concerns About Case Detection

The methodological limitations of lay-administered instruments in ascertaining the incidence and prevalence of schizophrenia in community-based studies are notorious. Unless the individuals then have validating assessments by clinicians, it is very difficult to distinguish a low-prevalence disorder such as schizophrenia from false positives that result from "respondent misunderstanding, schizotypal traits, drug-induced states, and culturally sanctioned magical or religious beliefs" (Kendler et al. 1996, p. 1022), as well as dissociative symptoms, affective psychoses, and other psychotic disorders. In a seminal study, Kendler and colleagues (1996) reported the results of a clinical reappraisal of the nonaffective psychosis diagnoses obtained on a national probability subsample (N=5,877) of the U.S. National Comorbidity Survey with the lay-administered CIDI. Follow-up interviews were conducted by mental health professionals and reviewed by a senior clinician. Whereas the CIDI algorithm yielded a lifetime U.S. prevalence of 1.3% for schizophrenia and schizophreniform disorder, clinical reappraisal reduced the national prevalence to 0.2%. The authors concluded that lifetime prevalence estimates of schizophrenia and other psychotic disorders in community samples "are strongly influenced by methods of assessment and diagnosis"; epidemiological surveys yielded estimates that "agreed poorly with clinical diagnoses" and "may require collection of extensive contextual information" in order to improve their accuracy (Kendler et al. 1996, p. 1022). As a result of these methodological limitations, more recent CIDI versions no longer include a schizophrenia module but instead include a nondiagnostic assessment of six psychotic symptoms and a screening question regarding receipt of a diagnosis of schizophrenia or psychosis by a clinician.

Cross-National Incidence, Prevalence, and Outcomes of Schizophrenia

The methodological problems discussed in the previous section raise concerns about the validity of epidemiological incidence and prevalence estimates that are obtained solely with lay-administered instruments. Luckily, other studies are available that yield epidemiological estimates that include some form of clinical validation, and these estimates can be compared with lay-administered community-based assessments. Two systematic reviews of incidence (McGrath et al. 2004) and prevalence (Saha et al. 2005) revealed that schizophrenia estimates range substantially not only across sites within a single country but across nations. The median annual incidence across 33 countries (N=176,056), for example, was 15.2 per 100,000 persons, but the 10%–90% quantile range was 7.7–43.0/100,000, a 5.6-fold difference across nations (McGrath et al. 2004). The median lifetime prevalence across 46 countries (N=154,140) was 4.0/1,000 persons, with a 7.6-fold range of 1.6–12.1/1,000 (Saha et al. 2005). Interestingly, method of case identification (i.e., lay-administered community-based surveys, clinical interviews, chart/case records) did not significantly affect the estimate distributions (McGrath et al. 2004). Another review of annual incidence noted a cross-national variation "greater than one order of magnitude, from a low estimate in the city of Vancouver of 0.04/1000/year to a high estimate in the city of Madras (now Chennai) of 0.58/1000/year" (Messias et al. 2007, p. 325). These more recent estimates confirm and expand on the cross-national incidence variation found in three large studies conducted by the World Health Organization (WHO): the International Pilot Study of Schizophrenia (World Health Organization 1973), the Determinants of Outcome Study (Sartorius et al. 1986), and the International Study of Schizophrenia (Hopper et al. 2007).

Longitudinal follow-up of individuals with schizophrenia conducted as part of these WHO studies revealed significant variability in outcomes, with better prognosis in low- and middle-income countries (LMICs) (e.g., India, Nigeria) than in high-income countries (HICs) (e.g., Denmark, the United States) (Leff et al. 1992; Sartorius et al. 1986). Individuals with schizophrenia in LMICs were significantly more likely to be asymptomatic or in remission and/or to have better social outcomes at 2-year and 5-year follow-ups than were participants in HICs. This pattern persisted even after adjusting for known risk factors for poorer schizophrenia outcome, such as male gender, gradual onset, and pattern of mental health service utilization (Leff et al. 1992). Possible explanations are largely sociocultural, such as worse conditions in HICs, including harsher economic competition, greater impact of stigma, higher expressed emotion, and smaller family networks to share in patient care (Leff et al. 1992; Messias et al. 2007). Nevertheless, many questions remain. For instance, outcomes varied substantially across different LMICs and HICs, underscoring local particularities; precise sociocultural and contextual factors associated with better outcomes have yet to be fully elucidated, and in any case, these factors appear to be changing with globalization. In addition, there is substantial evidence of human rights abuses and preventable early mortality of individuals with schizophrenia in LMICs as well as in HICs (Jablensky and Sartorius 2008; Patel et al. 2006). Cohen and colleagues (2008) noted that WHO studies did not account for differences in culturally specific understandings of disability, social functioning, occupational status, or the role of families; that patients in LMICs often sought care in highly specialized academic medical centers; and that the studies ignored variations in outcomes within countries. Clearly, for schizophrenia, as for all disorders, the incidence, prevalence, and outcome vary across societies, depending on a range of local biological, sociocultural, and other environmental and contextual factors (Messias et al. 2007).

Cultural Groupings Associated With Unique Expressions of Psychotic Disorders

Certain categories of people display variations in the manifestation of schizophrenia. This section discusses studies related to two groups of individuals: 1) immigrants and 2) racial and ethnic minorities. Our aim is not to suggest that the studies' findings relate to all immigrants or members of racial and ethnic minorities but to provide a firm conceptual grounding for clinicians as they customize their cultural assessments for individual patients.

Immigrants

Psychiatric researchers have long noted the association between migration status and the risk for developing psychosis. In the first meta-analysis on this issue, investigators calculated the relative risk of psychosis for migrants, compared with native-born populations, to be 2.7 for first-generation migrants and 4.5 for second-generation migrants (Cantor-Graae and Selten 2005). Subgroups of migrants seem to show greater risk for psychosis. For example, Black Caribbean groups in England have 4.7 higher odds of progressing to major psychotic disorders such as schizophrenia and bipolar disorder compared with native populations; this risk has been attributed to cumulative social disadvantage and adverse childhood events (Tortelli et al. 2015). The CFI presented in the next section can help clinicians assess their patients for migration status, social disadvantage, and adverse childhood events.

Notably, higher risk for schizophrenia persists even among the migrants' second-generation offspring. A review of studies across various geographical locations shows that the offspring of first-generation immigrants have 2.3 higher odds of developing a psychotic disorder compared with the offspring of native-born populations (Bourque et al. 2011). Considering that the Cantor-Graae and Selten's (2005) meta-analysis, mentioned in the preceding paragraph, showed that second-generation immigrants had 4.5 higher odds of developing a psychotic disorder, it is possible that differences are attributed to varying experiences of social adversity. Indeed, environmental factors such as socioeconomic deprivation and discrimination have been implicated in this risk (Ilić et al. 2017) Studies that apply big-data methods show roughly the same pattern of disorder prevalence. In a cohort study in Denmark that analyzed the records of over 1.8 million people born between 1971 and 2000, first-generation immigrants had 2.1 higher odds and foreign-born adoptees of Danish parents 2.5 higher odds of developing schizophrenia compared with the native Danish population (Cantor-Graae and Pedersen 2013). A Swedish study that examined the records of over 2.2 million individuals from 1992 to 1999 found that compared with native Swedes, first-generation Finnish immigrants had 2.2 higher odds, and their second-generation offspring 2.3 higher odds, of developing schizophrenia (Leão et al. 2006).

The risk for psychotic disorders appears to be higher for groups that experience social discrimination. In a 7-year prospective study of over 600 patients, Dutch investigators found a correlation between perceived experiences of high, medium, low, and very low discrimination and higher incidence rate ratios (IRRs) of a schizophrenia spectrum disorder in ethnic minority groups compared with the native population.

The following statistically significant IRRs were reported for particular nationalities after adjusting for age and gender: Moroccans, 4.0; Surinamese, 2.2; and Turks, 1.6. The IRRs were virtually no higher for those from Europe who may not be identified as obvious minorities on the basis of their appearance (i.e., "visible minorities") (Veling et al. 2007). Other researchers have challenged this study by noting that the incidence of schizophrenia among minorities was no greater than for the baseline native population when a thorough cultural assessment was used as a part of the diagnostic evaluation, eliciting a debate about the role of clinician bias in diagnosis (Zandi et al. 2010). Most of the studies on clinician bias have occurred in the United States, and these studies are discussed in the next subsection.

To this point, scientific studies have not been designed to evaluate the independent contributions of racial and ethnic minority status versus migration status to the risk of developing a psychotic disorder. The fact that risk of psychotic disorder continues in second-generation offspring has led some to conjecture that it is minority status rather than immigration that is the determining factor (Veling 2013). In fact, it is significant that social integration is associated with a remission of symptoms for people across race and ethnicity, even when antipsychotic medications are discontinued after a first psychotic episode (Bowtell et al. 2018). In addition, the incidence of psychotic disorder among first- and second-generation immigrants to the Netherlands is significantly increased compared with native Dutch individuals when the immigrant resides in a neighborhood with a low proportion of members of their same ethnic origin (low-ethnic-density neighborhoods); in high-ethnic-density neighborhoods, by contrast, the incidence for immigrants was not significantly different from that for the native Dutch, and this finding was consistent across immigrants from Morocco, Suriname, and Turkey (Veling et al. 2008). These data therefore indicate that immigrants who are less socially integrated—defined as not having educational opportunities, gainful employment, or close social associates such as family and friends—in their countries of resettlement may be at higher risk for psychotic disorder. The CFI can help clinicians elucidate how immigrants perceive their process of acculturation and social integration.

One line of research has tried to predict which immigrant groups are most at risk. Data appear most robust for individuals who migrate from low-income to high-income countries (Matheson et al. 2014). For example, in Cantor-Graae and Selten's (2005) meta-analysis, the relative risk of schizophrenia for migrants from developing versus developed countries was 3.3. Risk also varies by country, possibly due to local characteristics of adaptation, social integration, and discrimination: IRRs of psychotic disorder among first- and second-generation migrants are higher in England (2.8 and 3.7, respectively) than in the Netherlands (2.5 and 3.0) or Scandinavian countries (2.3 and 1.8), and the lowest IRRs are observed in Israel (1.5 and 1.1). Those immigrants experiencing the greatest risk for psychosis have the darkest skin color, highlighting the role of social discrimination for visible minorities from LMICs (Bourque et al. 2011; Cantor-Graae and Selten 2005). At the same time, individuals from more socioeconomically disadvantaged countries may present with significant symptom burdens and rates of disability due to long durations of untreated psychosis (Farooq et al. 2009), and symptoms that went unrecognized in their countries of origin could be responsible for illness presentations after migration. Finally, age at migration also appears to be associated with developing a psychotic disorder; a Dutch study has shown that individuals ages 0–4 years at the time of migration had 2.96 higher odds of a psychotic disorder, and risk decreased with older age at migration: 5–9 years, odds ratio (OR)=2.31; 10–14 years, OR=1.51; >29 years, OR=1.0 (Veling et al. 2011). The same pattern has been found for mood and anxiety disorders among specific ethnic subgroups of Latino immigrants to the United States (Fernández et al. 2016), suggesting that similar risk factors may be operating across various disorders and population groups.

Racial and Ethnic Minorities

Several types of psychotic disorder variability, in relation to racial and ethnic minority status, have been the subject of research. We discuss the following types of variation across racially or ethnically defined social groups with respect to schizophrenia and related disorders: 1) symptom manifestations of the disorder; 2) routes of entry into mental health care, specifically the role of coercion or involuntariness; 3) rates of diagnosis, including the possibility of clinician bias; and 4) quality of mental health care, including pharmacotherapy.

Symptom Manifestations of Schizophrenia

Variations in the phenomenology of schizophrenia and related disorders have been found among social groups, even when using the umbrella U.S. race and ethnicity categories. In one study of 351 patients (198 whites, 88 blacks, and 65 Latinos) with schizophrenia or schizoaffective disorder, scores on the Positive and Negative Syndrome Scale for schizophrenia were examined in total, by subscale, and for individual items (Barrio et al. 2003); an analysis of individual items showed that blacks had higher rates of suspiciousness and hallucinatory behavior, whites had higher rates of excitement, and Latinos scored higher than both groups on somatic concerns. Another study that compared 63 white and 53 Mexican American patients with schizophrenia showed that Mexican Americans were more likely to report somatic symptoms and whites reported more persecutory or supernatural delusions (Weisman et al. 2000). A third study based on clinical record review of 133 middle-aged and older inpatients with a severe psychotic disorder found differences in subtypes of hallucinations and delusions (Yamada et al. 2006). White patients (n=52) were most likely to exhibit grandiosity content in their delusions, African Americans (n=31) exhibited more generalized paranoia as part of persecutory delusions, and Latinos (n=50) reported more religious and family-related content in their visual hallucinations and more auditory command voices. Also, Latino patients' persecutory hallucinations tended to focus on a specific source of harm (e.g., friends/family) rather than a generalized one, as was the case with African Americans (Yamada et al. 2006). These data confirm a longstanding tenet within cultural psychiatry and psychiatric anthropology that culture indeed molds the patterning of symptom expressions (Kleinman 1988).

Routes of Entry Into Mental Health Care

A more established line of research has examined variations in how racial and ethnic minorities experience care within the medical system. In some instances, the role of coercion within the health system is apparent. For example, a meta-analysis of seven studies from Canada and England found that compared with white patients, black patients have 2.11 higher odds of being referred to care for first-episode psychosis through police involvement and lower odds (OR=0.7) of being referred by a general practitioner (Anderson et al. 2014a). In England, African Caribbean men had over 3.5 higher odds of being involuntarily admitted than white patients experiencing first-episode psychosis, and the odds were over fourfold greater for Black African patients (Mann et al. 2014). The CFI presented in the next section can help clinicians ask patients about adverse experiences with health care and about whether such experiences influence perceptions of help seeking for the current illness.

Rates of Schizophrenia Diagnosis, Including Role of Clinician Bias

Once racial and ethnic minorities enter the health care system, they are more likely to be diagnosed with schizophrenia than their white counterparts. One meta-analysis of 55 studies with well-defined probability samples showed that black patients in England and Canada received diagnoses of schizophrenia more frequently than white patients (OR=2.42), even in a subset of studies in which structured instruments were used (OR=1.77); studies with a greater proportion of white patients or lower patient age showed the greatest differences in rates of schizophrenia diagnosis (Olbert et al. 2018). This tendency toward higher rates of diagnosis varies among racial and ethnic minorities in single-country studies. For example, in the United States, blacks and Latinos are at greater risk than whites of receiving a diagnosis of psychotic disorder: OR=3–4 for blacks and OR=3 for Latinos (Schwartz and Blankenship 2014). A systematic literature review of incidence rates in England over a 60-year period found the following significantly elevated relative risks for a psychotic disorder when minorities were compared with whites: Black Caribbeans, 5.6; Black Africans, 4.7; and South Asians, 2.4 (Kirkbride et al. 2012). Several reasons have been examined for these differences in rates, which are most pronounced among persons of African descent.

An important clue regarding varied incidence rates comes from longitudinal data on diagnostic practice, which show greater instability of schizophrenia diagnoses over sequential hospitalizations among African American and Latino inpatients than among whites (Chen et al. 1996). Studies have investigated the possibility that affective psychoses or ambiguous symptoms (e.g., nonpsychotic wariness, perceptual alterations, intense spiritual experiences) may be more frequently misdiagnosed as schizophrenia among racial and ethnic minorities than among whites, possibly due to clinician bias, contributing to greater diagnostic instability and higher rates of schizophrenia diagnoses (Gara et al. 2012). Typical evidence for clinician bias comes from Strakowski and colleagues' (1997) study in a psychiatric emergency department, in which significantly lower agreement was found between clinician and SCID diagnoses of schizophrenia among African American than among white patients (35% vs. 54%; adjusted OR=2.7). Two main causes of disagreement were identified: "information variance" (difference in the availability of clinical information) and "criterion variance" (misapplication of diagnostic criteria). Although no racial difference was found in the proportion of the disagreement due to the criterion variance (24% in both groups), the contribution of information variance to misdiagnosis was much higher among African Americans than among whites (40% vs. 22%; adjusted OR=2.8), after adjustments for clinical and demographic covariates. Missing information on affective signs and symptoms led to a clinician diagnosis of schizophrenia or psychosis not otherwise specified for 55% of the patients with information variance (Strakowski et al. 1997). These studies suggest that differential assessment information related to patient race is a potential driver of schizophrenia misdiagnosis, especially for individuals with affective psychosis.

Other possible explanations for racial and ethnic differences in schizophrenia diagnoses include 1) more severe manic, affective, and psychotic episodes—including auditory hallucinations and mood-incongruent delusions—among African Americans and Latinos than among whites (Haeri et al. 2011; Mukherjee et al. 1983); 2) greater manifestation of mistrust and guardedness by African Americans with depression, which may be misinterpreted by clinicians as persecutory delusions typical of schizophrenia (Whaley 1997); and 3) longer durations of untreated psychosis, which could lead to worse outcomes when compared with majority populations. However, systematic reviews show no racial or ethnic differences in durations of untreated psychosis (Anderson et al. 2014b).

Quality of Mental Health Care

The treatment and course of schizophrenia are also likely to differ for racial and ethnic minorities. The data on disparities are most robust for black patients (Olbert et al. 2018), who compared with white patients have higher rates of hospitalization (Rost et al. 2011), higher doses of antipsychotics (Arnold et al. 2004), and more frequent prescriptions of long-acting injections (Aggarwal et al. 2012). There do not appear to be racial or ethnic disparities in the general use versus nonuse of antipsychotics, but African Americans and Latinos have 0.62 and 0.77, respectively, lower odds than whites of being treated with newer antipsychotics (Puyat et al. 2013). In this context of unequal treatment, research has often found lower medication adherence among racial and ethnic minorities with schizophrenia and bipolar disorder, related to fears of addiction and higher stigma about taking medications regularly for mental disorders (García et al. 2016). Differential rates of medication adherence may affect symptom remission scores. In one study of 137 white patients compared with 62 black patients receiving treatment for first-episode psychosis, black patients experienced less improvement in positive symptoms, bizarre behavior, avolition, anhedonia, functional performance, and affective symptoms due to statistically significant differences in medication adherence (Li et al. 2011). The CFI can help clinicians uncover cultural concerns about addiction to medications or stigma as barriers to treatment adherence.

Summary

Much remains unknown about cross-cultural variations in the risk for developing a psychotic disorder and in outcomes from care. Although certain patient-level causes have been identified, such as adverse childhood experiences, decreased acculturation, and socioeconomic discrimination, clinician-level bias may also play a role. The next section explores how the CFI can be used to elicit patient- and clinician-level factors to improve diagnostic accuracy and treatment adherence for all patients.

DSM-5 Cultural Formulation Interview and the Cultural Assessment of Schizophrenia

Studies suggest that accurate cultural assessments can prevent the misdiagnosis of psychotic disorders. Clinical researchers who staff McGill University's Cultural Consultation Service (CCS) have identified the usefulness of the cultural formulation approach in correcting diagnoses among ethnic minority and immigrant patients whose symptom presentations were unfamiliar to clinicians. In a landmark study, use of the cultural formulation approach for case reassessment of 323 patients referred over a 10-year period resulted in 34 of 70 cases (49%) with a referral diagnosis of a psychotic disorder being rediagnosed as a nonpsychotic disorder, and 12 of 253 cases (5%) with a referral diagnosis of a nonpsychotic disorder being rediagnosed as a psychotic disorder (Adeponle et al. 2012). The CCS draws on 60 cultural and linguistic brokers, 1.5-hour clinical assessments, and a 2-hour case conference. The approach of the CCS may not be reproducible in most settings, so the CFI was created for DSM-5 through systematic literature reviews, expert consensus, and field trial testing for clinicians to conduct a standardized cultural assessment with patients from any background with a psychotic disorder.

The CFI is a cultural assessment tool that can help clinicians process their biases as countertransference reactions to avoid misdiagnoses of psychotic disorders. The CFI comprises three categories of semistructured interviews that facilitate a cultural assessment: a 16-item patient questionnaire that is known as the "core" standard version, a CFI–Informant Version to elicit collateral information from caregivers, and 12 supplementary modules to inquire about topics introduced in the core CFI and to assess cultural factors that may be unique to specific populations (e.g., immigrants, refugees). The core CFI is reproduced in Table 4–1. The CFI, the CFI–Informant Version, and 12 supplementary modules are available online at https://www.psychiatry.org/psychiatrists/practice/dsm/educational-resources/assessment-measures.

TABLE 4–1.   DSM-5 Cultural Formulation Interview (CFI)

Supplementary modules used to expand each CFI subtopic are noted in parentheses.

GUIDE TO INTERVIEWER	INSTRUCTIONS TO THE INTERVIEWER ARE ITALICIZED.
The following questions aim to clarify key aspects of the presenting clinical problem from the point of view of the individual and other members of the individual's social network (i.e., family, friends, or others involved in current problem). This includes the problem's meaning, potential sources of help, and expectations for services.	*INTRODUCTION FOR THE INDIVIDUAL:* I would like to understand the problems that bring you here so that I can help you more effectively. I want to know about **your** experience and ideas. I will ask some questions about what is going on and how you are dealing with it. Please remember there are no right or wrong answers.

CULTURAL DEFINITION OF THE PROBLEM

CULTURAL DEFINITION OF THE PROBLEM

(Explanatory Model, Level of Functioning)

Elicit the individual's view of core problems and key concerns. *Focus on the individual's own way of understanding the problem.* *Use the term, expression, or brief description elicited in question 1 to identify the problem in subsequent questions (e.g., "your conflict with your son").*	1. What brings you here today? *IF INDIVIDUAL GIVES FEW DETAILS OR ONLY MENTIONS SYMPTOMS OR A MEDICAL DIAGNOSIS, PROBE:* People often understand their problems in their own way, which may be similar to or different from how doctors describe the problem. How would *you* describe your problem?

TABLE 4–1. **DSM-5 Cultural Formulation Interview (CFI)** *(continued)*

Supplementary modules used to expand each CFI subtopic are noted in parentheses.

GUIDE TO INTERVIEWER	INSTRUCTIONS TO THE INTERVIEWER ARE *ITALICIZED.*
Ask how individual frames the problem for members of the social network.	2. Sometimes people have different ways of describing their problem to their family, friends, or others in their community. How would you describe your problem to them?
Focus on the aspects of the problem that matter most to the individual.	3. What troubles you most about your problem?

CULTURAL PERCEPTIONS OF CAUSE, CONTEXT, AND SUPPORT

CAUSES
(Explanatory Model, Social Network, Older Adults)

This question indicates the meaning of the condition for the individual, which may be relevant for clinical care.	4. Why do you think this is happening to you? What do you think are the causes of your [PROBLEM]?
Note that individuals may identify multiple causes, depending on the facet of the problem they are considering.	*PROMPT FURTHER IF REQUIRED:* Some people may explain their problem as the result of bad things that happen in their life, problems with others, a physical illness, a spiritual reason, or many other causes.
Focus on the views of members of the individual's social network. These may be diverse and vary from the individual's.	5. What do others in your family, your friends, or others in your community think is causing your [PROBLEM]?

STRESSORS AND SUPPORTS
(Social Network, Caregivers, Psychosocial Stressors, Religion and Spirituality, Immigrants and Refugees, Cultural Identity, Older Adults, Coping and Help Seeking)

Elicit information on the individual's life context, focusing on resources, social supports, and resilience. May also probe other supports (e.g., from co-workers, from participation in religion or spirituality).	6. Are there any kinds of support that make your [PROBLEM] better, such as support from family, friends, or others?
Focus on stressful aspects of the individual's environment. Can also probe, e.g., relationship problems, difficulties at work or school, or discrimination.	7. Are there any kinds of stresses that make your [PROBLEM] worse, such as difficulties with money, or family problems?

ROLE OF CULTURAL IDENTITY
(Cultural Identity, Psychosocial Stressors, Religion and Spirituality, Immigrants and Refugees, Older Adults, Children and Adolescents)

	Sometimes, aspects of people's background or identity can make their [PROBLEM] better or worse. By **background** or **identity**, I mean, for example, the communities you belong to, the languages you speak, where you or your family are from, your race or ethnic background, your gender or sexual orientation, or your faith or religion.

TABLE 4–1.   **DSM-5 Cultural Formulation Interview (CFI) *(continued)***

Supplementary modules used to expand each CFI subtopic are noted in parentheses.

GUIDE TO INTERVIEWER	INSTRUCTIONS TO THE INTERVIEWER ARE *ITALICIZED.*
Ask the individual to reflect on the most salient elements of his or her cultural identity. Use this information to tailor questions 9–10 as needed.	8. For you, what are the most important aspects of your background or identity?
Elicit aspects of identity that make the problem better or worse. *Probe as needed (e.g., clinical worsening as a result of discrimination due to migration status, race/ ethnicity, or sexual orientation).*	9. Are there any aspects of your background or identity that make a difference to your [PROBLEM]?
Probe as needed (e.g., migration-related problems; conflict across generations or due to gender roles).	10. Are there any aspects of your background or identity that are causing other concerns or difficulties for you?

CULTURAL FACTORS AFFECTING SELF-COPING AND PAST HELP SEEKING

SELF-COPING
(Coping and Help Seeking, Religion and Spirituality, Older Adults, Caregivers, Psychosocial Stressors)

Clarify self-coping for the problem.	11. Sometimes people have various ways of dealing with problems like [PROBLEM]. What have you done on your own to cope with your [PROBLEM]?

PAST HELP SEEKING
(Coping and Help Seeking, Religion and Spirituality, Older Adults, Caregivers, Psychosocial Stressors, Immigrants and Refugees, Social Network, Clinician-Patient Relationship)

Elicit various sources of help (e.g., medical care, mental health treatment, support groups, work-based counseling, folk healing, religious or spiritual counseling, other forms of traditional or alternative healing). *Probe as needed (e.g., "What other sources of help have you used?").* *Clarify the individual's experience and regard for previous help.*	12. Often, people look for help from many different sources, including different kinds of doctors, helpers, or healers. In the past, what kinds of treatment, help, advice, or healing have you sought for your [PROBLEM]? *PROBE IF DOES NOT DESCRIBE USEFULNESS OF HELP RECEIVED:* What types of help or treatment were most useful? Not useful?

BARRIERS
(Coping and Help Seeking, Religion and Spirituality, Older Adults, Psychosocial Stressors, Immigrants and Refugees, Social Network, Clinician-Patient Relationship)

Clarify the role of social barriers to help seeking, access to care, and problems engaging in previous treatment. *Probe details as needed (e.g., "What got in the way?").*	13. Has anything prevented you from getting the help you need? *PROBE AS NEEDED:* For example, money, work or family commitments, stigma or discrimination, or lack of services that understand your language or background?

TABLE 4–1.	**DSM-5 Cultural Formulation Interview (CFI)** *(continued)*

Supplementary modules used to expand each CFI subtopic are noted in parentheses.

GUIDE TO INTERVIEWER	INSTRUCTIONS TO THE INTERVIEWER ARE *ITALICIZED.*

CULTURAL FACTORS AFFECTING CURRENT HELP SEEKING

PREFERENCES
(Social Network, Caregivers, Religion and Spirituality, Older Adults, Coping and Help Seeking)

Clarify individual's current perceived needs and expectations of help, broadly defined.	Now let's talk some more about the help you need.
Probe if individual lists only one source of help (e.g., "What other kinds of help would be useful to you at this time?").	14. What kinds of help do you think would be most useful to you at this time for your [PROBLEM]?
Focus on the views of the social network regarding help seeking.	15. Are there other kinds of help that your family, friends, or other people have suggested would be helpful for you now?

CLINICIAN-PATIENT RELATIONSHIP
(Clinician-Patient Relationship, Older Adults)

Elicit possible concerns about the clinic or the clinician-patient relationship, including perceived racism, language barriers, or cultural differences that may undermine goodwill, communication, or care delivery.	Sometimes doctors and patients misunderstand each other because they come from different backgrounds or have different expectations.
Probe details as needed (e.g., "In what way?"). Address possible barriers to care or concerns about the clinic and the clinician-patient relationship raised previously.	16. Have you been concerned about this and is there anything that we can do to provide you with the care you need?

Source. Reprinted from American Psychiatric Association: *Diagnostic and Statistical Manual of Mental Disorders,* 5th Edition, Arlington, VA, American Psychiatric Association, 2013, pp. 752–754. Copyright © 2013 American Psychiatric Association. Used with permission.

The DSM-5 Gender and Cross-Cultural Issues Study Group adopted an evidence-based method to create the CFI from the DSM-IV Outline for Cultural Formulation by 1) conducting a comprehensive literature review of 140 publications in seven languages; 2) field-testing the core CFI with 321 patients, 75 clinicians, and 86 family members in six countries; and 3) revising this field test version into the final version included in DSM-5 based on feedback from patients, clinicians, and family members (Lewis-Fernández et al. 2017). For nearly 6 months in 2011 and again in 2012, a draft of the CFI was posted on the American Psychiatric Association's DSM-5 website to elicit comments from the public in recognition that cultural assessments interest multiple stakeholders such as patients, clinicians, and service administrators (Aggarwal et al. 2016a).

Following this active solicitation of feedback from diverse groups of people, the CFI was designed for use with any patient in any mental health setting. On average, the CFI takes about 20 minutes to complete (Lewis-Fernández et al. 2017). Hence, a clinician could initiate a new relationship with a patient right from the intake evaluation, using a culturally informed approach. However, DSM-5 specifies that the CFI may be helpful at any point in the treatment, not just during the initial session. The

CFI may be most helpful when problems in assessment arise from differences in the cultural, religious, or socioeconomic backgrounds of the clinician and patient; when there is uncertainty about the fit between official diagnostic criteria and cultural variations; when it is difficult to judge illness severity or impairment; when patients and clinicians disagree on treatment planning; or when patients do not adhere to treatments or attend appointments (American Psychiatric Association 2013). Each of these themes has been discussed earlier in this chapter, and the CFI may equip patients with solutions to these problems.

The core and informant versions of the CFI include instructions to clinicians on the left side of the page and questions on the right so that clinicians understand the point of each question and its clinical use. The CFI–Informant Version can be used to obtain collateral information or used when the patient cannot interact effectively during the interview, such as with young children or individuals with cognitive impairments due to dementia, substance intoxication, or florid psychosis. There are two types of supplementary modules: 1) those expanding sections of the core CFI and 2) those addressing the cultural needs of certain populations (Table 4–2). The semistructured nature of these interviews and the diversity of topics allow clinicians to customize their cultural assessments as situations warrant.

In the remainder of this chapter, we discuss how the core CFI can assist clinicians with uncovering the cultural variations in psychotic disorders. The core CFI has four domains. The first domain, Cultural Definition of the Problem, poses three questions. Question 1—"What brings you here today?"—initiates the patient interview with a nonjudgmental open-ended question in which the patient can help to set the agenda. For example, some patients may report that they hear voices or see things that others cannot experience, whereas others may list somatic concerns. If patients provide few details or only mention biomedical information, the follow-up elucidation with probe question is "People often understand their problems in their own way, which may be similar to or different from how doctors describe the problem. How would *you* describe your problem?" As a normalizing statement followed by a question, the probe can bridge the cultural gap between patients and clinicians in understandings of illness. Question 2 reads, "Sometimes people have different ways of describing their problem to their family, friends, or others in their community. How would you describe your problem to them?" This question operationalizes the definition of culture presented in DSM-5 by asking clinicians to understand how cultural systems of knowledge and concepts are learned and transmitted in social groups. Question 3 asks, "What troubles you most about your problem?" As we noted earlier, many subpopulations experience psychotic symptoms such as hearing voices that do not rise to the level of clinical impairment, and this question helps clinicians determine the manifesting problem's impact on quality of life and level of functioning.

Questions 4–10 are in the second domain, Cultural Perceptions of Cause, Context, and Support. Questions 4–7 elicit the patient's illness explanations by asking about the causes and the social stressors and supports—topics of interest to cultural psychiatrists because accessing patients' understandings of health and illness can be a window into their social worlds in order to help plan treatments (Kirmayer 2007). Question 4 is "Why do you think this is happening to you? What do you think are the causes of your [PROBLEM]?" Some patients may report that they have no problem at all, which may happen if they do not see their experiences of psychosis as problem-

TABLE 4–2. **Supplementary modules to the DSM-5 core Cultural Formulation Interview**

1. Explanatory Model
2. Level of Functioning
3. Social Network
4. Psychosocial Stressors
5. Spirituality, Religion, and Moral Traditions
6. Cultural Identity
7. Coping and Help-Seeking
8. Patient-Clinician Relationship
9. School-Age Children and Adolescents
10. Older Adults
11. Immigrants and Refugees
12. Caregivers

atic. Others may understand their illness to be the result of interpersonal stressors, adverse life events, or genetic inheritance. To make patients feel safe in disclosing their perceptions about the cause of illness, a follow-up prompt is this: "Some people may explain their problem as the result of bad things that happen in their life, problems with others, a physical illness, a spiritual reason, or many other causes." Question 5 expands the inquiry to include close associates as a way of recognizing that culture is transmitted within social groups: "What do others in your family, your friends, or others in your community think is causing your [PROBLEM]?" With this question, clinicians can ascertain whether the patient's responses seem to correspond with the views of others within his or her cultural subgrouping. Question 6 asks, "Are there any kinds of support that make your [PROBLEM] better, such as support from family, friends, or others?" Question 7 is "Are there any kinds of stresses that make your [PROBLEM] worse, such as difficulties with money, or family problems?" Questions 6 and 7 are intended to place the individual in ecological context by clarifying important types of social supports and stressors.

The discussion then turns to cultural identity. An introduction to this section of the second domain helps clinicians avoid overgeneralizing based on stereotypes. The introduction is as follows:

> Sometimes, aspects of people's background or identity can make their [PROBLEM] better or worse. By *background* or *identity*, I mean, for example, the communities you belong to, the languages you speak, where you or your family are from, your race or ethnic background, your gender or sexual orientation, or your faith or religion.

Question 8 then asks the patient directly about background or identity: "For you, what are the most important aspects of your background or identity?" DSM-5 acknowledges that most individuals belong to multiple cultures through which they construct unique identities, and this question lets patients nominate a cultural identity so that clinicians do not mistakenly make assumptions based on a group affiliation such as race or ethnicity (Aggarwal 2011). Question 9 asks the patient to consider how this identity relates to the current problem: "Are there any aspects of your background or identity that make a difference to your [PROBLEM]?" This question helps clinicians with integrating cultural information through diagnostic and treatment planning. Finally, Question 10 asks patients to consider cultural factors that may not seem evident but that could, nevertheless, impact care, such as problems with migration, gender roles, or intergenerational conflict: "Are there any aspects of your background or identity that are causing other concerns or difficulties for you?" Here, clinicians can explore whether adverse life experiences, decreased acculturation, socioeconomic discrimination, or migration relates to the experience of psychosis.

The third and fourth domains address culturally informed ideas about treatment preferences. The third domain is Cultural Factors Affecting Self-Coping and Past Help Seeking. Question 11 is "Sometimes people have various ways of dealing with problems like [PROBLEM]. What have you done on your own to cope with your [PROBLEM]?" Question 12 normalizes the possibility that patients may have sought help outside the biomedical system: "Often, people look for help from many different sources, including different kinds of doctors, helpers, or healers. In the past, what kinds of treatment, help, advice, or healing have you sought for your [PROBLEM]?" This question may be particularly helpful for patients who prefer not to seek mental health care because of concerns about stigma. To help patients identify successful modalities for the current illness episode, probe questions for Question 12 ask: "What types of help or treatment were most useful? Not useful?" Answers to these questions may help clinicians create treatment plans that incorporate previous forms of care that were helpful while avoiding those that were not. Question 13 asks about past barriers to treatment so that clinicians customize current treatments in a patient-centered way: "Has anything prevented you from getting the help you need?" A follow-up question lists examples of barriers: "For example, money, work or family commitments, stigma or discrimination, or lack of services that understand your language or background?" The final three questions belong to the fourth domain, Cultural Factors Affecting Current Help Seeking. Question 14 asks the patient about treatment preferences to get the help needed for the current illness: "What kinds of help do you think would be most useful to you at this time for your [PROBLEM]?" By asking patients about their treatment preferences, clinicians may be able to improve appointment and treatment adherence. Question 15 explores treatment preferences among close associates: "Are there other kinds of help that your family, friends, or other people have suggested would be helpful for you now?" With this question, clinicians can assess the extent to which others have an influence on the patient's ideas about treatment. Like Questions 2 and 5, this question addresses how health information is culturally transmitted among social groups. Finally, Question 16 broaches the topic of clinician bias and begins with an introduction: "Sometimes doctors and patients misunderstand each other because they come from different backgrounds or have different expectations. Have you been concerned about this and is there anything that we can do to provide you with the care you need?" The introduction normalizes patient concerns around intercultural differences rather than pretending that clinician bias does not exist. Whether or not the patient answers immediately, the question signals to patients that the current patient-clinician encounter is attuned to cultural safety and may provide a corrective experience to past adverse experiences with care.

Patients with psychotic symptoms were enrolled during the CFI field trial; however, the field trial version differs slightly from the final version in DSM-5. Only one study has been published on use of the CFI for patients with explicit psychosis. Muralidharan and colleagues (2017) completed a case series of the CFI with 12 patients in the Veterans Affairs hospital system, 7 with a diagnosis of schizophrenia or schizoaffective disorder, 4 with a diagnosis of bipolar disorder, and 1 with major depressive disorder with psychotic features. The investigators found that the CFI promoted recovery by encouraging patients to draw connections between their past experiences and present circumstances with their clinicians. More studies are therefore needed to characterize for which patients the CFI may or may not be useful, because patients in this sample were clinically stable.

Conclusion

This chapter provides a brief introduction to cultural variations in the presentation of psychotic disorders. While the study of cultural variations continues to delineate symptoms that are similar and different across social groups, our understanding of culture now assumes that individuals define their cultural identities as dynamic, ever-changing, and acquired rather than only inherited. Future research is needed to determine why certain groups such as immigrants and racial and ethnic minorities experience greater risk for developing psychotic disorders and to assess the role of clinician bias in potential misdiagnoses. The CFI is a practical tool that can elicit such variations in the manifestations of psychosis, minimize clinician biases, and standardize the way that cultural information is elicited for ongoing research.

Additional Resources

Video portrayals of the Cultural Formulation Interview (CFI) are also freely available at https://www.appi.org/Lewis-Fernandez. The videos show clinicians using the core CFI and the Supplementary Modules to the core CFI, such as Spirituality, Religion, and Moral Traditions and Older Adults, in various clinical settings. An online training module on the core CFI is also available from the Center of Excellence for Cultural Competence via www.nyculturalcompetence.org or by emailing cpihelp@nyspi.columbia.edu. Beyond just reading the CFI questions for practice, video instruction permits clinicians to see how the CFI is used as a form of behavior modeling (Aggarwal et al. 2016b).

References

Accreditation Council for Graduate Medical Education: CLER pathways to excellence, 2014. Available at: http://www.acgme.org/Portals/0/PDFs/CLER/CLER_Brochure.pdf. Accessed May 22, 2019.

Adeponle AB, Thombs BD, Groleau D, et al: Using the cultural formulation to resolve uncertainty in diagnoses of psychosis among ethnoculturally diverse patients. Psychiatr Serv 63(2):147–153, 2012 22302332

Aggarwal NK: Intersubjectivity, transference, and the cultural third. Contemp Psychoanal 47(2):204–223, 2011

Aggarwal NK: Hybridity and intersubjectivity in the clinical encounter: impact on the cultural formulation. Transcult Psychiatry 49(1):121–139, 2012 22218399

Aggarwal NK, Rosenheck RA, Woods SW, et al: Race and long-acting antipsychotic prescription at a community mental health center: a retrospective chart review. J Clin Psychiatry 73(4):513–517, 2012 22579151

Aggarwal NK, Cedeño K, Guarnaccia P, et al: The meanings of cultural competence in mental health: an exploratory focus group study with patients, clinicians, and administrators. Springerplus 5:384, 2016a 27065092

Aggarwal NK, Lam P, Castillo EG, et al: How do clinicians prefer cultural competence training? Findings from the DSM-5 Cultural Formulation Interview field trial. Acad Psychiatry 40(4):584–591, 2016b 26449983

Aggarwal NK, Like R, Kopelowicz A, et al: Has the time come for a cultural psychiatry fellowship in the USA? Acad Psychiatry 40(6):928–931, 2016c 27472932

American Board of Psychiatry and Neurology: Psychiatry core competencies outline. ABPN Board of Directors, July 22, 2011. Available at https://www.abpn.com/wp-content/uploads/2015/02/2011_core_P_MREE.pdf. Accessed May 22, 2019.

American Psychiatric Association: Diagnostic and Statistical Manual of Mental Disorders, 4th Edition. Washington, DC, American Psychiatric Association, 1994

American Psychiatric Association: Diagnostic and Statistical Manual of Mental Disorders, 5th Edition. Arlington, VA, American Psychiatric Association, 2013

Anderson KK, Flora N, Archie S, et al: A meta-analysis of ethnic differences in pathways to care at the first episode of psychosis. Acta Psychiatr Scand 130(4):257–268, 2014a 24580102

Anderson KK, Flora N, Archie S, et al: Race, ethnicity, and the duration of untreated psychosis: a systematic review. Soc Psychiatry Psychiatr Epidemiol 49(7):1161–1174, 2014b 24213521

Arnold LM, Strakowski SM, Schwiers ML, et al: Sex, ethnicity, and antipsychotic medication use in patients with psychosis. Schizophr Res 66(2–3):169–175, 2004 15061250

Association of American Medical Colleges: Assessing change: evaluating cultural competence education and training, 2015. Available at: https://www.aamc.org/media/33226/download. Accessed October 10, 2019.

Barrio C, Yamada AM, Atuel H, et al: A tri-ethnic examination of symptom expression on the Positive and Negative Syndrome Scale in schizophrenia spectrum disorders. Schizophr Res 60(2–3):259–269, 2003 12591588

Boroffka A: Emil Kraepelin (1856–1926). Transcult Psychiatry 27(3):228–237, 1990

Bourque F, van der Ven E, Malla A: A meta-analysis of the risk for psychotic disorders among first- and second-generation immigrants. Psychol Med 41(5):897–910, 2011 20663257

Bowtell M, Ratheesh A, McGorry P, et al: Clinical and demographic predictors of continuing remission or relapse following discontinuation of antipsychotic medication after a first episode of psychosis: a systematic review. Schizophr Res 197:9–18, 2018 29146020

Cantor-Graae E, Pedersen CB: Full spectrum of psychiatric disorders related to foreign migration: a Danish population-based cohort study. JAMA Psychiatry 70(4):427–435, 2013 23446644

Cantor-Graae E, Selten J-P: Schizophrenia and migration: a meta-analysis and review. Am J Psychiatry 162(1):12–24, 2005 15625195

Chen YR, Swann AC, Burt DB: Stability of diagnosis in schizophrenia. Am J Psychiatry 153(5):682–686, 1996 8615415

Cohen A, Patel V, Thara R, et al: Questioning an axiom: better prognosis for schizophrenia in the developing world? Schizophr Bull 34(2):229–244, 2008 17905787

Cohen CI, Marino L: Racial and ethnic differences in the prevalence of psychotic symptoms in the general population. Psychiatr Serv 64(11):1103–1109, 2013 23904054

Devylder JE, Oh HY, Yang LH, et al: Acculturative stress and psychotic-like experiences among Asian and Latino immigrants to the United States. Schizophr Res 150(1):223–228, 2013 23932446

Farooq S, Large M, Nielssen O, et al: The relationship between the duration of untreated psychosis and outcome in low-and-middle income countries: a systematic review and meta analysis. Schizophr Res 109(1–3):15–23, 2009 19233621

Fernández RL, Morcillo C, Wang S, et al: Acculturation dimensions and 12-month mood and anxiety disorders across U.S. Latino subgroups in the National Epidemiologic Survey of Alcohol and Related Conditions. Psychol Med 46(9):1987–2001, 2016 27087570

Gara MA, Vega WA, Arndt S, et al: Influence of patient race and ethnicity on clinical assessment in patients with affective disorders. Arch Gen Psychiatry 69(6):593–600, 2012 22309972

García S, Martínez-Cengotitabengoa M, López-Zurbano S, et al: Adherence to antipsychotic medication in bipolar disorder and schizophrenic patients: a systematic review. J Clin Psychopharmacol 36(4):355–371, 2016 27307187

Geltman D, Chang G: Hallucinations in Latino psychiatric outpatients: a preliminary investigation. Gen Hosp Psychiatry 26(2):153–157, 2004 15038934

Haeri S, Williams J, Kopeykina I, et al: Disparities in diagnosis of bipolar disorder in individuals of African and European descent: a review. J Psychiatr Pract 17(6):394–403, 2011 22108396

Hopper K, Harrison G, Janca A, et al (eds): Recovery From Schizophrenia: An International Perspective. New York, Oxford University Press, 2007

Ilić B, Švab V, Sedić B, et al: Mental health in domesticated immigrant population—a systematic review. Psychiatr Danub 29(3):273–281, 2017 28949308

Jablensky A, Sartorius N: What did the WHO studies really find? Schizophr Bull 34(2):253–255, 2008 18203759

Jayasuriya L: Constructions of culture and identity in contemporary social theorising. Int J Cult Ment Health 1:30–43, 2008

Kapur S, Phillips AG, Insel TR: Why has it taken so long for biological psychiatry to develop clinical tests and what to do about it? Mol Psychiatry 17(12):1174–1179, 2012 22869033

Kendler KS, Gallagher TJ, Abelson JM, et al: Lifetime prevalence, demographic risk factors, and diagnostic validity of nonaffective psychosis as assessed in a U.S. community sample. The National Comorbidity Survey. Arch Gen Psychiatry 53(11):1022–1031, 1996 8911225

Kirkbride JB, Errazuriz A, Croudace TJ, et al: Incidence of schizophrenia and other psychoses in England, 1950–2009: a systematic review and meta-analyses. PLoS One 7(3):e31660, 2012 22457710

Kirmayer L: The fate of culture in DSM-IV. Transcult Psychiatry 35:339–342, 1998

Kirmayer L: Cultural psychiatry in historical perspective, in Textbook of Cultural Psychiatry. Edited by Bhugra D, Bhui K. Cambridge, UK, Cambridge University Press, 2007, pp 3–19

Kleinman A: Rethinking Psychiatry: From Cultural Category to Personal Experience. New York, Free Press, 1988

Kraepelin E: Vergleichende Psychiatrie (1904), English translation. Transcult Psychiatry 11:108–112, 1974

Leão TS, Sundquist J, Frank G, et al: Incidence of schizophrenia or other psychoses in first- and second-generation immigrants: a national cohort study. J Nerv Ment Dis 194(1):27–33, 2006 16462552

Leff J, Sartorius N, Jablensky A, et al: The International Pilot Study of Schizophrenia: five-year follow-up findings. Psychol Med 22(1):131–145, 1992 1574549

Lewis-Fernández R, Horvitz-Lennon M, Blanco C, et al: Significance of endorsement of psychotic symptoms by US Latinos. J Nerv Ment Dis 197(5):337–347, 2009 19440107

Lewis-Fernández R, Aggarwal NK, Lam PC, et al: Feasibility, acceptability and clinical utility of the Cultural Formulation Interview: mixed-methods results from the DSM-5 international field trial. Br J Psychiatry 210(4):290–297, 2017 28104738

Li H, Eack SM, Montrose DM, et al: Longitudinal treatment outcome of African American and Caucasian patients with first episode psychosis. Asian J Psychiatr 4(4):266–271, 2011 23051160

Linscott RJ, van Os J: An updated and conservative systematic review and meta-analysis of epidemiological evidence on psychotic experiences in children and adults: on the pathway from proneness to persistence to dimensional expression across mental disorders. Psychol Med 43(6):1133–1149, 2013 22850401

Littlewood R: Psychiatry's culture. Int J Soc Psychiatry 42(4):245–268, 1996 9023608

Mann F, Fisher HL, Johnson S: A systematic review of ethnic variations in hospital admission and compulsory detention in first-episode psychosis. J Ment Health 23(4):205–211, 2014 25054369

Matheson SL, Shepherd AM, Carr VJ: How much do we know about schizophrenia and how well do we know it? Evidence from the Schizophrenia Library. Psychol Med 44(16):3387–3405, 2014 25065407

McGrath J, Saha S, Welham J, et al: A systematic review of the incidence of schizophrenia: the distribution of rates and the influence of sex, urbanicity, migrant status and methodology. BMC Med 2:13, 2004 15115547

McGrath JJ, Saha S, Al-Hamzawi A, et al: The bidirectional associations between psychotic experiences and DSM-IV mental disorders. Am J Psychiatry 173(10):997–1006, 2016 26988628

Messias E, Chen C-Y, Eaton WW: Epidemiology of schizophrenia: review of findings and myths. Psychiatr Clin North Am 30(3):323–338, 2007 17720026

Mischoulon D, Lagomasino IT, Harmon C: Atypical psychotic symptoms in a Hispanic population: diagnostic dilemmas and implications for treatment. Psychiatry (Edgmont) 2(10):38–46, 2005 21120089

Mukherjee S, Shukla S, Woodle J, et al: Misdiagnosis of schizophrenia in bipolar patients: a multiethnic comparison. Am J Psychiatry 140(12):1571–1574 1983 6650685

Muralidharan A, Schaffner RM, Hack S, et al: "I got to voice what's in my heart": participation in the Cultural Formulation Interview—perspectives of consumers with psychotic disorders. J Psychosoc Rehabil Ment Health 4:35–43, 2017

National Quality Forum: NQF endorses healthcare disparities and cultural competency measures. August 10, 2012. Available at: http://www.qualityforum.org/News_And _Resources/Press_Releases/2012/NQF_Endorses_Healthcare_Disparities_and_Cultural _Competency_Measures.aspx. Accessed May 22, 2019.

Olbert CM, Nagendra A, Buck B: Meta-analysis of black vs. white racial disparity in schizophrenia diagnosis in the United States: do structured assessments attenuate racial disparities? J Abnorm Psychol 127(1):104–115, 2018 29094963

Olfson M, Lewis-Fernández R, Weissman MM, et al: Psychotic symptoms in an urban general medicine practice. Am J Psychiatry 159(8):1412–1419, 2002 12153836

Patel V, Cohen A, Thara R, Gureje O: Is the outcome of schizophrenia really better in developing countries? Br J Psychiatry 28(2):149–152, 2006 16810400

Puyat JH, Daw JR, Cunningham CM, et al: Racial and ethnic disparities in the use of antipsychotic medication: a systematic review and meta-analysis. Soc Psychiatry Psychiatr Epidemiol 48(12):1861–1872, 2013 23942793

Rost K, Hsieh YP, Xu S, et al: Potential disparities in the management of schizophrenia in the United States. Psychiatr Serv 62(6):613–618, 2011 21632729

Saha S, Chant D, Welham J, McGrath J: A systematic review of the prevalence of schizophrenia. PLoS Med 2(5): e141, 2005 15916472

Sartorius N, Jablensky A, Korten A, et al: Early manifestations and first-contact incidence of schizophrenia in different cultures: a preliminary report on the initial evaluation phase of the WHO Collaborative Study on Determinants of Outcome of Severe Mental Disorders. Psychol Med 16(4):909–928, 1986 3493497

Schwartz RC, Blankenship DM: Racial disparities in psychotic disorder diagnosis: a review of empirical literature. World J Psychiatry 4(4):133–140, 2014 25540728

Strakowski SM, Hawkins JM, Keck PE Jr: The effects of race and information variance on disagreement between psychiatric emergency service and research diagnoses in first-episode psychosis. J Clin Psychiatry 58(10):457–463; quiz 464-5. 1997 9375599

Terracciano A, Abdel-Khalek AM, Adám N, et al: National character does not reflect mean personality trait levels in 49 cultures. Science 310(5745):96–100, 2005 16210536

Tortelli A, Errazuriz A, Croudace T, et al: Schizophrenia and other psychotic disorders in Caribbean-born migrants and their descendants in England: systematic review and meta-analysis of incidence rates, 1950–2013. Soc Psychiatry Psychiatr Epidemiol 50(7):1039–1055, 2015 25660551

van Os J, Linscott RJ, Myin-Germeys I, et al: A systematic review and meta-analysis of the psychosis continuum: evidence for a psychosis proneness-persistence-impairment model of psychotic disorder. Psychol Med 39(2):179–195, 2009 18606047

Vega WA, Sribney WM, Miskimen TM, et al: Putative psychotic symptoms in the Mexican American population: prevalence and co-occurrence with psychiatric disorders. J Nerv Ment Dis 194(7):471–477, 2006 16840842

Veling W: Ethnic minority position and risk for psychotic disorders. Curr Opin Psychiatry 26(2):166–171, 2013 23286992

Veling W, Selten JP, Susser E, et al: Discrimination and the incidence of psychotic disorders among ethnic minorities in the Netherlands. Int J Epidemiol 36(4):761–768, 2007 17517810

Veling W, Susser E, van Os J, et al: Ethnic density of neighborhoods and incidence of psychotic disorders among immigrants. Am J Psychiatry 165(1):66–73, 2008 18086750

Veling W, Hoek HW, Selten JP, Susser E: Age at migration and future risk of psychotic disorders among immigrants in the Netherlands: a 7-year incidence study. Am J Psychiatry 168(12):1278–1285, 2011 22193672

Weisman AG, López SR, Ventura J, et al: A comparison of psychiatric symptoms between Anglo-Americans and Mexican-Americans with schizophrenia. Schizophr Bull 26(4):817–824, 2000 11087014

Whaley AL: Ethnicity/race, paranoia, and psychiatric diagnoses: clinician bias versus sociocultural differences. J Psychopathol Behav Assess 19:1–20, 1997

World Health Organization: The International Pilot Study of Schizophrenia. Geneva, World Health Organization, 1973

Yamada AM, Barrio C, Morrison SW, et al: Cross-ethnic evaluation of psychotic symptom content in hospitalized middle-aged and older adults. Gen Hosp Psychiatry 28(2):161–168, 2006 16516067

Zandi T, Havenaar JM, Smits M, et al: First contact incidence of psychotic disorders among native Dutch and Moroccan immigrants in the Netherlands: influence of diagnostic bias. Schizophr Res 119(1–3):27–33, 2010 20332065

PART II

Etiology and Pathophysiology

CHAPTER 5

Causes

Matcheri S. Keshavan, M.D.

Paulo L. Lizano, M.D., Ph.D.

Seth W. Perry, Ph.D.

Konasale M. Prasad, M.D.

Julio Licinio, M.D., Ph.D.

Schizophrenia and related disorders are common, are highly disabling, and have substantive morbidity and mortality. Estimates of schizophrenia prevalence have been historically and regionally quite variable, typically falling in the range of 0.3%–0.8% (Charlson et al. 2018; McGrath et al. 2008; Messias et al. 2007), with incidence rates generally roughly one-tenth of prevalence rates, reflecting the chronic nature of the disorder (Messias et al. 2007), and a lifetime morbid risk of about 0.7% (Owen et al. 2016). Owen and colleagues (2016) have suggested that what helped spur the field to new insights regarding the importance of environmental and genetic risk factors in schizophrenia etiology was an evolving appreciation of the highly variant schizophrenia epidemiology, with sometimes substantial differences in prevalence, incidence, or risk observed across geography, sex, or other variables that could not be accounted for by diagnostic or methodological differences.

The causes of schizophrenia are complex and heterogeneous, with a multitude of potential risk and protective factors (Radua et al. 2018). A large body of literature points to genetic and environmental risk factors and their interactions (Tandon et al. 2008; van Os et al. 2008). In a review of this extensive literature, it is important to note some key caveats. First, most of what we know about causality comes from epidemiological data wherein guidelines exist about how to evaluate the strength of causal relationships (Hill 1965). These guidelines include strength of association between a putative causal factor and the effect, consistency of the observations between populations and studies, specificity of the relationship (no other explanation for the relationship), temporality (cause precedes the effect), dose effect (the greater the exposure, the higher the association), the availability of a plausible mechanism (subject to what is known), and laboratory or experimental data showing the causal effect (e.g., animal models). These strict criteria are rarely met in toto in medicine, including for well-accepted causal associations such as that between cigarette smoking and cancer and even less so for complex, multidetermined conditions such as schizophrenia. However, they offer a framework with which to evaluate the emerging literature on the etiology of schizophrenia.

Second, a distinction needs to be made between risk indicators and risk factors. In a recent large umbrella review, Radua et al. (2018) considered 55 systematic reviews and meta-analyses involving 683 individual studies and 170 risk or protective factors implicated in psychotic disorders. They came to the conclusion that only emergence of an ultrahigh-risk state and being Black Caribbean in England were convincing risk factors. However, premorbid antecedents such as the ultrahigh-risk state are *risk indicators* and thus are not the same as actual *risk factors* (such as genetic factors, trauma, or substance abuse) that may cause these antecedents in the first place.

Third, causal factors rarely work in isolation. For example, factors such as social defeat, social isolation, substance abuse, and discrimination in health care may mediate the impact of ethnic minority status on schizophrenia risk.

Finally, a distinction needs to be made between cause (etiology) and mechanism (pathophysiology). Thus, while discussing causal factors, we do not delve into pathways of pathogenesis such as inflammation, oxidative stress, alterations in brain circuitries, or neurochemistry. These topics are examined in other chapters of this volume.

Genetic Factors

Is Schizophrenia Familial?

Family studies have shown that biological relatives of patients with schizophrenia show higher risk for the disorder than the general population, proportional to the proximity of the relationship and number of affected relatives. Such relationships do not appear to be entirely a direct consequence of the proportion of shared genes. For instance, first-degree relatives (siblings, parents, and offspring) share approximately 50% of their genes with their ill relative, second-degree relatives (e.g., aunts, uncles, grandparents, nieces, nephews, and half siblings) share approximately 25% of their genes, and third-degree relatives (e.g., cousins) share approximately 13% of their genes. However, their risk for schizophrenia decreases by greater proportions (Table 5–1).

Although familiality alone is not sufficient to establish the genetic contributions to these disorders, familial relationship incontrovertibly plays a major role in modulating risk for schizophrenia; this is often termed "vertical" transmission. There have been attempts to examine "horizontal" transmission associated with familial relationships to make a case for environmental factors. These attempts largely failed to show such relationships, suggesting that familial aggregation is more likely to be due to genetic factors (Crow and Done 1986).

What Are the Relative Contributions of Genetic and Environmental Factors?

Twin studies allow estimation of the etiological variance contributed by shared genetic factors and environmental factors. Because monozygotic (MZ) twins share 100% of

TABLE 5–1.   **Risk of schizophrenia among family members of an affected individual**

	Percentage of genes shared	Schizophrenia risk
Identical twins	100%	48%
First-degree relatives	50%	
Fraternal twins		17%
Offspring		13%
Siblings		9%
Parents		6%
Second-degree relatives	25%	
Half siblings		6%
Grandchildren		5%
Nephews/nieces		4%
Aunts/uncles		2%
Third-degree relatives	12.5%	
First cousins		2%
General population		1%

Source. Adapted from Gottesman 1991.

their DNA and dizygotic (DZ) twins share about 50% of their DNA, differences in risk for schizophrenia among MZ twins versus DZ twins may be a measure of the differential contributions of genetic and environmental factors to that risk. In addition, twin studies show that the concordance rate of schizophrenia is about 40%–50% in MZ twins and around 15% in DZ twins, suggesting that even when the genes are fully shared, environmental factors play a major role. Epigenetic alterations of shared genes among MZ twins may also contribute to this discrepancy. Heritability, on the other hand, is a population concept that represents the portion of the measure (i.e., the phenotype) of interest that may be attributable to the effects of genes. Schizophrenia is highly heritable: a meta-analysis of 12 twin studies showed, for example, an MZ/DZ ratio of 0.92/0.52, and heritability of 81% (Sullivan et al. 2003). Shared environmental effects were also significant but smaller. Together, these findings, along with current estimates that less than one-third of schizophrenia risk arises from the sum of risks contributed by known gene variants, have given rise to the search for "missing heritability."

A limitation of twin studies is that MZ twins also share their environment more than DZ twins. Adoption studies address this by examining children of schizophrenia probands who were adopted at birth by families with no history of schizophrenia and comparing children of nonschizophrenia probands who were adopted away at birth. The basic premise of these studies is that individuals who shared genetic risk but not family environment would show higher risk compared with individuals who shared family environment but not genetic risk. The assumption is that if a genetic component of a disorder exists, then biological parents and their adopted-away children should show higher risk for schizophrenia. Several adoption studies have shown that children of parents with schizophrenia have substantially increased risk for the disorder, as shown by significantly more schizophrenia in the adopted-away offspring of schizophrenia probands (Ingraham and Kety 2000).

Twin studies (and family studies) are also useful in characterizing *endophenotypes*, which, as proposed by Gottesman and colleagues (Gottesman and Gould 2003; Gould and Gottesman 2006; Hasler et al. 2006; Lenzenweger 2013), are stable, heritable, quantitative trait-like abnormalities that co-occur with psychiatric illnesses at higher frequencies in first-degree biological relatives than they do in the general population. Gottesman and Gould (2003) also proposed that the identification of endophenotypes would aid the search for underlying susceptibility genes for the disorder in question. Several endophenotypes have been proposed over the last two decades (Braff et al. 2008), including cognitive deficits and brain volume abnormalities (Prasad and Keshavan 2008; Stone and Seidman 2016).

How Do We Search for the Risk Genes?

Traditional approaches for identifying implicated genes have included linkage analysis and association studies. Linkage analysis seeks to investigate the loci, *where* the risk genes may be located, on *regions* of chromosomes that tend to travel together within the families due to recombination events during meiosis I of the germ cells. Linkage analysis is performed on affected sibling pairs, other relatives, small nuclear families, or larger pedigrees (Glatt et al. 2007). Several chromosomal regions such as 1, 2q, 3q, 4q, 5q, 6p, 6q, 8p, 10p, 13q, 15q, and 22q (p refers to the short arm, and q refers to the long arm of chromosomes) have been linked to schizophrenia risk (Levinson 2003; Tsuang et al. 2011). However, many of these linkage loci could not be replicated independently. The number of genes within these loci could vary from a few to several thousand genes, thus posing further challenges to precisely identifying the exact causal genetic variant.

In contrast to linkage studies, genetic association studies inform about *what* genetic variations may underlie risk for neuropsychiatric disorders. There are three approaches involved in association studies. If a chromosome location has been implicated (by linkage analysis) to contain a risk gene for a psychotic disorder, a *positional candidate gene* approach is used by testing the functional impact of variants of the potentially contributing gene. Some of the strongly implicated positional candidate genes include the neuregulin gene *NRG1* and the Notch receptor 4 gene *NOTCH4*. *Functional candidate genes* may be selected based on a priori knowledge of a gene's biological function that may impact the trait or disease in question. Examples include genes that code for the dopamine receptors (*DRD3*) and genes coding for serotonin receptors (*HTR24*) (Joyce and Millan 2007; Tsuang et al. 2011). Genome-wide association studies (GWAS) employ a case-control design that tests tagged single nucleotide polymorphisms (SNPs) from all regions of the human genome for association with a disorder. It involves comparing the number of common variants (i.e., typically variants that occur in ≥5% of the population) among those with the disorder versus those without and making the appropriate adjustment for the large number of statistical tests performed. GWAS have strongly pointed to the human leukocyte antigen (HLA) locus, suggesting dysregulation of the immune system as a possible factor in schizophrenia etiology. Below, we highlight other genes that have been implicated in schizophrenia by GWAS.

DNA sequencing refers to determining the precise order of nucleotides in the genome or in a particular gene of interest. Two types of sequencing exist: *whole-genome sequencing*, which attempts to sequence the entire genome, and *exome sequencing*, which focuses on the protein coding sequences. DNA sequencing studies have identified several "neurofunctional" genes (i.e., genes affecting brain-related functions believed to contribute to schizophrenia pathology) (Merico et al. 2015) that encode for proteins related to synaptic function, voltage-gated calcium ion channels (Fromer et al. 2014), and the activity-regulated cytoskeleton-associated scaffold protein complex, which plays a role in synaptic plasticity and is essential to learning and memory (Schizophrenia Working Group of the Psychiatric Genomics Consortium 2014).

How Do We "Connect the Dots" Between Genes and Pathophysiology?

Schizophrenia is currently viewed as a disorder of disrupted connectivity across diverse neural circuitries, resulting from diverse pathophysiological processes (see Chapter 6, "Pathophysiological Theories," and Chapter 7, "Neurobiology"). It remains unclear at this time which of these processes is primary to the cause of the illness and which processes are downstream consequences of a cascading pathogenetic process that may begin early in development. Although it is possible that all these processes may converge onto a final pathophysiological end result that we call "schizophrenia," it is more likely that different subgroups of the illness may have distinct pathophysiological processes and perhaps distinct causes. This latter view is supported by the enormous genetic heterogeneity observed in psychotic disorders.

The large phenotypic heterogeneity of schizophrenia (Tsuang 1975) makes a single causative gene, or a few genes of major effect, highly unlikely. More likely scenarios include a large number of common genetic variations of small effect (polygenic inheritance), rare genes of large effect, and copy number variations (CNVs) (Rees et al. 2015) (Figure 5–1).

A large-scale genome-wide association study showed 108 schizophrenia-associated genetic loci involving 341 protein-coding genes reaching genome-wide significance (Schizophrenia Working Group of the Psychiatric Genomics Consortium 2014). Among these genetic loci were genes related to previously implicated theories of schizophrenia pathophysiology—that is, several glutamatergic genes and one dopaminergic gene (*DRD2*) (Table 5–2). More recent GWAS and related extensions of this approach have confirmed previously implicated genes, identified new neurofunctional targets, and provided novel biological insights into schizophrenia pathophysiology. Another large genome-wide association study of 11,260 cases and 24,542 control subjects identified 145 loci, 50 of which were novel and 33 of which were determined to contain candidate causal genes (Pardiñas et al. 2018). These clustered into the following six independent gene sets associated with schizophrenia: targets of the fragile X mental retardation protein; abnormal behavior; abnormal nervous system electrophysiology; voltage-gated calcium channel complexes; abnormal long-term potentiation; and the 5-HT$_{2C}$ receptor complex (Pardiñas et al. 2018). A few of the more novel or consistent targets from these and other GWAS are highlighted in Table 5–2, and readers can refer to the references noted for more detailed discussions.

Data from GWAS can also be combined with other genomics approaches to yield insights into the underlying biological mechanisms of schizophrenia. For example, by combining data from GWAS with expression quantitative trait loci analyses, Dobbyn and colleagues (2018) "identified a number of candidate genes for which genetic vari-

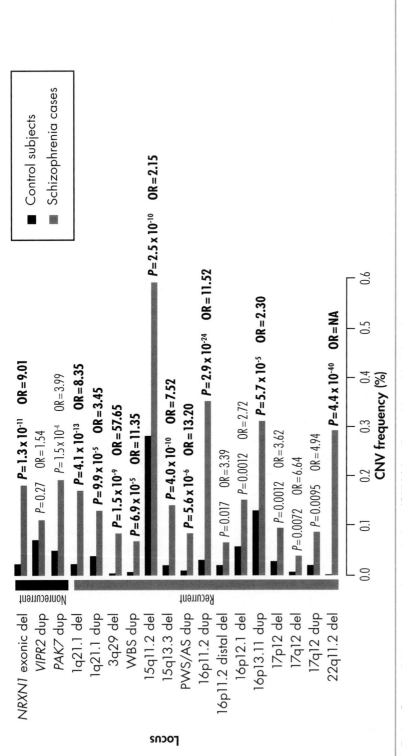

FIGURE 5–1.   Some of the copy number variations (CNVs) implicated in schizophrenia.

P values were generated with a two-sided Fisher's exact test. P values that survived correction for multiple testing (recurrent CNVs $P<4.1\times10^{-4}$; nonrecurrent CNVs $P<2.5\times10^{-6}$) are highlighted in bold. del=deletions; dup=duplications; $NRXN1$=neurexin; OR=odds ratio; $PAK7$=nonspecific serine/threonine protein kinase; PWS/AS=Prader-Willi syndrome/Angelman syndrome; $VIPR2$=vasoactive intestinal peptide receptor 2; WBS=Williams-Beuren syndrome. CNV frequencies in schizophrenia cases and control subjects were taken from Rees et al. 2014b, apart from $PAK7$ duplications, 17q12 duplications, and 16p12.1 deletions, which were taken from Morris et al. 2014, Szatkiewicz et al. 2014, and Rees et al. 2014a, respectively.

Source.   This figure and its legend are reprinted, with slight modifications to the legend, from Rees et al. 2015 under the Creative Commons Attribution License (CC BY) (https://creativecommons.org/licenses/by/3.0/).

TABLE 5–2. **Notable genetic associations in large-scale genome-wide association studies relevant to pathophysiological models of schizophrenia**

Pathophysiological model	Genetic association
Dopaminergic neurotransmission	*DRD2*
Glutamatergic neurotransmission	*CLCN3, GRIA1, GRIN2A, GRM3, SRR*
Ca^{2+}, ion channels, signal transduction	*CACNA1C, CACNA1D, CACNA1I, CACNB2, HCN1, KCNB1, RIMS1,*
G-protein-coupled receptor signaling	*GPR98, GRM3* (and *DRD2* above)
Other synaptic function and plasticity	*ARC, CNTN4, MAGI2, NMDAR, SNAP91*
Neurodevelopment	*FXR1, FYN, SATB2, SLC39A8,*
Immune function	Major histocompatibility complex (MHC) genes: *HLA-DQB1, HLA-DRA, HLA-DRB1*
	Complement genes: *C4A, C4B*
	FMR1
	PTGS2

Note. *ARC*=activity-regulated cytoskeleton-associated protein; *C4A*=complement component 4A; *C4B*=complement component 4B; *CACNA1C*=calcium voltage-gated channel subunit alpha1 C; *CACNA1D*=calcium voltage-gated channel subunit alpha1 D; *CACNA1I*=calcium voltage-gated channel subunit alpha1 I; *CACNB2*=calcium voltage-gated channel auxiliary subunit beta 2; *CLCN3*=chloride voltage-gated channel 3; *CNTN4*=contactin 4; *DRD2*=dopamine receptor D2; *FMR1*=fragile X mental retardation 1; *FXR1*=FMR1 autosomal homolog 1; *FYN*=FYN proto-oncogene, Src family tyrosine kinase; *GPR98*=G protein-coupled receptor 98; *GRIA1*=glutamate ionotropic receptor AMPA type subunit 1; *GRIN2A*=glutamate ionotropic receptor NMDA type subunit 2A; *GRM3*=glutamate metabotropic receptor 3; *HCN1*=hyperpolarization activated cyclic nucleotide gated potassium channel 1; *HLA-DRA*=major histocompatibility complex, class II, DR alpha; *HLA-DQB1*=major histocompatibility complex, class II, DQ beta 1; *HLA-DRB1*=major histocompatibility complex, class II, DR beta 1; *KCNB1*=potassium voltage-gated channel subfamily B member 1; *MAGI2*=membrane-associated guanylate kinase inverted 2; *NMDAR*=N-methyl-D-aspartate receptor; *PTGS2*=prostaglandin-endoperoxide synthase 2; *RIMS1*=regulating synaptic membrane exocytosis 1; *SATB2*=special AT-rich sequence-binding protein 2; *SLC39A8*=solute carrier family 39 member 8; *SNAP91*=synaptosome-associated protein 91; *SRR*=serine racemase.
Source. Adapted from Li et al. 2017; Lin et al. 2016; Pardiñas et al. 2018; Ripke et al. 2013; Schizophrenia Working Group of the Psychiatric Genomics Consortium 2014.

ation for expression co-localizes with genetic variation for schizophrenia risk" (p. 1180), including the iron-responsive element–binding protein 2 gene *IREB2* and signal transducer and activator of transcription 6 gene *STAT6*, among others, which suggests that the implicated genes may play a causal role in schizophrenia. Gusev and colleagues (2018) integrated schizophrenia data from GWAS with expression data from brain, blood, and adipose tissues in a transcriptome-wide association study to identify multiple novel gene targets implicated in schizophrenia, such as the mitogen-activated protein kinase 3 gene *MAPK3*. They found that total brain expression of *MAPK3* was associated with schizophrenia and that *MAPK3* induced neurodevelopmental changes in zebra fish (Pardiñas et al. 2018), making *MAPK3* an attractive target for further investigation. In another fascinating study using a combination of analyses of GWAS and single-cell RNA sequencing, Skene and colleagues (2018) reported that the common genetic findings for schizophrenia mapped most consistently "to just four of 24 main brain cell types: MSNs [medium spiny neurons], pyramidal cells in hippocampal CA1, pyramidal cells in somatosensory cortex, and cortical interneurons," suggesting that "these discrete cell types are central to the etiology of schizophrenia" (p. 8).

Recent developments also suggest that several de novo mutations may also contribute to schizophrenia risk. De novo mutations can arise from mutations occurring in the germ cell for the first time in one of the parents. Alternatively, such mutations can occur in the fertilized egg during embryogenesis. It is too early to comment on what proportion of patients with schizophrenia carry de novo mutations compared with the mutations transmitted by the parents. Overall, such emerging data could partly address missing heritability.

One series of observations has generated particular attention and "connects the dots" with previous theories and observations. First, based on the fact that schizophrenia's typical onset is during adolescence, Feinberg (1982–1983) initially suggested aberrant periadolescent pruning of synapses (too much pruning, too little pruning, or pruning of the wrong synapses) as underlying the pathogenesis of schizophrenia. We (Keshavan et al. 1994) subsequently suggested an exaggerated pruning of synapses in this illness. Although there is no direct evidence of excessive pruning, there are several compelling observations that indirectly support this view, such as decreased dendritic spine density in postmortem brains of patients with schizophrenia (Glantz and Lewis 2000) compared with healthy subjects and individuals with major depressive disorder. As mentioned earlier, GWAS have replicated the association of the HLA region in relation to risk for schizophrenia. The HLA region is highly complex and gene dense, and further studies by Sekar and colleagues (2016) showed that a CNV within the HLA region accounted for a portion of the risk for schizophrenia. Interestingly, Stephan and colleagues (2012) had shown that complement proteins, known components of the innate immune system, were repurposed for another role—that is, tagging the synapses for phagocytosis—and therefore in synaptic pruning processes during adolescence (Sekar et al. 2016). Complement component 4 genes *C4A* and *C4B* that share 99% sequence homology are part of this gene location, and individuals with higher copy numbers of the *C4A* long form (*C4AL*) showed a stronger association with schizophrenia. Sekar and colleagues also found that both *C4A* and *C4B* messenger RNA (mRNA) levels were elevated in five selected regions of the brains of patients with schizophrenia compared with healthy control subjects; approximately 40% higher expression was reported. Complement-deficient mice have decreased synaptic pruning during brain development (Stevens et al. 2007). A recent study using phosphorus magnetic resonance spectroscopy on patients with schizophrenia and control subjects showed that increasing *C4A* copy numbers were associated with greater neuropil contraction, suggesting a gene dosage effect on the possibility of increased synaptic pruning (Prasad et al. 2018). Taken together, these observations point to the possibility of identifying subgroups of psychotic disorders in which a known set of risk genes works via a known pathophysiological mechanism to produce an observable illness phenotype.

A continuing challenge in understanding the causes of psychotic disorders is that many biological findings (Tamminga et al. 2014) and the implicated susceptibility genes overlap across psychotic disorders but also across psychotic, affective, and developmental disorders (Cross-Disorder Group of the Psychiatric Genomics Consortium 2013). For this reason, the Research Domain Criteria (RDoC) approaches (Insel 2014) are important to advance the field by examining data across multiple disorders and also to capture the continuous variation between health and disease. Recent studies such as the Bipolar-Schizophrenia Network on Intermediate Phenotypes (B-SNIP) are beginning to show that it is possible to identify biological subtypes that cut across DSM psychotic disorders and may show better validation by external validators such as neuroimaging data (Pearlson et al. 2016). Transdiagnostic overlaps are seen in gene expression as well. For example, transcriptomic profiling of molecular brain-based phenotypes identified shared polygenic overlap underlying a substantial proportion of cross-disorder expression across autism, schizophrenia, bipolar disorder, depression, and alcoholism (Gandal et al. 2018).

Environmental Risk Factors

Environmental risk factors have been relatively ignored in the investigations of the neurobiology of schizophrenia. Research from the last few decades suggests that genetic factors do not explain all of the variance associated with the onset of schizophrenia. Although schizophrenia is highly heritable, the contribution of genetic factors varies considerably depending on the type of genetic factor involved. For example, common variants such as SNPs contribute 4%–9% of the variance, whereas rare CNVs can contribute up to 30% of the variance. Even among MZ twins, who share 100% of their genes, the risk for schizophrenia is about 40%–50%. These data suggest that a sizable portion of the etiological variance is not explained by genetic factors and that schizophrenia is the result of an interaction between multiple genetic and environmental factors.

Ronald Fisher proposed more than 100 years ago that multiple genetic factors of small effects in the context of environmental factors can explain the role of genetic factors in non-Mendelian heritable traits (Kendler 2015). This conceptualization is the forerunner of the current multifactorial polygenic threshold (MFPT) model. Despite such a comprehensive conceptualization, there are many challenges in investigating the MFPT model. For example, modeling the interactions among several genetic factors of small effects (gene-gene interactions) and among multiple genetic and environmental factors (gene-environment interactions) can be very complicated and require very large sample sizes. This challenge is made even more complicated by the identification of an increasing number of variants of small effects through GWAS. Ripke and colleagues (2013) reported that about 8,300 common SNPs collectively could account for approximately 32% of the variance. Although CNVs contribute to a larger proportion of the etiological variance, because of their rarity, the proportion of affected individuals carrying such CNVs can be very small. Thus, the overall contribution of known genetic factors is considerably lower than the total heritability estimates of approximately 80% for schizophrenia; this disparity is often referred to as the missing heritability.

Notwithstanding very promising data from GWAS, the significance of associated genetic variants for clinical manifestations and for refining the diagnosis or developing novel treatments is questioned based on unknown pathophysiological significance of identified variants (Ebstein 2018). This is due primarily to the location of tag SNPs included in the GWAS in the intronic regions (which are generally noncoding regions for proteins) and because gene annotation is incomplete. *Gene annotation* refers to the process of precisely identifying the location of genes and all of their coding regions and determining the function(s) of these genes. Furthermore, the associated SNP itself may not be etiologically significant, but other SNPs that are in linkage disequilibrium with the significant SNP may be the ones contributing to etiology. Thus, additional work is required even after replicating the association of an SNP in genome-wide associated investigations. To partly circumvent this, a summated risk score, called the polygenic risk score (PGRS), was developed. Recent studies show that the PGRS does not reliably relate to gene expression changes in postmortem brain samples of patients with schizophrenia (Curtis 2018), although associations with several endophenotypes are reported. It can therefore be surmised that the impact of genetic factors may be modulated by environmental factors, both protective and risk conferring. This makes a case for more intensively studying the environmental factors.

There are several challenges in examining environmental factors as well. First, the number of known associated environmental factors has been increasing, thus widening the analytical space. The number of environmental factors and their variability across the globe can be statistically overwhelming. Second, environmental factors may also interact with each other, further complicating the analyses. Various environmental factors found to be associated with schizophrenia are presented in Table 5–3; some of these factors (presented in no particular order) are discussed in the following subsections.

Obstetric Complications

A variety of obstetric complications, including preeclampsia, bleeding, Rh incompatibility, diabetes, asphyxia, uterine atony, emergency cesarean section, and other obstetric abnormalities that lead to low birth weight, congenital malformations, and a small head circumference, have been associated with schizophrenia, with an odds ratio (OR) of 2 in one meta-analysis (Geddes and Lawrie 1995). Among these obstetric complications, emergency cesarean section and placental abruption may have the largest effect sizes. It is hard to consistently attribute risk to a single obstetric complication because obstetric events may be linked with each other. For example, gestational diabetes may increase risk for preeclampsia, which can in turn increase risk for birth complications (Clarke et al. 2006). Low birth weight among boys is related to higher risk for schizophrenia. Mechanisms that contribute to higher risk for schizophrenia appear to be hypoxia-induced changes in critical brain regions, such as the hippocampus. Although the majority of patients with schizophrenia may not have had complications at birth, a Swedish study reported a decreasing incidence of schizophrenia with improving maternal health care (Söderlund et al. 2015). Improved maternal health care, reduced perinatal and maternal infections, better maternal nutrition, and fewer obstetric complications might have contributed to such decreased incidence.

Prenatal Stress

Prenatal stress has been examined extensively in relation to risk for schizophrenia. Maternal exposure to stressors such as serious illness, war, and famine has been associated with increased risk for schizophrenia (Hoek et al. 1998; Levine et al. 2016), although causal relationships are far from clear. These associations have been explored

TABLE 5–3. **Environmental risk factors implicated in schizophrenia**

Environmental factor	Associations with schizophrenia	Comments on associations	Key references
Seasonality of birth	Approximately 5%–8% winter birth excess in schizophrenia patients, suggesting increased risk; may be relatively specific to schizophrenia	Seasonality of birth is one of the most replicated findings. Neurobiological underpinnings are unclear; implications for treatment development are uncertain. Shifting seasonality patterns make selection of control subjects difficult.	Torrey et al. 1997
Obstetric complications	Increased risk with complications involving hypoxia	Obstetric complications are interlinked with each other. A large portion of schizophrenia patients do not report obstetric complications.	Geddes and Lawrie 1995
Maternal infections	Increased risk with first- and second-trimester infections	Prenatal exposure to influenza, *Toxoplasma gondii*, and herpes simplex virus type 2 are associated with higher risk for schizophrenia.	Brown 2006
Postnatal infection	Increased risk with serious infections requiring hospitalization	Population study using birth registers showed that serious infections increased risk for schizophrenia both independently and through interaction with autoimmune disorders.	Benros et al. 2011
Substance use	Increased risk with cannabis in particular	Adolescent exposure to cannabis is associated with risk for schizophrenia. Interaction with *COMT* and *AKT1* variants is reported. Pooled OR of 2.3 is reported.	Semple et al. 2005
Nutrition	Increased risk with first- and second-trimester malnutrition, lower vitamin D and folate levels, higher level of homocysteine, and iron deficiencies	Dutch famine study reported twofold increased risk; finding was replicated in two Chinese famine studies. Relationship of vitamin D deficiency is more complex in that a curvilinear association (increased risk in lowest three quintiles and highest quintile, and lowest risk in the fourth-highest quintile) was reported in one study, but no significant association was reported in another study.	St Clair et al. 2005; Susser et al. 1996; Valipour et al. 2014

TABLE 5–3.	Environmental risk factors implicated in schizophrenia *(continued)*

Environmental factor	Associations with schizophrenia	Comments on associations	Key references
Autoimmune disorders	Increased risk and interaction with serious postnatal infection	Probable mechanism may be through inflammation. Autoantibodies to neuronal cell surface proteins could also lead to schizophrenia symptoms.	Benros et al. 2011
Childhood trauma	Increased risk with varieties of trauma before age 16 years	Evidence is still weak. More studies are needed.	Brown 2011
Urban birth and residence	Increased risk with urban birth in a dose-dependent fashion	Risk association was consistently replicated, but reasons are uncertain. Urbanicity may be a proxy for other environmental factors, such as exposure to infections, drugs, stress, and trauma.	Pedersen and Mortensen 2001
Social status	Increased risk with lower social status	Two recent studies appear to show higher risk in relation to low social status at birth.	Wicks et al. 2005
Stress	Increased risk with repeated and severe stress	Prenatal stress in particular may be a risk factor.	Morgan and Fisher 2007
Minority status	Elevated risk for ethnic minorities	Risk association is unclear because migration status may partly contribute.	Cantor-Graae and Selten 2005
Immigration	Elevated risk for recent immigrants	Risk association is seen even among second-generation immigrants.	Radua et al. 2018
Inadequate social support	Increased risk	Poor social support may increase stress.	Veling et al. 2008
Advanced paternal age	Rising risk with increasing paternal age	Advanced paternal age is one of the most replicated associations with risk for schizophrenia.	Miller et al. 2011

Note. AKT1=AKT serine/threonine kinase 1; *COMT*=catechol O-methyltransferase; OR=odds ratio.

in both ecological and cohort studies. Maternal stress during pregnancy has been linked to changes in corticosteroids and to the consequent association with small-for-gestational-age births.

Infectious Agents

Infectious agents are prototypical examples of discretely defined environmental factors. Prenatal and postnatal exposures to infections have been examined using ecological as well as birth cohort data. Researchers have investigated early prenatal exposure in children conceived during the influenza epidemic in 1957 and found a higher prevalence of schizophrenia among subjects who were in utero during the second trimester when the epidemic occurred than in those who were not in utero (Mednick et al. 1988). These associations were replicated in populations from Great Britain, Japan, and Australia, but not in studies of larger populations with more precise case ascertainment strategies. Overall, data show that influenza exposure in the first half of pregnancy may be associated with three times the risk for schizophrenia (Brown 2012). Similarly, exposures to rubella, *Toxoplasma gondii*, and herpes simplex virus (HSV) type 2 have been linked to higher risk for schizophrenia.

Postnatal exposures to HSV type 1 have consistently been associated with cognitive impairments observed in schizophrenia, suggesting that some infections may add to poor outcomes even if they do not elevate the risk for schizophrenia (Prasad et al. 2012). Future studies evaluating the role of infectious agents can provide opportunities for examining gene-environment interactions (Kim et al. 2007; Prasad et al. 2010).

Cannabis Use

Adolescent cannabis use has been identified as a risk factor for schizophrenia, a finding that has been replicated in multiple analyses. Early evidence came from a 1987 study, which reported nearly six times the risk for schizophrenia among heavy cannabis users compared with nonusers (Andréasson et al. 1987). Results from a study in Dunedin, New Zealand, suggested that the risk was four times higher for users (Arseneault et al. 2004). Evidence of an association has also been reported from Germany, Sweden, and the Netherlands, although the estimates are variable. Often, it is suspected that individuals who are at risk of converting to psychosis may use cannabis to alleviate the symptoms of psychosis. Interaction with certain genetic variants, such as catechol O-methyltransferase *COMT* and AKT serine/threonine kinase 1 (*AKT1*) variants, has been reported, indicating that gene-environment interactions may contribute to variability in risk estimates (Caspi et al. 2005; Morgan et al. 2016).

Malnutrition

The Dutch (Susser et al. 1996) and Chinese (St Clair et al. 2005) famine studies mentioned in Table 5–3 have been followed up by investigating deficiencies of specific nutrients. For example, a meta-analysis showed a vitamin D deficiency in nearly two-thirds of patients with schizophrenia, a deficiency that was associated with an OR of 2.16 for schizophrenia (Valipour et al. 2014). Prenatal protein deprivation in animals was associated with interesting changes in the brain, including altered dendritic architecture with associated decrease in sensorimotor gating. Postmortem neuropathology of patients with schizophrenia has provided replicated data on altered dendritic architecture, specifically dendritic spine loss. Micronutrient deficiencies of folate and iron, as well as elevations of homocysteine, have also been related to an elevated risk for schizophrenia.

Autoimmune Disorders

Autoimmune disorders represent a group of immunological conditions in which the immune system mounts an aberrant "defense" against healthy tissues that are misidentified as "foreign." Autoimmune disorders have been associated with an increased risk for schizophrenia (Benros et al. 2011). Specifically, type 1 diabetes, celiac disease, autoimmune thyroid diseases, and systemic lupus erythematosus have ranked high in contributing to risk for schizophrenia. Interestingly, even a family history of autoimmune disorders is associated with elevated risk for schizophrenia. An exception to this is rheumatoid arthritis, which is associated with decreased risk for schizophrenia. A likely pathway connecting autoimmune disorders with schizophrenia may be inflammation in the brain. There have also been inconsistent reports of autoantibodies mounted against neuronal surface receptors such as N-methyl-D-aspartate (NMDA), α-amino-3-hydroxy-5-methyl-4-isoxazolepropionic acid (AMPA), γ-aminobutyric acid, type A (GABA$_A$), contactin-associated protein-like 2 (CASPR2), leucine-rich, glioma inactivated 1 (LGI1), and dipeptidyl peptidase-like protein 6 (DPPX), and against metabotropic cell-surface receptors such as dopamine D$_2$ receptor and metabotropic glutamate receptor 5 (mGluR5). Given that genetic variations that alter these receptors are reported, it is likely that the antibodies are mounted against altered proteins of these receptors. However, overall findings are variable, and the relationship between autoantibodies and schizophrenia needs further investigation.

Childhood Trauma

Childhood trauma of various kinds has been associated with the risk for schizophrenia. However, most studies investigating this relationship have been conducted using small sample sizes. Overall, a threefold to sevenfold increase in risk for schizophrenia has been found when the trauma occurred before age 16 years. Studies have differed in their inclusion of different types of trauma, with some focusing solely on childhood sexual abuse and others including additional varieties of trauma. Currently, the evidence for establishing a causal link between childhood trauma and risk for psychosis is growing but modest (Brown 2011; van Winkel et al. 2013).

Urban Birth

An association between urban birth and elevated risk for schizophrenia has been reported in many population cohort studies. Interestingly, a dose-response relationship has been seen between the degree of urbanicity and the risk for psychosis. Subsequent urban residence for a person born in a rural area is also associated with greater risk for schizophrenia. Factors that have been proposed to underlie such elevated risk include overcrowding, increased stress, and infections; however, none of these have been conclusively proven to be causal. A recent study suggested that such associations of urbanicity and schizophrenia may be found in developed countries but not in developing countries (DeVylder et al. 2018).

Socioeconomic Status

Socioeconomic status has long been associated with schizophrenia, although the nature of the relationship remains unresolved. The direction of a possibly causal connection is unclear: it could be due to either social causation or social drift, with the former explanation implying that low socioeconomic status is a causative factor for schizophrenia, and the latter suggesting that individuals with schizophrenia gravitate toward low socioeconomic status due to job loss and other financial hardships sustained while living in more affluent neighborhoods. Although this controversy has not been fully resolved, there is some evidence of a modest increase in the risk for schizophrenia when lower social class at birth was considered among the factors (Harrison et al. 2001; Wicks et al. 2005).

Immigration

Immigrant status has been studied as a risk factor for schizophrenia from as early as 1932, when Norwegian immigrants to the United States were found to have double the rate of schizophrenia compared with native-born Americans (Odegaard 1932). These risks are shown to be higher in both first-generation and second-generation immigrants. Another key finding was that immigrants moving from developing to developed countries had higher risk of the disease compared with immigrants from developed countries who moved to another developed country. Individuals with darker skin color had higher risk when they migrated to countries inhabited by white-skinned people. Although racial discrimination has been proposed as an explanation for this, other hypothesized factors include vitamin D deficiency.

Advanced Paternal Age

Advanced paternal age was initially observed in 1958 as a risk factor for schizophrenia in offspring, but it was not until 1979 that the separate contributions of maternal and paternal age could be teased apart (Malaspina et al. 2001). A more sophisticated study found that offspring of fathers ages 45–49 years had twice the risk for schizophrenia, and offspring of fathers age 50 years and older had three times the risk compared with children of fathers who were age 25 years or younger (Wohl and Gorwood 2007). Although precise mechanisms are unclear, accumulation of several point mutations during the replications of spermatogonial stem cells and epigenetic changes related to methylation, demethylation, and histone modifications have been proposed.

Summary

In sum, the ORs for risk for schizophrenia contributed by the environmental factors discussed in this section are significant but not substantively large. At this time, it is not clearly known what combination of environmental factors and genetic factors eventually leads to the onset of schizophrenia. The likely interactive effect of multiple environmental factors suggests that a composite measure such as a "polyenviromic" score (similar to the polygenic scores) may have more predictive validity of clinical value than separate risk factors considered individually (Padmanabhan et al. 2017). Additionally, the precise mechanisms through which environmental factors contribute to schizophrenia are unknown. They appear to eventually affect neurotransmitter systems and neural circuitries often implicated in schizophrenia, but environmental factors seem to be diverse. Stress, fetal hypoxia, inflammation, and nutritional deficiencies may be putative neurobiological mechanisms through which these factors could lead to psychosis.

It is likely that each individual with schizophrenia has a different combination of these environmental factors, which would explain the observed clinical and neurobiological heterogeneity. Thus, it is possible that schizophrenia as currently defined may be a final common manifestation of various combinations of genetic and environmental factors, providing rich opportunities for biological dissection into separate diseases.

Epigenetics

Epigenetics is challenging traditional inheritance paradigms. Its focus involves several mechanisms that provide regulatory information to a genome without altering its primary nucleotide sequence, thus resulting in heritable gene expression changes and nonheritable long-term transcriptional alterations (Allis et al. 2007). Epigenetics consists of interacting molecular mechanisms, including 1) DNA methylation, 2) histone modifications, and 3) noncoding RNA (ncRNA)–mediated regulation of gene expression through dynamic changes to promoters, distal regulatory regions, imprinting, and X-chromosome inactivation that occur during development or cellular differentiation (Allis et al. 2007; Avner and Heard 2001; Bourc'his and Bestor 2004; Colantuoni et al. 2011; Kouzarides 2007; Meissner et al. 2008; Numata et al. 2012; Tadokoro et al. 2007).

Epigenetic control is particularly important in the human brain due to dynamic gene expression changes during fetal/infant life that become more stable with time (Colantuoni et al. 2011; Numata et al. 2012). It is possible that dysregulation of this coordinated gene expression through epigenetic mechanisms may play a vital role in the pathogenesis of schizophrenia (Grayson and Guidotti 2013) and could disturb the formation of essential brain circuits. The environment also plays a major role in the regulation of epigenetic mechanisms, which can result in changes in specific tissue and cell types (Allis et al. 2015; Bettscheider et al. 2012). Additionally, exogenous factors similar to those implicated in the development of schizophrenia have been associated with altering DNA methylation levels, both at specific loci and globally. These factors include changes in diet (Heijmans et al. 2008), early life stress (Bahari-Javan et al. 2017; Luoni et al. 2016), obstetric complications (Ursini et al. 2016; Zucchi et al. 2013), infections (Labouesse et al. 2015; Richetto et al. 2017), and exposure to cigarette smoking (Breitling et al. 2011) and arsenic (Reichard et al. 2007).

DNA Methylation in Schizophrenia

DNA methylation occurs from the conversion of cytosine to 5-methylcytosine in areas with a high concentration of guanine (CpG islands), which is catalyzed by DNA methyltransferases using S-adenosylmethionine as the methyl group source (Allis et al. 2007). These islands are particularly enriched along gene promoters, so the pattern of cytosine methylation may affect the gene expression by either activating or repressing transcription (Allis and Jenuwein 2016). DNA methylation is important for epigenetic regulation of gene expression; alternative splicing; promoter usage; orchestrating tissue differentiation and development during fetal life, childhood, and adolescence; and guiding functional activity in adulthood (Maunakea et al. 2010; Wagner et al. 2014).

Several genome-wide studies of DNA methylation in the postmortem brains of patients with schizophrenia have identified differentially methylated positions related to neuronal differentiation, development, dopaminergic gene expression, and interneuron physiology (Aberg et al. 2014; Ruzicka et al. 2015; Viana et al. 2017). Several papers have shown that the DNA sequence itself plays a large role in the maintenance of DNA methylation (Bird 2011; Lienert et al. 2011; Schilling et al. 2009), providing one potential mechanism for the clinical associations of SNPs from large GWAS. For example, a survey of approximately 450,000 genome-wide CpG sites in fetal cortical brain tissue revealed a fourfold enrichment in GWAS of schizophrenia risk loci among DNA methylation quantitative trait loci (mQTLs) associated with nearby differential DNA methylation (Hannon et al. 2016). A concurrent study by Jaffe et al. (2016) using a similar CpG array in the brain tissue of healthy control volunteers across the life span reported that approximately 60% of the significant loci identified in the large schizophrenia genome-wide association study may function as mQTL. The same study compared DNA methylation differences in the brain between individuals with schizophrenia and control subjects and found 2,104 differential CpGs between the populations that were strongly associated with the prenatal-postnatal but not the adolescence-adult neurodevelopmental periods, suggesting that individuals with schizophrenia may harbor different epigenetic signatures (Jaffe et al. 2016).

Histone Modification in Schizophrenia

Histones undergo posttranslational modifications such as acetylation, methylation, phosphorylation, and SUMOylations (Bowman and Poirier 2015; Emre and Berger 2006), and they regulate the accessibility of transcription machinery to DNA through histone acetyltransferases, deacetylases, methyltransferases, and demethylases (Islam et al. 2011; Song et al. 2016). In schizophrenia, less is known regarding histone modification because this mechanism has only recently become of interest (Aston et al. 2004). However, histone methylation has been implicated as a general biological process involved in schizophrenia pathogenesis (Network and Pathway Analysis Subgroup of Psychiatric Genomics Consortium 2015; Singh et al. 2016; Takata et al. 2016), specifically SET domain containing 1A, histone lysine methyltransferase (*SETD1A*), a component of a histone methyltransferase complex that produces mono-, di-, and trimethylated histone H3 at lysine 4 (H3K4me, H3K4me2, and H3K4me3), which is generally known to mark the transcription start sites of active genes. In the study by Singh et al. (2016), the authors demonstrated that all heterozygous carriers for *SETD1A* have a rare loss-of-function variant, which meet the criteria for a schizophrenia diagnosis, and this variant could be classified as a novel susceptibility gene.

Noncoding RNA in Schizophrenia

There are several types of ncRNAs, including short (with <200 base pairs) and long (with >200 base pairs) ncRNAs, which are located throughout the human genome (Allis et al. 2015; Esteller 2011). The most widely studied among the ncRNAs are the microRNAs (miRNAs); there are about 2,500 catalogued human miRNAs (Petrov et al. 2015). Each miRNA can bind to hundreds of different messenger RNAs (mRNAs), which collectively results in the regulation of more than 60% of protein-coding genes in humans (Esteller 2011). Short ncRNAs bind to complementary sequences within the mRNA transcript, which in turn affects protein translation through mRNA degradation or by physically obstructing the translation by ribosomes (Carthew and Sontheimer 2009; Kosik 2006). Long ncRNAs regulate transcription through transcription factor inhibition (Burenina et al. 2017; Long et al. 2017), alternative mRNA splicing (Yoon et al. 2013), chromatin interaction (Sawyer and Dundr 2017; Wang et al. 2017), and mRNA stability via binding to complementary transcripts or removing miRNA (Rashid et al. 2016; Yoon et al. 2013). There is a growing realization of the importance of ncRNA in the development and maintenance of the central nervous system (Fineberg et al. 2009) and of the contribution ncRNA to disorders of the nervous system (Millan 2013).

There is an increasing body of literature showing that miRNAs play a major role in the pathophysiology of schizophrenia (Beveridge et al. 2010; Moreau et al. 2011; Santarelli et al. 2011). Furthermore, an expanding body of evidence suggests that long ncRNAs are important contributors to schizophrenia (Chen et al. 2016; Hu et al. 2016).

Human postmortem studies report diverse changes in protein and coding-RNA expression in different parts of the brain in subjects with schizophrenia (Clark et al. 2006; Dean et al. 2005; Martins-de-Souza et al. 2009; Pennington et al. 2008; Perkins et al. 2007; Scarr et al. 2018). Several subsequent studies have reported changes in various miRNAs in areas of the frontal (Banigan et al. 2013; Moreau et al. 2011; Santarelli et al. 2011) and temporal (Beveridge et al. 2010) cortices, which neuroimaging studies suggest are affected in schizophrenia (Dirnberger et al. 2014; Kim et al. 2017; Wojtalik et al. 2017). In silico pathway analysis and in vitro studies suggest that miRNAs altered in schizophrenia are able to regulate the expression of several schizophrenia candidate genes involved in important neurotransmitter signaling and neurodevelopmental pathways (Beveridge et al. 2010; Kim et al. 2010; Miller et al. 2012). Also, several transcriptome-wide array studies have reported altered long ncRNA expression profiles in both the periphery and the central nervous system of subjects with schizophrenia (Chen et al. 2016; Cui et al. 2017; Hu et al. 2016; Kim et al. 2010; Ren et al. 2015).

Conclusion

Promises and Challenges

What is currently known about the etiology of schizophrenia may already be yielding better approaches to diagnosis, treatment, and prediction. Using a combination of risk markers and indicators in individuals at clinical or familial high risk for schizophrenia, it is possible to predict conversion to psychotic disorders with a moderately high level of specificity (Carrión et al. 2016; Padmanabhan et al. 2017). The observation that a substantial minority of patients with schizophrenia have rare large-effect gene mutations or CNVs points to the value of genetic counseling (Gershon and Alliey-Rodriguez 2013). Several leads are now emerging that suggest the value of pharmacogenetic prediction of side effects (e.g., agranulocytosis with clozapine) and efficacy of antipsychotics, which may be increasingly used in clinical practice (Zai et al. 2018).

Understanding the causal factors in psychotic disorders is clearly critical for developing innovative therapeutic targets and potentially better diagnosis and treatments for complex illnesses such as schizophrenia. It is possible, using large-scale schizophrenia data sets from GWAS, to identify potential "druggable" genes that encode proteins, some of which are already targets of currently approved medications for other medical illnesses (e.g., glaucoma, epilepsy, hypertension) (Lencz and Malhotra 2015). Some of the 20 identified genes were previously of interest in the study of neuropsychiatric disorders; these genes include the dopamine receptor D2 gene *DRD2*, calcium voltage-gated channel subunit alpha1 C gene *CACNA1C*, glutamate ionotropic receptor NMDA type subunit 2A gene *GRIN2A*, and hyperpolarization activated cyclic nucleotide gated potassium channel 1 gene *HCN1*. GWAS also help to characterize disease-gene networks in order to elucidate drug-disease relationships. Kauppi et al. (2018) recently examined protein interactomes to map antipsychotic drug targets to gene networks related to schizophrenia. They observed that antipsychotic drug targets overlapped with the core disease-gene network module consisting of multiple pathways not limited to dopamine. Other risk genes not connected to antipsychotics may be targets for novel compounds that can address unmet needs in schizophrenia treatment, such as cognitive and negative symptoms.

Several challenges remain, however. These include the lack of specific or satisfactory treatments, and the scarcity of actionable biomarkers or laboratory tests for early detection, outcome prediction, and treatment selection. Much of the heritability of psychotic disorders must still be delineated. Even the identified liability genes have relatively small effect sizes, which together account for only a modest proportion of the genetic risk. The majority of the genes implicated in schizophrenia are in noncoding regions of DNA (i.e., intergenic or intronic), whose functional significance remains unclear. A large part of the missing heritability may also be because of unknown gene-gene interactions (epistasis). Developing new treatments has been slow for the reasons elucidated above and also due to the lengthy drug development process and diminishing investment by industry in psychopharmacological research (Keshavan et al. 2017).

Paths Ahead

Several recent initiatives promise to circumvent some of these roadblocks to progress. Progress toward bridging the missing heritability will benefit from the National Institute of Mental Health's PsychENCODE initiative (Akbarian et al. 2015), which seeks to characterize the function of noncoding genomic elements in cell- and tissue-specific samples in the brain in health and neuropsychiatric disease. New bioinformatics and analytical tools are beginning to elucidate the interactions between genomic data and environmental and other "omic" (proteome, epigenome, interactome) data to better understand disease biology. Increasing understanding of molecular and genetic interconnectedness helps delineation of disease pathways caused by networks of genes, offering better therapeutic targets than single gene products (Gebicke-Haerter 2016). Finally, the induced pluripotent stem cells from patient populations can yield neuronal cell-based phenotypes to model human illness and generate in vitro biomarkers for disease identification and treatment development (Haggarty et al. 2016).

All of these translational and transformative advances have the potential to help accelerate the journey from the genome to the clinic, reverse the stagnation of new treatment development, improve lives, and combat the stigma associated with serious mental illnesses.

References

Aberg KA, McClay JL, Nerella S, et al: Methylome-wide association study of schizophrenia: identifying blood biomarker signatures of environmental insults. JAMA Psychiatry 71(3):255–264, 2014 24402055

Akbarian S, Liu C, Knowles JA, et al; PsychENCODE Consortium: The PsychENCODE project. Nat Neurosci 18(12):1707–1712, 2015 26605881

Allis CD, Jenuwein T: The molecular hallmarks of epigenetic control. Nat Rev Genet 17(8):487–500, 2016 27346641

Allis CD, Jenuwein T, Reinberg D: Overview and concepts, in Epigenetics. Edited by Allis CD, Jenuwein T, Reinberg D, et al. Cold Spring Harbor, NY, Cold Spring Harbor Laboratory Press, 2007, pp 23–62

Allis CD, Caparros M-L, Jenuwein T, et al: Overview and concepts, in Epigenetics, 2nd Edition. Edited by Allis CD, Caparros M-L, Jenuwein T, et al. Cold Spring Harbor, NY, Cold Spring Harbor Laboratory Press, 2015, pp 47–115

Andréasson S, Allebeck P, Engström, Rydberg U: Cannabis and schizophrenia: a longitudinal study of Swedish conscripts. Lancet 2(8674) 1483–1486, 1987 2892048

Arseneault L, Cannon M, Whitton J, Murray RM: Causal association between cannabis and psychosis: examination of the evidence. Br J Psychiatry 184:110–117, 2004 14754822

Aston C, Jiang L, Sokolov BP: Microarray analysis of postmortem temporal cortex from patients with schizophrenia. J Neurosci Res 77(6):858–866, 2004 15334603

Avner P, Heard E: X-chromosome inactivation: counting, choice and initiation. Nat Rev Genet 2(1):59–67, 2001 11253071

Bahari-Javan S, Varbanov H, Halder R, et al: HDAC1 links early life stress to schizophrenia-like phenotypes. Proc Natl Acad Sci USA 114(23):E4686–E4694, 2017 28533418

Banigan MG, Kao PF, Kozubek JA, et al: Differential expression of exosomal microRNAs in prefrontal cortices of schizophrenia and bipolar disorder patients. PLoS One 8(1):e48814, 2013 23382797

Benros ME, Nielsen PR, Nordentoft M, et al: Autoimmune diseases and severe infections as risk factors for schizophrenia: a 30-year population-based register study. Am J Psychiatry 168(12):1303–1310, 2011 22193673

Bettscheider M, Kuczynska A, Almeida O, et al: Optimized analysis of DNA methylation and gene expression from small, anatomically defined areas of the brain. J Vis Exp (65):e3938, 2012 22824867

Beveridge NJ, Gardiner E, Carroll AP, et al: Schizophrenia is associated with an increase in cortical microRNA biogenesis. Mol Psychiatry 15(12):1176–1189, 2010 19721432

Bird A: Putting the DNA back into DNA methylation. Nat Genet 43(11):1050–1051, 2011 22030606

Bourc'his D, Bestor TH: Meiotic catastrophe and retrotransposon reactivation in male germ cells lacking Dnmt3L. Nature 431(7004):96–99, 2004 15318244

Bowman GD, Poirier MG: Post-translational modifications of histones that influence nucleosome dynamics. Chem Rev 115(6):2274–2295, 2015 25424540

Braff DL, Greenwood TA, Swerdlow NR, et al; Investigators of the Consortium on the Genetics of Schizophrenia: Advances in endophenotyping schizophrenia. World Psychiatry 7(1):11–18, 2008 18458787

Breitling LP, Yang R, Korn B, et al: Tobacco-smoking-related differential DNA methylation: 27K discovery and replication. Am J Hum Genet 88(4):450–457, 2011 21457905

Brown AS: Prenatal infection as a risk factor for schizophrenia. Schizophr Bull 32(2):200–202, 2006 16469941

Brown AS: The environment and susceptibility to schizophrenia. Prog Neurobiol 93(1):23–58, 2011 20955757

Brown AS: Epidemiologic studies of exposure to prenatal infection and risk of schizophrenia and autism. Dev Neurobiol 72(10):1272–1276, 2012 22488761

Burenina OY, Oretskaya TS, Kubareva EA: Non-coding RNAs as transcriptional regulators in eukaryotes. Acta Naturae 9(4):13–25, 2017 29340213

Cantor-Graae E, Selten JP: Schizophrenia and migration: a meta-analysis and review. Am J Psychiatry 162(1):12–24, 2005 15625195

Carrión RE, Cornblatt BA, Burton CZ, et al: Personalized prediction of psychosis: external validation of the NAPLS-2 Psychosis Risk Calculator with the EDIPPP Project. Am J Psychiatry 173(10):989–996, 2016 27363511

Carthew RW, Sontheimer EJ: Origins and Mechanisms of miRNAs and siRNAs. Cell 136(4):642–655, 2009 19239886

Caspi A, Moffitt TE, Cannon M, et al: Moderation of the effect of adolescent-onset cannabis use on adult psychosis by a functional polymorphism in the catechol-O-methyltransferase gene: longitudinal evidence of a gene X environment interaction. Biol Psychiatry 57(10):1117–1127, 2005 15866551

Charlson FJ, Ferrari AJ, Santomauro DF, et al: Global epidemiology and burden of schizophrenia: findings from the Global Burden of Disease Study 2016. Schizophr Bull 44(6):1195–1203, 2018 29762765

Chen S, Sun X, Niu W, et al: Aberrant expression of long non-coding RNAs in schizophrenia patients. Med Sci Monit 22:3340–3351, 2016 27650396

Clark D, Dedova I, Cordwell S, et al: A proteome analysis of the anterior cingulate cortex gray matter in schizophrenia. Mol Psychiatry 11(5):459–470, 423, 2006 16491132

Clarke MC, Harley M, Cannon M: The role of obstetric events in schizophrenia. Schizophr Bull 32(1):3–8, 2006 16306181

Colantuoni C, Lipska BK, Ye T, et al: Temporal dynamics and genetic control of transcription in the human prefrontal cortex. Nature 478(7370):519–523, 2011 22031444

Cross-Disorder Group of the Psychiatric Genomics Consortium: Identification of risk loci with shared effects on five major psychiatric disorders: a genome-wide analysis. Lancet 381(9875):1371–1379, 2013 23453885

Crow TJ, Done DJ: Age of onset of schizophrenia in siblings: a test of the contagion hypothesis. Psychiatry Res 18(2):107–117, 1986 3014586

Cui X, Niu W, Kong L, et al: Can lncRNAs be indicators for the diagnosis of early onset or acute schizophrenia and distinguish major depressive disorder and generalized anxiety disorder? A cross validation analysis. Am J Med Genet B Neuropsychiatr Genet 174(4):335–341, 2017 28371072

Curtis D: Polygenic risk score for schizophrenia is not strongly associated with the expression of specific genes or gene sets. Psychiatr Genet 28(4):59–65, 2018 29672343

Dean B, Keriakous D, Thomas E, et al: Understanding the pathology of schizophrenia: the impact of high-throughput screening of the genome and proteome in postmortem CNS. Cur Psychiatry Rev 1(1):1–9, 2005

DeVylder JE, Kelleher I, Lalane M, et al: Association of urbanicity with psychosis in low- and middle-income countries. JAMA Psychiatry 75(7):678–686, 2018 29799917

Dirnberger G, Fuller R, Frith C, Jahanshahi M: Neural correlates of executive dysfunction in schizophrenia: failure to modulate brain activity with task demands. Neuroreport 25(16):1308–1315, 2014 25275638

Dobbyn A, Huckins LM, Boocock J, et al; CommonMind Consortium: Landscape of conditional eQTL in dorsolateral prefrontal cortex and co-localization with schizophrenia GWAS. Am J Hum Genet 102(6):1169–1184, 2018 29805045

Ebstein RP: Has the gloom lifted on genome-wide association studies? Biol Psychiatry 83(7):544–545, 2018 29506653

Emre NC, Berger SL: Histone post-translational modifications regulate transcription and silent chromatin in Saccharomyces cerevisiae. Ernst Schering Res Found Workshop (57):127–153, 2006 16568953

Esteller M: Non-coding RNAs in human disease. Nat Rev Genet 12(12):861–874, 2011 22094949

Feinberg I: Schizophrenia: caused by a fault in programmed synaptic elimination during adolescence? J Psychiatr Res 17(4):319–334, 1982–1983 7187776

Fineberg SK, Kosik KS, Davidson BL: MicroRNAs potentiate neural development. Neuron 64(3):303–309, 2009 19914179

Fromer M, Pocklington AJ, Kavanagh DH, et al: De novo mutations in schizophrenia implicate synaptic networks. Nature 506(7487):179–184, 2014 24463507

Gandal MJ, Haney JR, Parikshak NN, et al; CommonMind Consortium; PsychENCODE Consortium; iPSYCH-BROAD Working Group: Shared molecular neuropathology across major psychiatric disorders parallels polygenic overlap. Science 359(6376):693–697, 2018 29439242

Gebicke-Haerter PJ: Systems psychopharmacology: a network approach to developing novel therapies. World J Psychiatry 6(1):66–83, 2016 27014599

Geddes JR, Lawrie SM: Obstetric complications and schizophrenia: a meta-analysis. Br J Psychiatry 167(6):786–793, 1995 8829748

Gershon ES, Alliey-Rodriguez N: New ethical issues for genetic counseling in common mental disorders. Am J Psychiatry 170(9):968–976, 2013 23897273

Glantz LA, Lewis DA: Decreased dendritic spine density on prefrontal cortical pyramidal neurons in schizophrenia. Arch Gen Psychiatry 57(1):65–73, 2000 10632234

Glatt SJ, Faraone SV, Tsuang MT: Genetic risk factors for mental disorders: general principles and state of the science, in Recognition and Prevention of Major Mental and Substance Use Disorders. Edited by Tsuang MT, Stone WS, Lyons MJ. Washington, DC, American Psychiatric Publishing, 2007, pp 3–20

Gottesman II: Schizophrenia Genesis: The Origins of Madness. New York, WH Freeman/Times Books/Henry Holt, 1991

Gottesman II, Gould TD: The endophenotype concept in psychiatry: etymology and strategic intentions. Am J Psychiatry 160(4):636–645, 2003 12668349

Gould TD, Gottesman II: Psychiatric endophenotypes and the development of valid animal models. Genes Brain Behav 5(2):113–119, 2006 16507002

Grayson DR, Guidotti A: The dynamics of DNA methylation in schizophrenia and related psychiatric disorders. Neuropsychopharmacology 38(1):138–166, 2013 22948975

Gusev A, Mancuso N, Won H, et al: Transcriptome-wide association study of schizophrenia and chromatin activity yields mechanistic disease insights. Nat Genet 50(4):538–548, 2018 29632383

Haggarty SJ, Silva MC, Cross A, et al: Advancing drug discovery for neuropsychiatric disorders using patient-specific stem cell models. Mol Cell Neurosci 73:104–115, 2016 26826498

Hannon E, Spiers H, Viana J, et al: Methylation QTLs in the developing brain and their enrichment in schizophrenia risk loci. Nat Neurosci 19(1):48–54, 2016 26619357

Harrison G, Gunnell D, Glazebrook C, et al: Association between schizophrenia and social inequality at birth: case-control study. Br J Psychiatry 179:346–350, 2001 11581116

Hasler G, Drevets WC, Gould TD, et al: Toward constructing an endophenotype strategy for bipolar disorders. Biol Psychiatry 60(2):93–105, 2006 16406007

Heijmans BT, Tobi EW, Stein AD, et al: Persistent epigenetic differences associated with prenatal exposure to famine in humans. Proc Natl Acad Sci USA 105(44):17046–17049, 2008 18955703

Hill AB: The environment and disease: association or causation? Proc R Soc Med 58:295–300, 1965 14283879

Hoek HW, Brown AS, Susser E: The Dutch famine and schizophrenia spectrum disorders. Soc Psychiatry Psychiatr Epidemiol 33(8):373–379, 1998 9708024

Hu J, Xu J, Pang L, et al: Systematically characterizing dysfunctional long intergenic non-coding RNAs in multiple brain regions of major psychosis. Oncotarget 7(44):71087–71098, 2016 27661005

Ingraham LJ, Kety SS: Adoption studies of schizophrenia. Am J Med Genet 97(1):18–22, 2000

Insel TR: The NIMH Research Domain Criteria (RDoC) Project: precision medicine for psychiatry. Am J Psychiatry 171(4):395–397, 2014 24687194

Islam AB, Richter WF, Lopez-Bigas N, et al: Selective targeting of histone methylation. Cell Cycle 10(3):413–424, 2011 21270517

Jaffe AE, Gao Y, Deep-Soboslay A, et al: Mapping DNA methylation across development, genotype and schizophrenia in the human frontal cortex. Nat Neurosci 19(1):40–47, 2016 26619358

Joyce JN, Millan MJ: Dopamine D3 receptor agonists for protection and repair in Parkinson's disease. Curr Opin Pharmacol 7(1):100–105, 2007 17174156

Kauppi K, Rosenthal SB, Lo MT, et al: Revisiting antipsychotic drug actions through gene networks associated with schizophrenia. Am J Psychiatry 175(7):674–682, 2018 29495895

Kendler KS: A joint history of the nature of genetic variation and the nature of schizophrenia. Mol Psychiatry 20(1):77–83, 2015 25134695

Keshavan MS, Anderson S, Pettegrew JW: Is schizophrenia due to excessive synaptic pruning in the prefrontal cortex? The Feinberg hypothesis revisited. J Psychiatr Res 28(3):239–265, 1994 7932285

Keshavan MS, Lawler AN, Nasrallah HA, et al: New drug developments in psychosis: challenges, opportunities and strategies. Prog Neurobiol 152:3–20, 2017 27519538

Kim AH, Reimers M, Maher B, et al: MicroRNA expression profiling in the prefrontal cortex of individuals affected with schizophrenia and bipolar disorders. Schizophr Res 124(1–3):183–191, 2010 20675101

Kim G-W, Kim Y-H, Jeong G-W: Whole brain volume changes and its correlation with clinical symptom severity in patients with schizophrenia: a DARTEL-based VBM study. PLoS One 12(5):e0177251, 2017 28520743

Kim JJ, Shirts BH, Dayal M, et al: Are exposure to cytomegalovirus and genetic variation on chromosome 6p joint risk factors for schizophrenia? Ann Med 39(2):145–153, 2007 17453677

Kosik KS: The neuronal microRNA system. Nat Rev Neurosci 7(12):911–920, 2006 17115073

Kouzarides TB: SL chromatin modifications and their mechanism of action, in Epigenetics. Edited by Allis CD, Jenuwein T, Reinberg D, et al. Cold Spring Harbor, NY, Cold Spring Harbor Laboratory Press, 2007, pp 191–210

Labouesse MA, Dong E, Grayson DR, et al: Maternal immune activation induces GAD1 and GAD2 promoter remodeling in the offspring prefrontal cortex. Epigenetics 10(12):1143–1155, 2015 26575259

Lencz T, Malhotra AK: Targeting the schizophrenia genome: a fast track strategy from GWAS to clinic. Mol Psychiatry 20(7):820–826, 2015 25869805

Lenzenweger MF: Thinking clearly about the endophenotype-intermediate phenotype-biomarker distinctions in developmental psychopathology research. Dev Psychopathol 25(4 Pt 2):1347–1357, 2013 24342844

Levine SZ, Levav I, Pugachova I, et al: Transgenerational effects of genocide exposure on the risk and course of schizophrenia: a population-based study. Schizophr Res 176(2–3):540–545, 2016 27401532

Levinson DF: Molecular genetics of schizophrenia: a review of the recent literature. Curr Opin Psychiatry 16(2):157–170, 2003

Li Z, Chen J, Yu H, et al: Genome-wide association analysis identifies 30 new susceptibility loci for schizophrenia. Nat Genet 49(11):1576–1583, 2017 28991256

Lienert F, Wirbelauer C, Som I, et al: Identification of genetic elements that autonomously determine DNA methylation states. Nat Genet 43(11):1091–1097, 2011 21964573

Lin J-R, Cai Y, Zhang Q, et al: Integrated post-GWAS analysis sheds new light on the disease mechanisms of schizophrenia. Genetics 204(4):1587–1600, 2016 27754856

Long Y, Wang X, Youmans DT, et al: How do lncRNAs regulate transcription? Sci Adv 3(9):eaao2110, 2017 28959731

Luoni A, Massart R, Nieratschker V, et al: Ankyrin-3 as a molecular marker of early life stress and vulnerability to psychiatric disorders. Transl Psychiatry 6(11):e943, 2016 27824361

Malaspina D, Harlap S, Fennig S, et al: Advancing paternal age and the risk of schizophrenia. Arch Gen Psychiatry 58(4):361–367, 2001 11296097

Martins-de-Souza D, Gattaz WF, Schmitt A, et al: Proteome analysis of schizophrenia patients Wernicke's area reveals an energy metabolism dysregulation. BMC Psychiatry 9:17, 2009 19405953

Maunakea AK, Nagarajan RP, Bilenky M, et al: Conserved role of intragenic DNA methylation in regulating alternative promoters. Nature 466(7303):253–257, 2010 20613842

McGrath J, Saha S, Chant D, et al: Schizophrenia: a concise overview of incidence, prevalence, and mortality. Epidemiol Rev 30:67–76, 2008 18480098

Mednick SA, Machon RA, Huttunen MO, et al: Adult schizophrenia following prenatal exposure to an influenza epidemic. Arch Gen Psychiatry 45(2):189–192, 1988 3337616

Meissner A, Mikkelsen TS, Gu H, et al: Genome-scale DNA methylation maps of pluripotent and differentiated cells. Nature 454(7205):766–770, 2008 18600261

Merico D, Zarrei M, Costain G, et al: Whole-genome sequencing suggests schizophrenia risk mechanisms in humans with 22q11.2 deletion syndrome. G3 (Bethesda) 5(11):2453–2461, 2015 26384369

Messias EL, Chen CY, Eaton WW: Epidemiology of schizophrenia: review of findings and myths. Psychiatr Clin North Am 30(3):323–338, 2007 17720026

Millan MJ: An epigenetic framework for neurodevelopmental disorders: from pathogenesis to potential therapy. Neuropharmacology 68:2–82, 2013 23246909

Miller B, Messias E, Miettunen J, et al: Meta-analysis of paternal age and schizophrenia risk in male versus female offspring. Schizophr Bull 37(5):1039–1047, 2011 20185538

Miller BH, Zeier Z, Xi L, et al: MicroRNA-132 dysregulation in schizophrenia has implications for both neurodevelopment and adult brain function. Proc Natl Acad Sci USA 109(8):3125–3130, 2012 22315408

Moreau MP, Bruse SE, David-Rus R, et al: Altered microRNA expression profiles in postmortem brain samples from individuals with schizophrenia and bipolar disorder. Biol Psychiatry 69(2):188–193, 2011 21183010

Morgan C, Fisher H: Environment and schizophrenia: environmental factors in schizophrenia: childhood trauma—a critical review. Schizophr Bull 33(1):3–10, 2007 17105965

Morgan CJA, Freeman TP, Powell J, et al: AKT1 genotype moderates the acute psychotomimetic effects of naturalistically smoked cannabis in young cannabis smokers. Transl Psychiatry 6:e738, 2016 26882038

Morris DW, Pearson RD, Cormican P, et al; International Schizophrenia Consortium, SGENE+ Consortium; Wellcome Trust Case Control Consortium 2: An inherited duplication at the gene p21 protein-activated kinase 7 (PAK7) is a risk factor for psychosis. Hum Mol Genet 23(12):3316–3326, 2014 24474471

Network and Pathway Analysis Subgroup of Psychiatric Genomics Consortium: Psychiatric genome-wide association study analyses implicate neuronal, immune and histone pathways. Nat Neurosci 18(2):199–209, 2015 25599223

Numata S, Ye T, Hyde TM, et al: DNA methylation signatures in development and aging of the human prefrontal cortex. Am J Hum Genet 90(2):260–272, 2012 22305529

Odegaard O: Emigration and insanity: a study of mental disease among the Norwegian-born population of Minnesota. Acta Psychiatr Neurol Suppl (4):11–206, 1932

Owen MJ, Sawa A, Mortensen PB: Schizophrenia. Lancet 388(10039):86–97, 2016 26777917

Padmanabhan JL, Shah JL, Tandon N, et al: The "polyenviromic risk score": aggregating environmental risk factors predicts conversion to psychosis in familial high-risk subjects. Schizophr Res 181:17–22, 2017 28029515

Pardiñas AF, Holmans P, Pocklington AJ, et al: Common schizophrenia alleles are enriched in mutation-intolerant genes and in regions under strong background selection. Nat Genet 50(3):381–389, 2018 29483656

Pearlson GD, Clementz BA, Sweeney JA, et al: Does biology transcend the symptom-based boundaries of psychosis? Psychiatr Clin North Am 39(2):165–174, 2016 27216897

Pedersen CB, Mortensen PB: Evidence of a dose-response relationship between urbanicity during upbringing and schizophrenia risk. Arch Gen Psychiatry 58(11):1039–1046, 2001 11695950

Pennington K, Beasley CL, Dicker P, et al: Prominent synaptic and metabolic abnormalities revealed by proteomic analysis of the dorsolateral prefrontal cortex in schizophrenia and bipolar disorder. Mol Psychiatry 13(12):1102–1117, 2008 17938637

Perkins DO, Jeffries CD, Jarskog LF, et al: microRNA expression in the prefrontal cortex of individuals with schizophrenia and schizoaffective disorder. Genome Biol 8(2):R27, 2007 17326821

Petrov AI, Kay SJE, Gibson R, et al; RNAcentral Consortium: RNAcentral: an international database of ncRNA sequences. Nucleic Acids Res 43(Database issue):D123–D129, 2015 25352543

Prasad KM, Keshavan MS: Structural cerebral variations as useful endophenotypes in schizophrenia: do they help construct "extended endophenotypes"? Schizophr Bull 34(4):774–790, 2008 18408230

Prasad KM, Bamne MN, Shirts BH, et al: Grey matter changes associated with host genetic variation and exposure to herpes simplex virus 1 (HSV1) in first episode schizophrenia. Schizophr Res 118(1–3):232–239, 2010 20138739

Prasad KM, Watson AM, Dickerson FB, et al: Exposure to herpes simplex virus type 1 and cognitive impairments in individuals with schizophrenia. Schizophr Bull 38(6):1137–1148, 2012 22490995

Prasad KM, Chowdari KV, D'Aiuto LA, et al: Neuropil contraction in relation to complement C4 gene copy numbers in independent cohorts of adolescent-onset and young adult-onset schizophrenia patients-a pilot study. Transl Psychiatry 8(1):134, 2018 30026462

Radua J, Ramella-Cravaro V, Ioannidis JPA, et al: What causes psychosis? An umbrella review of risk and protective factors. World Psychiatry 17(1):49–66, 2018 29352556

Rashid F, Shah A, Shan G: Long non-coding RNAs in the cytoplasm. Genomics Proteomics Bioinformatics 14(2):73–80, 2016 27163185

Rees E, Walters JTR, Chambert KD, et al; Wellcome Trust Case Control Consortium: CNV analysis in a large schizophrenia sample implicates deletions at 16p12.1 and SLC1A1 and duplications at 1p36.33 and CGNL1. Hum Mol Genet 23(6):1669–1676, 2014a 24163246

Rees E, Walters JTR, Georgieva L, et al: Analysis of copy number variations at 15 schizophrenia-associated loci. Br J Psychiatry 204(2):108–114, 2014b 24311552

Rees E, O'Donovan MC, Owen MJ: Genetics of schizophrenia. Curr Opin Behav Sci 2:8–14, 2015

Reichard JF, Schnekenburger M, Puga A: Long term low-dose arsenic exposure induces loss of DNA methylation. Biochem Biophys Res Commun 352(1):188–192, 2007 17107663

Ren Y, Cui Y, Li X, et al: A co-expression network analysis reveals lncRNA abnormalities in peripheral blood in early onset schizophrenia. Prog Neuropsychopharmacol Biol Psychiatry 63:1–5, 2015 25967042

Richetto J, Massart R, Weber-Stadlbauer U, et al: Genome-wide DNA methylation changes in a mouse model of infection-mediated neurodevelopmental disorders. Biol Psychiatry 81(3):265–276, 2017 27769567

Ripke S, O'Dushlaine C, Chambert K, et al; Multicenter Genetic Studies of Schizophrenia Consortium; Psychosis Endophenotypes International Consortium; Wellcome Trust Case Control Consortium 2: Genome-wide association analysis identifies 13 new risk loci for schizophrenia. Nat Genet 45(10):1150–1159, 2013 23974872

Ruzicka WB, Subburaju S, Benes FM: Circuit- and diagnosis-specific DNA methylation changes at γ-aminobutyric acid-related genes in postmortem human hippocampus in schizophrenia and bipolar disorder. JAMA Psychiatry 72(6):541–551, 2015 25738424

Santarelli DM, Beveridge NJ, Tooney PA, et al: Upregulation of dicer and microRNA expression in the dorsolateral prefrontal cortex Brodmann area 46 in schizophrenia. Biol Psychiatry 69(2):180–187, 2011 21111402

Sawyer IA, Dundr M: Chromatin loops and causality loops: the influence of RNA upon spatial nuclear architecture. Chromosoma 126(5):541–557, 2017 28593374

Scarr E, Udawela M, Dean B: Changed frontal pole gene expression suggest altered interplay between neurotransmitter, developmental, and inflammatory pathways in schizophrenia. NPJ Schizophr 4(1):4, 2018 29463818

Schilling E, El Chartouni C, Rehli M: Allele-specific DNA methylation in mouse strains is mainly determined by cis-acting sequences. Genome Res 19(11):2028–2035, 2009 19687144

Schizophrenia Working Group of the Psychiatric Genomics Consortium: Biological insights from 108 schizophrenia-associated genetic loci. Nature 511(7510):421–427, 2014 25056061

Sekar A, Bialas AR, de Rivera H, et al; Schizophrenia Working Group of the Psychiatric Genomics Consortium: Schizophrenia risk from complex variation of complement component 4. Nature 530(7589):177–183, 2016 26814963

Semple DM, McIntosh AM, Lawrie SM: Cannabis as a risk factor for psychosis: systematic review. J Psychopharmacol 19(2):187–194, 2005 15871146

Singh T, Kurki MI, Curtis D, et al; Swedish Schizophrenia Study; INTERVAL Study; DDD Study; UK10 K Consortium: Rare loss-of-function variants in SETD1A are associated with schizophrenia and developmental disorders. Nat Neurosci 19(4):571–577, 2016 26974950

Skene NG, Bryois J, Bakken TE, et al; Major Depressive Disorder Working Group of the Psychiatric Genomics Consortium: Genetic identification of brain cell types underlying schizophrenia. Nat Genet 50(6):825–833, 2018 29785013

Söderlund J, Wicks S, Jörgensen L, et al: Comparing cohort incidence of schizophrenia with that of bipolar disorder and affective psychosis in individuals born in Stockholm County 1955–1967. Psychol Med 45(16):3433–3439, 2015 26189466

Song Y, Wu F, Wu J: Targeting histone methylation for cancer therapy: enzymes, inhibitors, biological activity and perspectives. J Hematol Oncol 9(1):49, 2016 27316347

St Clair D, Xu M, Wang P, et al: Rates of adult schizophrenia following prenatal exposure to the Chinese famine of 1959-1961. JAMA 294(5):557–562, 2005 16077049

Stephan AH, Barres BA, Stevens B: The complement system: an unexpected role in synaptic pruning during development and disease. Annu Rev Neurosci 35(1):369–389, 2012 22715882

Stevens B, Allen NJ, Vazquez LE, et al: The classical complement cascade mediates CNS synapse elimination. Cell 131(6):1164–1178, 2007 18083105

Stone WS, Seidman LJ: Neuropsychological and structural imaging endophenotypes in schizophrenia, in Developmental Psychopathology, Vol 2: Developmental Neuroscience. Edited by Cicchetti D. Hoboken, NJ, Wiley, 2016, pp 931–965

Sullivan PF, Kendler KS, Neale MC: Schizophrenia as a complex trait: evidence from a meta-analysis of twin studies. Arch Gen Psychiatry 60(12):1187–1192, 2003 14662550

Sussser E, Neugebauer R, Hoek HW, et al: Schizophrenia after prenatal famine: further evidence. Arch Gen Psychiatry 53(1):25–31, 1996 8540774

Szatkiewicz JP, O'Dushlaine C, Chen G, et al: Copy number variation in schizophrenia in Sweden. Mol Psychiatry 19(7):762–773, 2014 24776740

Tadokoro Y, Ema H, Okano M, et al: De novo DNA methyltransferase is essential for self-renewal, but not for differentiation, in hematopoietic stem cells. J Exp Med 204(4):715–722, 2007 17420264

Takata A, Ionita-Laza I, Gogos JA, et al: De novo synonymous mutations in regulatory elements contribute to the genetic etiology of autism and schizophrenia. Neuron 89(5):940–947, 2016 26938441

Tamminga CA, Pearlson G, Keshavan M, et al: Bipolar and Schizophrenia Network for Intermediate Phenotypes: outcomes across the psychosis continuum. Schizophr Bull 40 (suppl 2):S131–S137, 2014 24562492

Tandon R, Keshavan MS, Nasrallah HA: Schizophrenia, "just the facts" what we know in 2008, 2: epidemiology and etiology. Schizophr Res 102(1–3):1–18, 2008 18514488

Torrey EF, Miller J, Rawlings R, et al: Seasonality of births in schizophrenia and bipolar disorder: a review of the literature. Schizophr Res 28(1):1–38, 1997 9428062

Tsuang MT: Heterogeneity of schizophrenia. Biol Psychiatry 10(4):465–474, 1975 1100126

Tsuang MT, Faraone SV, Glatt SJ: Schizophrenia: The Facts, 3rd Edition. New York, Oxford University Press, 2011

Ursini G, Cavalleri T, Fazio L, et al: BDNF rs6265 methylation and genotype interact on risk for schizophrenia. Epigenetics 11(1):11–23, 2016 26889735

Valipour G, Saneei P, Esmaillzadeh A: Serum vitamin D levels in relation to schizophrenia: a systematic review and meta-analysis of observational studies. J Clin Endocrinol Metab 99(10):3863–3872, 2014 25050991

van Os J, Rutten BP, Poulton R: Gene-environment interactions in schizophrenia: review of epidemiological findings and future directions. Schizophr Bull 34(6):1066–1082, 2008 18791076

van Winkel R, van Nierop M, Myin-Germeys I, van Os J: Childhood trauma as a cause of psychosis: linking genes, psychology, and biology. Can J Psychiatry 58(1):44–51, 2013 23327756

Veling W, Hoek HW, Mackenbach JP: Perceived discrimination and the risk of schizophrenia in ethnic minorities: a case-control study. Soc Psychiatry Psychiatr Epidemiol 43(12):953–959, 2008 18575790

Viana J, Hannon E, Dempster E, et al: Schizophrenia-associated methylomic variation: molecular signatures of disease and polygenic risk burden across multiple brain regions. Hum Mol Genet 26(1):210–225, 2017 28011714

Wagner JR, Busche S, Ge B, et al: The relationship between DNA methylation, genetic and expression inter-individual variation in untransformed human fibroblasts. Genome Biol 15(2):R37, 2014 24555846

Wang C, Wang L, Ding Y, et al: LncRNA structural characteristics in epigenetic regulation. Int J Mol Sci 18(12):E2659, 2017 29292750

Wicks S, Hjern A, Gunnell D, et al: Social adversity in childhood and the risk of developing psychosis: a national cohort study. Am J Psychiatry 162(9):1652–1657, 2005 16135624

Wohl M, Gorwood P: Paternal ages below or above 35 years old are associated with a different risk of schizophrenia in the offspring. Eur Psychiatry 22(1):22–26, 2007 17142012

Wojtalik JA, Smith MJ, Keshavan MS, et al: A systematic and meta-analytic review of neural correlates of functional outcome in schizophrenia. Schizophr Bull 43(6):1329–1347, 2017 28204755

Yoon JH, Abdelmohsen K, Gorospe M: Posttranscriptional gene regulation by long noncoding RNA. J Mol Biol 425(19):3723–3730, 2013 23178169

Zai CC, Tiwari AK, Zai GC, et al: New findings in pharmacogenetics of schizophrenia. Curr Opin Psychiatry 31(3):200–212, 2018 29528898

Zucchi FC, Yao Y, Ward ID, et al: Maternal stress induces epigenetic signatures of psychiatric and neurological diseases in the offspring. PLoS One 8(2):e56967, 2013 23451123

CHAPTER 6

Pathophysiological Theories

Donald C. Goff, M.D.

An ideal pathophysiological model for schizophrenia would account for diverse findings from epidemiology, clinical observation, and laboratory measures. These sources of data include environmental and genetic risk factors; neurodevelopmental timing of illness onset; anatomical and functional findings across postmortem, neuroimaging, and electrophysiological studies; and clinical presentation, including pharmacological response. Importantly, it is unclear if such a model should attempt to explain schizophrenia as a single, discrete brain disorder or as multiple variants in brain development and function that converge at the level of clinical phenomenology but differ in their etiological pathways.

To address the heterogeneity of the illness—both the array of symptoms (positive, negative, cognitive, affective) within individuals and interindividual variability in presentation—various models have been proposed. One approach is to identify brain structures or circuits that may contribute to specific symptoms and to examine symptom complexes individually in relation to these structures or circuits. In another approach, the diverse effects of individual risk genes or of environmental events that may disrupt brain development can be studied in relation to the full range of symptoms of the illness, because these factors would not be expected to selectively involve single brain structures or circuits. In contrast, the "automobile mechanic" approach, in which a single brain structure is identified as the source of all pathology, is promising only if neurodevelopmental factors or patterns of genetic expression can be identified that would account for such regional selectivity (Forero et al. 2017; Ramsden et al. 2015). In another potential approach to modeling schizophrenia, symptoms may be viewed as reflecting homeostatic mechanisms within molecular networks that maintain equilibrium or that are constrained

I would like to thank Daphne Holt, M.D., Ph.D., Joshua Roffman, M.D., and Diana Perkins, M.D., for their invaluable editorial comments.

TABLE 6–1.   **Elements of pathophysiological models for schizophrenia**

Genetic Factors

    Common variants (small effect)

    Rare variants (larger effect)

Molecular Factors

    Dopamine

    Glutamate

    γ-Aminobutyric acid (GABA)

    Endocannabinoids

Key circuits

    Hippocampal, thalamic, prefrontal cortical, and nigrostriatal pathways

Environmental risk factors

    Inflammation

    Oxidative stress

    Hypoxia

by limitations on energy utilization. A final model posits that neuroplasticity, which is required for memory and adaptation to a changing environment, requires excitatory glutamatergic transmission, which, if excessive, may be excitotoxic. Under conditions of environmental stress and genetic vulnerability, a pathogenic shift in the balance of excitatory versus inhibitory tone may occur during brain development in individuals at risk for schizophrenia. An enduring challenge in constructing theories of pathophysiology is determining whether such abnormalities in brain development or function are primary causal factors or represent compensatory changes within circuits or within molecular networks. In this chapter, several existing models of schizophrenia are reviewed (Table 6–1) and evaluated for the degree to which they account for clinical findings, neurodevelopmental timing, genetics, and laboratory measures.

Genetic Models

Schizophrenia has long been considered to be principally a genetic disease (Table 6–2). Earlier twin studies found monozygotic concordance rates to be approximately 50% versus dizygotic concordance rates of approximately 20%, whereas more rigorous studies have found monozygotic concordance rates as low as 30% (Hilker et al. 2018). Estimates of hereditary risk range from 64% to 80%, with estimates of environmental contributions to risk ranging from 0% to 11% (Hilker et al. 2018; Lichtenstein et al. 2009; Sullivan et al. 2003). Single nucleotide polymorphism–based heritability is estimated at approximately 30%, although the 108 genetic loci that have achieved statistically significant association account for less than 4% of variability in risk (Schizophrenia Working Group of the Psychiatric Genomics Consortium 2014). Genetic loci identified by genome-wide association studies (GWAS) are involved in many biological functions but notably include genes related to dopamine D_2 receptor expression, glutamatergic neurotransmission, plasticity, and immune function (Schizophrenia Working Group of the Psychiatric Genomics Consortium 2014). However, individual loci that have been identified by GWAS

TABLE 6–2.   **Categories and activities of genes associated with schizophrenia**

Findings from studies of genetic variants

Dopamine transmission

Glutamate transmission

Calcium conductance

Pruning (complement activity)

Inflammation

Histone methylation

Activity-regulated cytoskeleton-associated scaffold protein of the postsynaptic density

Targets of fragile X mental retardation protein

Findings from studies of postmortem gene expression

Increased expression

  Genes associated with astrocytes

Decreased expression

  Genes associated with neuronal function

  Genes associated with synaptic function

have a median associated relative risk of only 1.08. Rare copy number variations (CNVs) have been associated with larger risk, but within families that share CNVs, risk is not specific for schizophrenia (Hoeffding et al. 2017; Malhotra and Sebat 2012). The relatively low degree of association that has been found in genetic studies of schizophrenia has been attributed to poor phenotyping, yet the lack of phenotypic specificity associated with CNVs suggests that risk genes may not "breed true" and that efforts at more selective diagnostic phenotypes may be misguided. Single rare disruptive mutations have implicated voltage-gated calcium channels, the activity-regulated cytoskeleton-associated scaffold protein of the postsynaptic density, and targets of fragile X mental retardation protein (FMRP) (Purcell et al. 2014). Additional biological processes implicated by common and rare variants include proteins associated with neurodevelopmental "pruning" and histone methylation. Genes involved in the expression of L-type calcium channels and associated intracellular pathways are strongly implicated in schizophrenia and in several other psychiatric disorders; these receptors have diverse effects on brain development, plasticity, neurogenesis, and regulation of synaptic transmission (Recillas-Morales et al. 2014), suggesting that this category of risk genes may place individuals at risk for psychiatric illness in general, although the specific expression of schizophrenia may require additional genetic or environmental factors. Similarly, FMRP has been linked to multiple neurodevelopmental syndromes; its targets include approximately 30% of the postsynaptic density proteome on neurons, including N-methyl-D-aspartate (NMDA) subunits (Darnell and Klann 2013). MicroRNAs that regulate expression of schizophrenia risk genes have also been implicated (Hauberg et al. 2016).

    Postmortem studies of differential cortical gene expression offer a potentially powerful approach to understanding the relationship between genetic load, environmental and epigenetic effects on gene expression, and brain localization of genetic variants (see lower portion of Table 6–2). Postmortem studies are potentially confounded by lifetime exposure to medication; experiments in animals have demonstrated that antipsychotic medication generally "normalizes" gene expression and therefore would be unlikely to account for many findings (Gandal et al. 2018). In addition, postmortem findings may be impacted by adverse environmental factors associated with the illness, such as cigarette smoking, substance abuse, and poor nutrition. Appropriate control groups can be included to address such factors. For example, in a recent study of differential gene expression in individuals with schizophrenia, autism, depression, bipolar disorder, and alcohol use disorder, compared with healthy control subjects, Gandal and colleagues (2018) found decreased expression of genes related to neuronal function (including mitochondrial energetics) and synaptic function and increased expression of astrocyte-related genes in schizophrenia. Gene expression patterns in schizophrenia were very similar to those in bipolar disorder and autism; however, genes related to microglia did not display differential expression in schizophrenia as they did in autism (Gandal et al. 2018). In addition, analysis of methylation patterns in DNA provides a clue to epigenetic or environmental factors that may influence gene expression, although the correspondence between blood and brain methylation patterns is quite limited (Walton et al. 2016). For example, in a methylome-wide association study of DNA methylation biomarkers in blood, Aberg and colleagues (2014) found 25 methylation sites that differed significantly between subjects with schizophrenia and healthy control subjects, including sites associated with hypoxia and infection.

In summary, schizophrenia is a complex, polygenic disorder that results from interactions between a very large number of common genetic variants of small effect, rare variants of larger effect, and environmental factors. Currently, it is not possible to derive a single coherent molecular model for the illness based on genetic data; identification of rare disruptive mutations with large effect may lead to the recognition of genetic disorders with broad psychiatric phenomenology and very little specificity for schizophrenia. Network analysis may lead to models that predict interactive effects within relevant biological systems, such as neurodevelopment, calcium signaling, or synaptic function, that can define multiple pathways to schizophrenia. Because of a lack of reliable historical developmental data for subjects in genetic studies, the contribution of environmental factors has most likely been underestimated in these models and remains a serious deficit that may in part be remedied by analysis of epigenetic markers.

Strategies to address the relationships between genetic polymorphisms and environment include genetic engineering. Unfortunately, it is not clear that creating genetically engineered mice will help clarify the relative contributions of these factors because schizophrenia is a distinctly human disorder. Induced pluripotent stem cell biology may be a more productive avenue for the experimental manipulation of candidate genes. Fortunately, the correlation between genetic risk factors identified in large samples of patients by GWAS and differential gene expression in postmortem samples is quite high (Gandal et al. 2018), indicating that genetic analysis is a reliable basis upon which to model molecular contributions to circuit dysfunction in schizophrenia.

Molecular Models

Dopamine Models

Of the molecular models for schizophrenia (Table 6–3), the classic model posits excessive dopamine transmission based on the observations that repeated dosing with do-

TABLE 6–3.   **Molecular models for schizophrenia**

Dopamine

Increased striatal postsynaptic dopamine D_2 density (possibly only in high-affinity receptors)

Increased dopamine release in response to amphetamine

Increased presynaptic dopamine synthesis capacity (possibly due to decreased dopamine storage)

Glutamate

Increased sensitivity to N-methyl-D-aspartate (NMDA) receptor blockade

Possible decreased NMDA receptor activity on inhibitory interneurons

Possible increased glutamate transmission/toxicity at postsynaptic non-NMDA glutamate receptors

γ-Aminobutyric acid (GABA)

Decreased inhibitory GABAergic transmission

Compensatory increase in GAD_{67} and postsynaptic GABA receptors

Endocannabinoid

Increased CB_1 receptor density

Possible dysregulation of endocannabinoid regulation of inflammation and oscillatory integrity

Symptoms worsened by CB_1 agonists; possibly improved by cannabidiol

Note. CB_1=cannabinoid receptor type 1; GAD_{67}=glutamic acid decarboxylase 67.

pamine agonists can produce psychosis and that therapeutic potency of antipsychotic drugs highly correlates with antagonist affinity at dopamine D_2 receptors (Carlsson 1978). This model was subsequently modified by proposing a deficit of prefrontal cortical dopamine that contributes to cognitive impairment and negative symptoms and a reciprocal excess of mesolimbic dopamine activity to which are attributed psychotic symptoms (Davis et al. 1991). Postmortem studies are confounded by antipsychotic treatment, but these studies have found increased levels of tyrosine hydroxylase, the rate-limiting enzyme in dopamine synthesis, in the substantia nigra (Howes et al. 2013) and increased dimerization of striatal dopamine receptors (Wang et al. 2010). PET studies employing D_2 receptor antagonist ligands have consistently demonstrated increased ligand displacement at D_2/D_3 receptors in the associative striatum following amphetamine challenge in unmedicated subjects with schizophrenia compared with control subjects, suggesting excessive presynaptic dopamine release (Abi-Dargham et al. 1998). This excessive displacement strongly correlates with response to antipsychotic medication. In contrast, use of a high-affinity D_2/D_3 antagonist PET ligand revealed *decreased* displacement in nonstriatal regions in the prefrontal cortex, hippocampus, and midbrain, following amphetamine administration in subjects with schizophrenia, suggesting decreased dopamine release in other circuits, including mesolimbic pathways (Slifstein et al. 2015). This model was further complicated by results of a recent study in medication-free patients with schizophrenia that used a D_2 receptor agonist PET ligand and failed to find increased striatal displacement following amphetamine administration in subjects with schizophrenia (Frankle et al. 2018). Because dopamine and other D_2 agonists bind selectively to high-affinity D_2 receptors, whereas antagonists bind to both high- and low-affinity receptors, this finding, if replicated, suggests that the abnormality in schizophrenia could be due to an increase in the proportion of postsynaptic high-affinity D_2 receptors rather than an increase in presynaptic dopamine release following administration of amphetamine. Of note, mice that overexpress D_2 receptors in the striatum display cognitive and behavioral deficits and abnormal regulation of midbrain dopamine neuron firing consistent with schizophrenia (Drew et al. 2007; Kellendonk et al. 2006), lending support for this alternative interpretation. In addition, the relevance of amphetamine challenge as a test of dopamine release is unclear; amphetamine elevates synaptic dopamine by reversing the dopamine transporter but has multiple other effects as well, including actions at the trace amino acid receptor 1 (TAAR1). Importantly, Mizrahi and colleagues (Mizrahi et al. 2012; Tseng et al. 2018) used a psychosocial stressor rather than amphetamine challenge and found increased displacement of a D_2/D_3 receptor agonist PET ligand in the associative striatum and in the substantia nigra in medication-free individuals with schizophrenia.

PET studies with [^{18}F]-6-L-fluorodopa (fluorinated L-DOPA), a precursor of dopamine, have demonstrated increased presynaptic L-DOPA uptake in the associative striatum and midbrain in individuals with schizophrenia (McCutcheon et al. 2018), which also predicts response to antipsychotic treatment (Demjaha et al. 2012) and has been interpreted to represent excessive dopamine synthetic capacity. However, the enzyme responsible for uptake of L-DOPA, DOPA decarboxylase, is not a rate-limiting step in dopamine synthesis. In addition, activity of DOPA decarboxylase, which determines the rate of conversion from L-DOPA to dopamine, increases in the context of reduced levels of dopamine, as does activity of tyrosine hydroxylase, which determines the rate of dopamine synthesis (Meiser et al. 2013). Thus, whether increased uptake of [^{18}F]-6-L-fluorodopa represents an increase or decrease in presynaptic dopamine storage remains uncertain (Reith et al. 1994). PET studies in humans implicate nigrostriatal associative rather than limbic pathways, whereas animal models of schizophrenia have focused on regulation of ventral tegmental area (VTA) dopamine neuron firing and activity of mesolimbic pathways. This discrepancy between associative and limbic pathways may in part reflect the substantial difference in rodent versus primate anatomy: the VTA is proportionately much larger in rodents, and the demarcation of these two systems may be less clear in humans (Kesby et al. 2018). The associative striatum, which has been implicated in PET studies in schizophrenia, is defined by connections to frontal and parietal associative cortices and is primarily involved with goal-directed behavior and cognitive flexibility. In contrast, the limbic striatum is associated with reward and motivation. Dopamine release is associated with salience, reward, novelty detection, memory encoding, and attention—all processes that may be dysregulated in schizophrenia. Thus, dopamine may play a role in the pathophysiology of schizophrenia via multiple mechanisms.

Patients' responses to pharmacological treatment are highly variable and may provide clues to the molecular underpinnings of psychotic symptoms. Improvement of psychosis often is delayed for weeks after initiation of D_2 blockers and relapse may be delayed for months after discontinuation, suggesting that psychosis is not merely the consequence of excessive dopamine occupancy of D_2 receptors. One study demonstrated that D_2 blockade triggers complex alterations in gene expression in pathways associated with neuroplasticity and results in greater morphological complexity (Bowling et al. 2014); this evidence suggests that the role dopamine plays in psychosis may involve structural regulation of plasticity, not merely signaling related to novelty or reward.

Glutamate Models

As it became increasingly apparent that the dopamine model did not adequately account for the range of clinical findings and that drugs targeting D_2 receptors did not improve cognitive deficits or negative symptoms, a hypothesized dysregulation of glutamate transmission was added to the dopamine model of schizophrenia (Carlsson and Carlsson 1990; Goff and Coyle 2001). The strongest evidence has come from observations that phencyclidine and ketamine, which block glutamatergic NMDA receptor-gated channels, produce psychotic symptoms, negative symptoms, and memory impairment in healthy individuals, as well as transient psychotic relapse in remitted patients with schizophrenia (Javitt and Zukin 1991; Krystal et al. 1994). Furthermore, glutamate pathways have been implicated in genetic studies, including genes coding for NMDA receptor subunit expression and genes that belong to pathways involved in the phosphorylation and trafficking of NMDA receptors. In addition, anti-NMDA antibodies have been linked to schizophrenia, although the specificity is low and the phenotype usually includes neurological impairment (Kayser et al. 2013).

A prominent glutamatergic model for schizophrenia posits that hypofunction of NMDA receptors on inhibitory interneurons results in a deficit of inhibitory drive, excessive activation of non-NMDA glutamatergic receptors, and disruption of oscillatory synchrony (Cohen et al. 2015; Lisman et al. 2008). However, it is not clear that the putative deficit in NMDA receptor function in schizophrenia or the psychotomimetic effect of ketamine is limited to NMDA receptors on inhibitory interneurons. It has been shown that the experimental ablation of NMDA receptors on inhibitory interneurons in mice only produces behavioral effects if performed before adolescence (Belforte et al. 2010)—suggesting that a deficit in NMDA receptor function may have greater relevance to schizophrenia via its impact on neurodevelopment than on brain function in adulthood. In addition, NMDA receptors modulate midbrain dopamine neuron firing and ketamine increases striatal dopamine in response to amphetamine in healthy subjects (Kegeles et al. 2000), thus mimicking findings of dysregulated dopamine release in schizophrenia. However, effects of ketamine administration on dopamine concentrations in the absence of amphetamine challenge have been less consistent with patterns observed in schizophrenia (Rabiner 2007); for example, ketamine increases dopamine release in prefrontal cortex, not in the striatum (Verma and Moghaddam 1996). In genetically engineered mice, a reduction in NMDA receptors on GABAergic neurons early in development produced a pattern of increased dopamine release in response to amphetamine in nucleus accumbens and decreased release in prefrontal cortex (Nakao et al. 2019), suggesting that neurodevelopmental effects on inhibitory neuron function could account for the pattern of dopamine dysregulation in schizophrenia.

An important potential link between hypofunction of NMDA receptors, stress, and inflammation is kynurenic acid, a tryptophan metabolite that is synthesized in astrocytes and acts as an antagonist at NMDA and nicotinic muscarinic receptors while also modulating GABAergic and dopaminergic activity (Flores-Barrera et al. 2017; Schwarcz and Stone 2017). Kynurenic acid concentrations have been reported to be elevated in cerebrospinal fluid (CSF) and cortex in individuals with schizophrenia (Linderholm et al. 2012; Schwarcz et al. 2001). Despite strong evidence that disruption of NMDA receptor transmission produces cognitive, psychotic, and negative symptoms of schizophrenia, pharmacological interventions aimed at enhancing NMDA receptor function or reducing excessive glutamate activity at non-NMDA receptors have not produced consistent benefit in large replication trials (Goff 2015), and the predictive value of ketamine challenge for identifying therapeutic agents in schizophrenia remains unclear.

γ-Aminobutyric Acid Models

A third prominent molecular model for schizophrenia posits a deficit in GABAergic inhibitory transmission. Postmortem studies have reported decreased densities of cortical parvalbumin-positive and somatostatin-positive GABAergic inhibitory neurons (Lewis et al. 2012), decreased concentrations of γ-aminobutyric acid (GABA) (Kutay et al. 1989), and decreased concentrations of glutamic acid decarboxylase 67 (GAD_{67}), a key enzyme in the synthesis of GABA (Akbarian and Huang 2006). Decreased concentrations of GABA in CSF of subjects with schizophrenia were found to correlate inversely with symptoms (Orhan et al. 2018). Measurement of cortical GABA concentrations by proton magnetic resonance spectroscopy in subjects with schizophrenia has not produced consistent findings (Taylor and Tso 2015). However, administration of the GABA transport blocker tiagabine was associated with lower elevation of GABA concentrations measured by PET in medial temporal lobe of subjects with schizophrenia compared with healthy control subjects; GABA levels were inversely associated with psychotic symptoms in subjects with schizophrenia and were inversely associated with gamma-band oscillation power in healthy control subjects (Frankle et al. 2015). Earlier models hypothesized that the deficiency in parvalbumin-containing inhibitory interneurons was primary and reflected genetic and environmental factors early in the neurodevelopment of inhibitory interneurons (Volk and Lewis 2014). This deficit has been viewed as a driving factor responsible for early psychosis, particularly in the resulting hyperactivity of key hippocampal circuits (Schobel et al. 2009). However, more recent models have attributed diminished GABAergic transmission as secondary to a deficit in neurotrophic factors or NMDA receptor activation and, most recently, as a compensatory response to reduced excitatory inputs to inhibitory interneurons (Chung et al. 2016). A reduction in GABAergic transmission in hippocampus has also been linked to anxiety and depressive disorders (Möhler 2012) and can be reproduced in animal models by social isolation and other stressors, raising questions about the specificity of reduced GABA for schizophrenia and its status as a primary or compensatory effect (Filipović et al. 2018). Despite the strength of evidence linking reduced GABAergic transmission to schizophrenia, therapeutic targeting of GABAergic receptors has not produced consistent results (Miyamoto et al. 2012).

Endocannabinoid Models

A recent addition to molecular models of schizophrenia is centered on the endocannabinoid system, composed of cannabinoid receptors type 1 and 2 (CB_1 and CB_2) and the endogenous ligands 2-arachidonoylglycerol (2-AG) and anandamide. Broadly speaking, the endocannabinoid system mediates response to environmental stress by modulating homeostatic stress response circuits in the brain; it is involved in inflammation, neuroprotection, pain perception, and oscillatory synchronization. In particular, the endogenous endocannabinoid anandamide is elevated in response to stress and—via activity at multiple receptors, including CB_1, CB_2, G protein-coupled receptor 55 (GPR55), and transient receptor potential vanilloid 1 (TRPV1)—exerts stabilizing effects on inhibitory and excitatory transmission and inflammatory response (Ruggiero et al. 2017). CSF anandamide levels were found to be elevated 10-fold in first-episode psychosis patients who were not cannabis users, whereas CSF anandamide levels were not elevated in first-episode psychosis patients who used cannabis (Leweke et al. 2007). Because CSF anandamide levels were inversely associated with symptom severity, these findings suggest that anandamide may be part of an endogenous homeostatic mechanism that counters psychosis—a mechanism that is impaired by heavy cannabis use. Cannabidiol (CBD), a constituent of cannabis that does not activate CB_1 receptors, elevates anandamide levels by inhibiting fatty acid amide hydrolase, which metabolizes anandamide; the increase in anandamide concentrations with CBD treatment correlated with antipsychotic response (Leweke et al. 2012). Hence, CBD may attenuate psychotic symptoms by activating, via anandamide, an endogenous system that protects against stress. CBD has demonstrated antipsychotic efficacy in two randomized controlled trials (Leweke et al. 2012; McGuire et al. 2018). Whereas CBD may have antipsychotic properties, excessive activation of CB_1 receptors by synthetic cannabinoids (CB_1 agonists) or, in the laboratory, by infusion of the CB_1 partial agonist tetrahydrocannabinol (THC) produces psychotic symptoms, apathy, and cognitive impairment (Ruggiero et al. 2017). Heavy cannabis use has been associated with a higher risk for developing schizophrenia and earlier onset; persistent use of cannabis after onset of illness is associated with poorer outcomes (Manseau and Goff 2015). However, because both schizophrenia and heavy cannabis use may have risk genes in common, the degree to which the association represents a causal relationship remains unclear (Sherva et al. 2016).

Summary

It is clear that manipulation of dopamine, glutamate, and cannabinoid transmission can mimic symptoms of schizophrenia, and evidence is compelling for dysregulation of each of these transmitter systems, plus GABA, in schizophrenia. It is likely that in some individuals, highly selective disruption of just one of these molecular pathways is responsible for the illness, resulting from a rare mutation or from autoantibodies targeting a specific receptor. However, these neurotransmitters are all tightly interactive in homeostatic networks and are highly regulated in response to inflammation, hypoxia, or other environmental stressors, suggesting that the larger molecular network may be disrupted during development or during the vulnerable period of young adulthood as a result of multiple and additive genetic or environmental insults that result in dysregulation. This makes it difficult to determine whether abnormalities in biomarkers for these molecular pathways are primary or compensatory, although emergence of data from GWAS implicating some of these systems supports a more causal role.

Circuit Models

Several circuit models have been proposed to account for positive, negative, and cognitive symptoms in schizophrenia (Table 6–4). Key structures include temporal lobe (hippocampus and entorhinal cortex), midbrain dopamine neurons (substantia nigra and VTA), striatum (associative striatum and nucleus accumbens), thalamus, and frontal cortex. Because the hippocampus and thalamus are particularly vulnerable to early environmental stress and display prominent volume loss early in the course of illness, these two structures have been implicated as potential early drivers of psychosis. Hyperactivity in the hippocampal cornu ammonis subfield CA1 is a consistent finding in ultrahigh-risk (prodromal) and first-episode psychosis patients and is thought to reflect a deficit of inhibitory input and excessive glutamatergic transmission (Kraguljac et al. 2013; Schobel et al. 2013). Through a polysynaptic connection via the nucleus accumbens and ventral pallidum, heightened hippocampal output may dysregulate midbrain dopamine neuron firing (Grace and Gomes 2019). Excessive dopamine release from midbrain dopamine neurons in turn produces thalamic burst firing; the nucleus reuniens of the thalamus excites the CA1 subfield of the hippocampus, thereby producing a potential positive feedback loop (Lisman et al. 2010). Recent research has advanced the understanding of a thalamic role in attention and coordination of cortical processing of information relevant to schizophrenia pathology (Krol et al. 2018). The thalamic reticular nucleus (TRN) in particular has been linked to schizophrenia by risk genes that are differentially expressed in the TRN (Krol et al. 2018). In addition, the TRN plays a role in propagating sleep spindles and in modulating attention and sensory information processing. A deficit in sleep spindles has been one of the most compelling biomarker findings in schizophrenia and has been associated with psychotic symptoms (Ferrarelli et al. 2010; Wamsley et al. 2012). Individuals with schizophrenia also display deficits in local oscillatory activity, including generation of gamma and theta rhythms, and in long-range synchronization of oscillatory activity as measured by functional magnetic resonance imaging (fMRI) blood-oxygen-level-dependent (BOLD) signal covariance (Spellman and Gordon 2015). Deficits in synchronization of hippocampal theta and frontal cortical gamma rhythms have also been found in animal models of schizophrenia, indicating impaired communication between the two structures (Spellman and Gordon 2015). Disruptions of connectivity may reflect several mechanisms, including deficits in the balance of GABAergic inhibitory neurons and NMDA-mediated signaling, or loss of white matter integrity (Zeng et al. 2016), possibly due to impaired functioning of oligodendrocytes, or may reflect deficits in thalamic synchronization of cortical activation (Hwang et al. 2017).

Circuit Models for Psychosis

Positive symptoms are, by historical convention, the primary symptom complex that defines schizophrenia, and this complex is the only feature that is present in all individuals with this diagnosis. Key components thought to contribute to the formation and persistence of delusions include 1) abnormal salience, in which benign experiences or thoughts are associated with inappropriate affective valence (Kapur 2003); 2) errors in the processing of sensory input in which false representations of reality are incorporated into an individual's "schema"; and 3) an impairment in the system that monitors for a lack of correspondence between experience and expectations, known as "prediction error." In healthy individuals, the incongruity between a false belief or expectation and actual experience triggers a prediction error signal that results in the modification of the belief, thus preventing the establishment of delusions (Coltheart 2010). In addition to identifying ideas that do not comport with reality, prediction er-

TABLE 6–4.	Circuit models for schizophrenia

Psychosis

Abnormal salience

   Midbrain dopamine release, locus coeruleus, hippocampus

Memory/schema formation

   Hippocampal dentate gyrus and CA2/3 (pattern separation and completion)

   Prefrontal cortex (schematic representation of reality)

Prediction error

   Hippocampal CA1, anterior cingulate, ventromedial prefrontal cortex, thalamic dorsal medial nucleus

Negative symptoms

Reward anticipation and response

   Midbrain dopamine neurons, striatum

Computation of effort

   Midbrain dopamine neurons, anterior cingulate

Value representations

   Prefrontal cortex

Cognitive impairment

Long-term potentiation, inhibitory/excitatory balance, connectivity/synchronization

ror detection may also allow an individual to identify self-generated thoughts or sensations via corollary discharge (Crapse and Sommer 2008), a process mediated by transthalamic corticocortical circuits (Sherman 2016). In the case of an inappropriate prediction error signal (Shergill et al. 2005), internally generated thoughts may be interpreted as externally generated voices (hallucinations) or interpreted as the delusional experience of external control. Hippocampal circuits involved in pattern separation (dentate gyrus) and pattern completion (CA2/3 subfields) contribute to the initial processing of sensory input in which experience is categorized and linked to associated memories, and partial memories are completed based on past experience. It has been shown experimentally that disruption of this process can produce false memories (Ramirez et al. 2013) and that individuals with schizophrenia have significant and selective impairment in pattern separation (Das et al. 2014). The dentate gyrus is also involved in the association of mnemonic information with affective valence, which may account for the common linking of abnormal salience to delusions (Redondo et al. 2014).

Midbrain dopamine release provides a scalar signal to striatum and other structures regarding anticipated reward or punishment (Kempadoo et al. 2016), and in response to novelty or reward, dopamine release is associated with affective salience and enhanced memory encoding via activation of dopamine D_1 receptors, which facilitate hippocampal long-term potentiation. Studies have demonstrated that the locus coeruleus provides dopamine to the dorsal hippocampus (Kempadoo et al. 2016) and that locus coeruleus dopamine input to the hippocampal CA3 subfield is necessary for encoding of persistent memory in response to novelty (Wagatsuma et al. 2018). The detection of prediction error is attributed primarily to a "belief evaluation" function of the prefrontal cortex (Coltheart 2010; Corlett et al. 2010). Extinction generates a prediction error signal because expectation of an electric shock based on prior conditioning is not realized; a failure to activate the ventromedial prefrontal cortex in response to delayed extinction learning has been associated with delusions (Holt et al. 2009, 2012). However, many structures contribute to the identification of prediction error (Sheth et al. 2012), including the hippocampal CA1 subfield (Duncan et al. 2012) and anterior cingulate cortex (Sheth et al. 2012). Using "lesion network mapping," Darby and colleagues (2017) found that brain regions functionally connected to the right frontal cortex were associated with delusions, reflecting this region's role in detecting "expectation violation," whereas delusions associated with misidentification (Capgras syndrome) were associated with regions functionally connected to both the right frontal cortex and the left retrosplenial cortex, which detects "familiarity." Studies of brain lesions resulting from stroke that are associated with delusions have pointed toward the right inferior frontal gyrus, posterior temporoparietal region, and thalamus (Joyce 2018), whereas temporal lobe epilepsy remains a classic model for delusions, hallucinations, and negative symptoms (Nadkarni et al. 2007).

Circuit Models for Negative Symptoms

Negative symptoms, which consist of deficits in affective expression and in motivated behavior, are not present in all individuals with schizophrenia, nor are they restricted to schizophrenia, because they occur in other psychiatric and neurological disorders (Strauss and Cohen 2017). Although individuals with schizophrenia usually report hedonic pleasure in response to pleasurable activities, they often do not initiate action necessary to obtain rewarding experiences, possibly due to deficits in the recall of past hedonic experiences, deficits in learning from rewarding experiences, and a deficit in judging the necessary effort required to obtain reward (Strauss et al. 2014). Circuits that have been implicated in negative symptoms include dopaminergic transmission in the striatum that mediates reward anticipation and response, anterior cingulate and midbrain dopamine neurons involved in computation of effort requirements to obtain reward, prefrontal cortical circuits involved in updating and maintaining value representations, and prefrontal circuits that generate exploratory behavior in anticipation of uncertain reward (Strauss et al. 2014; Walton et al. 2018).

Circuit Models for Cognitive Deficits

Cognitive deficits in schizophrenia involve essentially all cognitive domains; this lack of selectivity suggests a diffuse brain process rather than pointing toward specific brain regions or circuits. The diffuse pattern of cognitive deficits exhibited by most individuals with the diagnosis of schizophrenia points to systemic involvement at the cellular, synaptic, microcircuit, or macrocircuit level. Potential mechanisms underlying these deficits are legion and in general terms include dysregulation of neuroplasticity including intracellular calcium conduction pathways, dysregulation of glutamatergic NMDA and L-type calcium channels, dysregulation of synaptic transmission, impaired long-term potentiation, and impaired memory consolidation via dysfunction in dendritic sprouting. Defects in connectivity may also play a role in cognitive inefficiency and may result from loss of white matter integrity and from disruption of oscillatory synchrony. Increasingly, dysfunction of thalamic regulation of cortical processing and memory consolidation has been proposed as playing a major role in attentional and memory impairments (Krol et al. 2018).

Summary

Just as establishing genetic profiles may provide insight into the multiple molecular pathways contributing to schizophrenia, delineation of circuit dysregulation may also provide clues to both molecular and neurodevelopmental factors that differ between individuals and hence may in part explain heterogeneity of symptom expression and of treatment response. Current evidence from postmortem studies suggests deficits at the level of microcircuits, whereas imaging has identified deficits in connectivity between brain regions, although the biological mechanisms responsible for patterns of covariance in fMRI BOLD signal are not clear. As tools from basic neuroscience characterize these circuit deficits and new therapeutic methods evolve that can be applied to patients, targeted treatment may follow, including manipulation at the level of both microcircuit and macrocircuit. For example, it may be possible in the future to develop techniques derived from basic laboratory science, including optogenetics, designer receptor activated by a designer drug (DREADD), and stem cell implantation. In addition, neuromodulatory devices utilizing magnetic, electrical, or ultrasound energy may allow greater precision in localization and, with closed-loop modulation of stimulation, may be able to specifically modulate dysregulated circuits.

Environmental and Developmental Risk Factors

Large variations, as great as fivefold, in the lifetime prevalence of schizophrenia between geographical regions and between demographic subgroups have been observed, suggestive of environmental risk factors (McGrath et al. 2008). Although the validity of some of the evidence is debated (Radua et al. 2018), environmental stressors during early neurodevelopment, childhood, and adolescence have been linked to schizophrenia (Table 6–5). Early in brain development—in utero—environmental stressors include maternal stress (Khashan et al. 2008), infections (Khandaker et al. 2013), and dietary deficiency (Brown and Susser 2005; Xu et al. 2009), as well as complications during labor and delivery (Brown 2011). Stressors in childhood and adolescence include psychological adversity (Varese et al. 2012), infections (Brown et al. 2004), immigrant status (Cantor-Graae and Pedersen 2007), and heavy cannabis use (Manseau and Goff 2015). In addition, paternal age has been associated with risk (Malaspina et al. 2001), possibly due to an increased incidence of spontaneous mutation. In support of the potential role of early environmental factors, disruption of brain development in animal models by maternal immune activation in utero, which releases maternal inflammatory cytokines during fetal brain development to mimic a viral infection (Knuesel et al. 2014), has been shown to decrease parvalbumin-expressing hippocampal inhibitory interneurons, increase hippocampal activity, increase striatal dopamine concentrations, disrupt white matter integrity, and disrupt synchrony between hippocampus and medial prefrontal cortex (Dickerson et al. 2010). Disruption of early brain development by administration of the toxin methylazoxymethanol acetate (Moore et al. 2006) or by ventral hippocampal lesions (Tseng et al. 2009) also produces deficits consistent with schizophrenia. Many environmental risk factors share activation of inflammatory and oxidative stress pathways, which are both closely linked to glutamatergic NMDA receptor function (Goff et al. 2016; Steullet et al. 2016). Results from GWAS have implicated an inflammatory component based on genes that play a role in inflammatory response (Carter 2009); for example, the major histocompatibility complex, which modulates several aspects of immune response, has been strongly linked to schizophrenia (Corvin and Morris 2014). Effects of inflammation during pregnancy appear to be mediated by the maternal inflammatory cytokine interleukin 6, which may activate microglia, stimulate release of free radicals, and disrupt inhibitory interneuron function and glutamatergic NMDA receptor signaling (Goff et al. 2016). Of note, risk genes that are linked to inflammation, oxidative stress, and cellular response to hypoxia are selectively expressed in the placenta and are more prevalent in cases of schizophrenia associated with environmental stress early in development (Ursini et al. 2018). Unlike autism, risk genes for schizophrenia are not preferentially expressed in the fetal brain (Birnbaum et al. 2014).

Early in development, NMDA receptor subunit composition favors increased transmission, which promotes formation of synapses while also increasing risk of excitotoxicity (Goff 2017). As neurodevelopment proceeds, the subunit composition of NMDA receptors changes, while the input from inhibitory interneurons increases to establish an optimal level of neuroplasticity and synchronization. Excessive inflammation and oxidative stress may disrupt this fine-tuning of microcircuits, resulting in deficient plasticity and desynchronization of theta and gamma oscillations. The increase in kynurenic acid in response to inflammation is one example of a compensatory decrease in NMDA transmission that may impair NMDA-mediated plasticity during brain development in order to protect against excitotoxicity. The relationship between inflammation, oxidative stress, and maintenance of excitatory versus inhibitory balance is also impacted by the cannabinoid system, which may account for the increased risk associated with heavy cannabis use in adolescence (Large et al. 2011). Whereas inflammation and oxidative stress may disrupt neuronal migration, synapse formation, inhibitory interneuron function, and oligodendrocyte function early in development, during adolescence and early adulthood, these factors may contribute to loss of gray matter and loss of white matter integrity. Early studies found increased microglial activation in schizophrenia, but recent studies have produced results consistent with decreased microglial activation in medication-naïve patients, raising the question of whether inflammation is primarily relevant during early neurodevelopment rather than at onset of illness (Plavén-Sigray et al. 2018). In addition, a recent study found that markers of inflammation and oxidative stress interacted with duration of untreated psychosis to predict hippocampal atrophy in first-episode psychosis, but levels of these biomarkers did not differ between patients and healthy control subjects (Goff et al. 2018), suggesting that individuals with the illness may differ in their vulnerability to oxidative stress and inflammation.

Cognitive decline may be an important characteristic defining developmental pathways to schizophrenia. Increasingly, studies have found differences in brain structure between individuals who appear to have deteriorated in cognitive functioning and individuals who are relatively cognitively intact or who appear to have been impaired from early in life (Keefe and Kahn 2017). The timing of this decline in cognitive functioning is not fully established—in most cases it precedes onset of psychotic symptoms, although a late-life decline has been noted in some studies (Kotov et al. 2017; Meier et al. 2014). Most evidence suggests a decline during adolescence, although evidence for earlier decline has also been reported. Gray matter loss, particularly in temporal lobe, prefrontal cortex, and thalamus, has been identified early in

TABLE 6–5.   **Environmental risk factors for schizophrenia**

Perinatal period
  Inflammation
  Maternal stress
  Malnutrition (folate deficiency)
  Complications during labor and delivery (hypoxia)
  Paternal age
Early childhood
  Stress/trauma/emigration
  Inflammation
Adolescence/young adulthood
  Cannabis use
  Psychosocial stressors

the course of illness and correlates with cognitive deficits and negative symptoms, whereas loss of white matter integrity may be more pronounced later in the course of illness (Cropley et al. 2017; Goff et al. 2018; Kotov et al. 2017; van Haren et al. 2011; Zeng et al. 2016). Whether changes in gray and white matter over time reflect a neurodegenerative progression of illness or medication effects remains the subject of debate (Goff et al. 2017).

An explanation for the developmental timing of psychosis onset remains unclear despite considerable research. Diffuse impairment of cognition usually is already present when psychosis (hallucinations and delusions) emerges, either abruptly in an initial full psychotic episode or as attenuated or intermittent psychosis in individuals who first enter a prodromal stage. Although hallucinations may be continuously experienced, delusions tend to consist of a single cognitive event in which a false schema is formed—subsequent experience is interpreted in terms of this single persistent false premise. Other aspects of delusional cognitive processing, such as paranoia or self-referential thinking (in which benign and unrelated phenomena are perceived as causally linked and as having special personal meaning), may also occur continuously. Onset of psychosis may be triggered by stress—particularly by the loss of one's social network—or by use of cannabis or other substances. From a neurodevelopmental perspective, onset of psychosis generally occurs years after the hormonal transitions of puberty and during a period in which myelination and synaptic pruning, which enhance the efficiency and distribution of cognitive functioning, are approaching completion.

Conclusion

No simple, comprehensive theory adequately integrates the many molecular, circuit-based, and epidemiological models for schizophrenia. At the level of molecular factors influencing microcircuit function, several themes emerge. One is the involvement of genes that modify components of neuronal signaling, including receptors and intracellular pathways associated with glutamatergic transmission and calcium transport. These systems fine-tune the delicate balance between excitation and inhibition and between potentially excitotoxic components of long-term potentiation and synchronization necessary for plasticity and connectivity versus components that protect against inflammation and oxidative stress that may limit plasticity in the developing brain. In addition, deficits in energetics involving mitochondrial function and cell metabolism may also contribute to dysfunction in the fine-tuning of microcircuits, particularly given the energy requirements of rapidly firing inhibitory interneurons. These deficits may represent a vulnerability to psychiatric illness or to cognitive deficits; the specific involvement of circuits involved in positive or negative symptoms may reflect a convergence of multiple factors, including the specific vulnerability of structures (e.g., the hippocampus, thalamus) to environmental injury and the neurodevelopmental stage during which disruption occurred. Currently, we are unable to differentiate between primary etiological factors and compensatory alterations in many clinical biomarkers, and the contribution of early environmental stressors remains poorly characterized, leaving us primarily with genetic risk factors. It is an appealing theory that most genetic risk factors are of small effect and relatively nonspecific and may primarily represent vulnerability to neurodevelopmental insults that depend on timing to determine the specific cell types and structures that are compromised. However, the vast amount of molecular, epidemiological, structural, and functional data must be analyzed without the assumption that schizophrenia is a single illness but rather with the assumption that multiple layers of interactive factors may additively affect circuits in patterns that we choose to call schizophrenia.

References

Aberg KA, McClay JL, Nerella S, et al: Methylome-wide association study of schizophrenia: identifying blood biomarker signatures of environmental insults. JAMA Psychiatry 71(3):255–264, 2014 24402055

Abi-Dargham A, Gil R, Krystal J, et al: Increased striatal dopamine transmission in schizophrenia: confirmation in a second cohort. Am J Psychiatry 155(6):761–767, 1998 9619147

Akbarian S, Huang HS: Molecular and cellular mechanisms of altered GAD1/GAD67 expression in schizophrenia and related disorders. Brain Res Brain Res Rev 52(2):293–304, 2006 16759710

Belforte JE, Zsiros V, Sklar ER, et al: Postnatal NMDA receptor ablation in corticolimbic interneurons confers schizophrenia-like phenotypes. Nat Neurosci 13(1):76–83, 2010 19915563

Birnbaum R, Jaffe AE, Hyde TM, et al: Prenatal expression patterns of genes associated with neuropsychiatric disorders. Am J Psychiatry 171(7):758–767, 2014 24874100

Bowling H, Zhang G, Bhattacharya A, et al: Antipsychotics activate mTORC1-dependent translation to enhance neuronal morphological complexity. Sci Signal 7(308):ra4, 2014 24425786

Brown AS: The environment and susceptibility to schizophrenia. Prog Neurobiol 93(1):23–58, 2011 20955757

Brown AS, Susser ES: Homocysteine and schizophrenia: from prenatal to adult life. Prog Neuropsychopharmacol Biol Psychiatry 29(7):1175–1180, 2005 16143442

Brown AS, Begg MD, Gravenstein S, et al: Serologic evidence of prenatal influenza in the etiology of schizophrenia. Arch Gen Psychiatry 61(8):774–780, 2004 15289276

Cantor-Graae E, Pedersen CB: Risk of schizophrenia in second-generation immigrants: a Danish population-based cohort study. Psychol Med 37(4):485–494, 2007 17202000

Carlsson A: Antipsychotic drugs, neurotransmitters, and schizophrenia. Am J Psychiatry 135(2):165–173, 1978 23684

Carlsson M, Carlsson A: Interactions between glutamatergic and monoaminergic systems within the basal ganglia—implications for schizophrenia and Parkinson's disease. Trends Neurosci 13(7):272–276, 1990 1695402

Carter CJ: Schizophrenia susceptibility genes directly implicated in the life cycles of pathogens: cytomegalovirus, influenza, herpes simplex, rubella, and Toxoplasma gondii. Schizophr Bull 35(6):1163–1182, 2009 18552348

Chung DW, Fish KN, Lewis DA: Pathological basis for deficient excitatory drive to cortical parvalbumin interneurons in schizophrenia. Am J Psychiatry 173(11):1131–1139, 2016 27444795

Cohen SM, Tsien RW, Goff DC, et al: The impact of NMDA receptor hypofunction on GABAergic neurons in the pathophysiology of schizophrenia. Schizophr Res 167(1–3):98–107, 2015 25583246

Coltheart M: The neuropsychology of delusions. Ann NY Acad Sci 1191:16–26, 2010 20392273

Corlett PR, Taylor JR, Wang XJ, et al: Toward a neurobiology of delusions. Prog Neurobiol 92(3):345–369, 2010 20558235

Corvin A, Morris DW: Genome-wide association studies: findings at the major histocompatibility complex locus in psychosis. Biol Psychiatry 75(4):276–283, 2014 24199664

Crapse TB, Sommer MA: Corollary discharge across the animal kingdom. Nat Rev Neurosci 9(8):587–600, 2008 18641666

Cropley VL, Klauser P, Lenroot RK, et al: Accelerated gray and white matter deterioration with age in schizophrenia. Am J Psychiatry 174(3):286–295, 2017 27919183

Darby RR, Laganiere S, Pascual-Leone A, et al: Finding the imposter: brain connectivity of lesions causing delusional misidentifications. Brain 140(2):497–507, 2017 28082298

Darnell JC, Klann E: The translation of translational control by FMRP: therapeutic targets for FXS. Nat Neurosci 16(11):1530–1536, 2013 23584741

Das T, Ivleva EI, Wagner AD, et al: Loss of pattern separation performance in schizophrenia suggests dentate gyrus dysfunction. Schizophr Res 159(1):193–197, 2014 25176349

Davis KL, Kahn RS, Ko G, et al: Dopamine in schizophrenia: a review and reconceptualization. Am J Psychiatry 148(11):1474–1486, 1991 1681750

Demjaha A, Murray RM, McGuire PK, et al: Dopamine synthesis capacity in patients with treatment-resistant schizophrenia. Am J Psychiatry 169(11):1203–1210, 2012 23034655

Dickerson DD, Wolff AR, Bilkey DK: Abnormal long-range neural synchrony in a maternal immune activation animal model of schizophrenia. J Neurosci 30(37):12424–12431, 2010 20844137

Drew MR, Simpson EH, Kellendonk C, et al: Transient overexpression of striatal D2 receptors impairs operant motivation and interval timing. J Neurosci 27(29):7731–7739, 2007 17634367

Duncan K, Ketz N, Inati SJ, et al: Evidence for area CA1 as a match/mismatch detector: a high-resolution fMRI study of the human hippocampus. Hippocampus 22(3):389–398, 2012 21484934

Ferrarelli F, Peterson MJ, Sarasso S, et al: Thalamic dysfunction in schizophrenia suggested by whole-night deficits in slow and fast spindles. Am J Psychiatry 167(11):1339–1348, 2010 20843876

Filipović D, Stanisavljević A, Jasnić N, et al: Chronic treatment with fluoxetine or clozapine of socially isolated rats prevents subsector-specific reduction of parvalbumin immunoreactive cells in the hippocampus. Neuroscience 371:384–394, 2018 29275206

Flores-Barrera E, Thomases DR, Cass DK, et al: Preferential disruption of prefrontal GABAergic function by nanomolar concentrations of the α7nACh negative modulator kynurenic acid. J Neurosci 37(33):7921–7929, 2017 28729445

Forero DA, Guio-Vega GP, González-Giraldo Y: A comprehensive regional analysis of genome-wide expression profiles for major depressive disorder. J Affect Disord 218:86–92, 2017 28460316

Frankle WG, Cho RY, Prasad KM, et al: In vivo measurement of GABA transmission in healthy subjects and schizophrenia patients. Am J Psychiatry 172(11):1148–1159, 2015 26133962

Frankle WG, Paris J, Himes M, et al: Amphetamine-induced striatal dopamine release measured with an agonist radiotracer in schizophrenia. Biol Psychiatry 83(8):707–714, 2018 29325847

Gandal MJ, Haney JR, Parikshak NN, et al; CommonMind Consortium; PsychENCODE Consortium; iPSYCH-BROAD Working Group: Shared molecular neuropathology across major psychiatric disorders parallels polygenic overlap. Science 359(6376):693–697, 2018 29439242

Goff DC: Drug development in schizophrenia: are glutamatergic targets still worth aiming at? Curr Opin Psychiatry 28(3):207–215, 2015 25710242

Goff DC: D-cycloserine in schizophrenia: new strategies for improving clinical outcomes by enhancing plasticity. Curr Neuropharmacol 15(1):21–34, 2017 26915421

Goff DC, Coyle JT: The emerging role of glutamate in the pathophysiology and treatment of schizophrenia. Am J Psychiatry 158(9):1367–1377, 2001 11532718

Goff DC, Romero K, Paul J, et al: Biomarkers for drug development in early psychosis: current issues and promising directions. Eur Neuropsychopharmacol 26(6):923–937, 2016 27005595

Goff DC, Falkai P, Fleischhacker WW, et al: The long-term effects of antipsychotic medication on clinical course in schizophrenia. Am J Psychiatry 174(9):840–849, 2017 28472900

Goff DC, Zeng B, Ardekani BA, et al: Association of hippocampal atrophy with duration of untreated psychosis and molecular biomarkers during initial antipsychotic treatment of first-episode psychosis. JAMA Psychiatry 75(4):370–378, 2018 29466532

Grace AA, Gomes FV: The circuitry of dopamine system regulation and its disruption in schizophrenia: insights into treatment and prevention. Schizophr Bull 45(1):148–157, 2019 29385549

Hauberg ME, Roussos P, Grove J, et al; Schizophrenia Working Group of the Psychiatric Genomics Consortium: Analyzing the role of microRNAs in schizophrenia in the context of common genetic risk variants. JAMA Psychiatry 73(4):369–377, 2016 26963595

Hilker R, Helenius D, Fagerlund B, et al: Heritability of schizophrenia and schizophrenia spectrum based on the nationwide Danish Twin Register. Biol Psychiatry 83(6):492–498, 2018 28987712

Hoeffding LK, Trabjerg BB, Olsen L, et al: Risk of psychiatric disorders among individuals with the 22q11.2 deletion or duplication: a Danish nationwide, register-based study. JAMA Psychiatry 74(3):282–290, 2017 28114601

Holt DJ, Lebron-Milad K, Milad MR, et al: Extinction memory is impaired in schizophrenia. Biol Psychiatry 65(6):455–463, 2009 18986648

Holt DJ, Coombs G, Zeidan MA, et al: Failure of neural responses to safety cues in schizophrenia. Arch Gen Psychiatry 69(9):893–903, 2012 22945619

Howes OD, Williams M, Ibrahim K, et al: Midbrain dopamine function in schizophrenia and depression: a post-mortem and positron emission tomographic imaging study. Brain 136 (Pt 11):3242–3251, 2013 24097339

Hwang K, Bertolero MA, Liu WB, et al: The human thalamus is an integrative hub for functional brain networks. J Neurosci 37(23):5594–5607, 2017 28450543

Javitt DC, Zukin SR: Recent advances in the phencyclidine model of schizophrenia. Am J Psychiatry 148(10):1301–1308, 1991 1654746

Joyce EM: Organic psychosis: the pathobiology and treatment of delusions. CNS Neurosci Ther 24(7):598–603, 2018 29766653

Kapur S: Psychosis as a state of aberrant salience: a framework linking biology, phenomenology, and pharmacology in schizophrenia. Am J Psychiatry 160(1):13–23, 2003 12505794

Kayser MS, Titulaer MJ, Gresa-Arribas N, et al: Frequency and characteristics of isolated psychiatric episodes in anti-N-methyl-d-aspartate receptor encephalitis. JAMA Neurol 70(9):1133–1139, 2013 23877059

Keefe RSE, Kahn RS: Cognitive decline and disrupted cognitive trajectory in schizophrenia. JAMA Psychiatry 74(5):535–536, 2017 28329400

Kegeles LS, Abi-Dargham A, Zea-Ponce Y, et al: Modulation of amphetamine-induced striatal dopamine release by ketamine in humans: implications for schizophrenia. Biol Psychiatry 48(7):627–640, 2000 11032974

Kellendonk C, Simpson EH, Polan HJ, et al: Transient and selective overexpression of dopamine D2 receptors in the striatum causes persistent abnormalities in prefrontal cortex functioning. Neuron 49(4):603–615, 2006 16476668

Kempadoo KA, Mosharov EV, Choi SJ, et al: Dopamine release from the locus coeruleus to the dorsal hippocampus promotes spatial learning and memory. Proc Natl Acad Sci USA 113(51):14835–14840, 2016 27930324

Kesby JP, Eyles DW, McGrath JJ, et al: Dopamine, psychosis and schizophrenia: the widening gap between basic and clinical neuroscience. Transl Psychiatry 8(1):30, 2018 29382821

Khandaker GM, Zimbron J, Lewis G, et al: Prenatal maternal infection, neurodevelopment and adult schizophrenia: a systematic review of population-based studies. Psychol Med 43(2):239–257, 2013 22717193

Khashan AS, Abel KM, McNamee R, et al: Higher risk of offspring schizophrenia following antenatal maternal exposure to severe adverse life events. Arch Gen Psychiatry 65(2):146–152, 2008 18250252

Knuesel I, Chicha L, Britschgi M, et al: Maternal immune activation and abnormal brain development across CNS disorders. Nat Rev Neurol 10(11):643–660, 2014 25311587

Kotov R, Fochtmann L, Li K, et al: Declining clinical course of psychotic disorders over the two decades following first hospitalization: evidence from the Suffolk County Mental Health Project. Am J Psychiatry 174(11):1064–1074, 2017 28774193

Kraguljac NV, White DM, Reid MA, et al: Increased hippocampal glutamate and volumetric deficits in unmedicated patients with schizophrenia. JAMA Psychiatry 70(12):1294–1302, 2013 24108440

Krol A, Wimmer RD, Halassa MM, et al: Thalamic reticular dysfunction as a circuit endophenotype in neurodevelopmental disorders. Neuron 98(2):282–295, 2018 29673480

Krystal JH, Karper LP, Seibyl JP, et al: Subanesthetic effects of the noncompetitive NMDA antagonist, ketamine, in humans: psychotomimetic, perceptual, cognitive, and neuroendocrine responses. Arch Gen Psychiatry 51(3):199–214, 1994 8122957

Kutay FZ, Pöğün S, Hariri NI, et al: Free amino acid level determinations in normal and schizophrenic brain. Prog Neuropsychopharmacol Biol Psychiatry 13(1–2):119–126, 1989 2748856

Large M, Sharma S, Compton MT, et al: Cannabis use and earlier onset of psychosis: a systematic meta-analysis. Arch Gen Psychiatry 68(6):555–561, 2011 21300939

Leweke FM, Giuffrida A, Koethe D, et al: Anandamide levels in cerebrospinal fluid of first-episode schizophrenic patients: impact of cannabis use. Schizophr Res 94(1–3):29–36, 2007 17566707

Leweke FM, Piomelli D, Pahlisch F, et al: Cannabidiol enhances anandamide signaling and alleviates psychotic symptoms of schizophrenia. Transl Psychiatry 2:e94, 2012 22832859

Lewis DA, Curley AA, Glausier JR, et al: Cortical parvalbumin interneurons and cognitive dysfunction in schizophrenia. Trends Neurosci 35(1):57–67, 2012 22154068

Lichtenstein P, Yip BH, Björk C, et al: Common genetic determinants of schizophrenia and bipolar disorder in Swedish families: a population-based study. Lancet 373(9659):234–239, 2009 19150704

Linderholm KR, Skogh E, Olsson SK, et al: Increased levels of kynurenine and kynurenic acid in the CSF of patients with schizophrenia. Schizophr Bull 38(3):426–432, 2012 20729465

Lisman JE, Coyle JT, Green RW, et al: Circuit-based framework for understanding neurotransmitter and risk gene interactions in schizophrenia. Trends Neurosci 31(5):234–242, 2008 18395805

Lisman JE, Pi HJ, Zhang Y, et al: A thalamo-hippocampal-ventral tegmental area loop may produce the positive feedback that underlies the psychotic break in schizophrenia. Biol Psychiatry 68(1):17–24, 2010 20553749

Malaspina D, Harlap S, Fennig S, et al: Advancing paternal age and the risk of schizophrenia. Arch Gen Psychiatry 58(4):361–367, 2001 11296097

Malhotra D, Sebat J: CNVs: harbingers of a rare variant revolution in psychiatric genetics. Cell 148(6):1223–1241, 2012 22424231

Manseau MW, Goff DC: Cannabinoids and schizophrenia: risks and therapeutic potential. Neurotherapeutics 12(4):816–824, 2015 26311150

McCutcheon R, Beck K, Jauhar S, et al: Defining the locus of dopaminergic dysfunction in schizophrenia: a meta-analysis and test of the mesolimbic hypothesis. Schizophr Bull 44(6):1301–1311, 2018 29301039

McGrath J, Saha S, Chant D, et al: Schizophrenia: a concise overview of incidence, prevalence, and mortality. Epidemiol Rev 30:67–76, 2008 18480098

McGuire P, Robson P, Cubala WJ, et al: Cannabidiol (CBD) as an adjunctive therapy in schizophrenia: a multicenter randomized controlled trial. Am J Psychiatry 175(3):225–231, 2018 29241357

Meier MH, Caspi A, Reichenberg A, et al: Neuropsychological decline in schizophrenia from the premorbid to the postonset period: evidence from a population-representative longitudinal study. Am J Psychiatry 171(1):91–101, 2014 24030246

Meiser J, Weindl D, Hiller K: Complexity of dopamine metabolism. Cell Commun Signal 11(1):34, 2013 23683503

Miyamoto S, Miyake N, Jarskog LF, et al: Pharmacological treatment of schizophrenia: a critical review of the pharmacology and clinical effects of current and future therapeutic agents. Mol Psychiatry 17(12):1206–1227, 2012 22584864

Mizrahi R, Addington J, Rusjan PM, et al: Increased stress-induced dopamine release in psychosis. Biol Psychiatry 71(6):561–567, 2012 22133268

Möhler H: The GABA system in anxiety and depression and its therapeutic potential. Neuropharmacology 62(1):42–53, 2012 21889518

Moore H, Jentsch JD, Ghajarnia M, et al: A neurobehavioral systems analysis of adult rats exposed to methylazoxymethanol acetate on E17: implications for the neuropathology of schizophrenia. Biol Psychiatry 60(3):253–264, 2006 16581031

Nadkarni S, Arnedo V, Devinsky O: Psychosis in epilepsy patients. Epilepsia 48 (suppl 9):17–19, 2007 18047594

Nakao K, Jeevakumar V, Jiang SZ, et al: Schizophrenia-like dopamine release abnormalities in a mouse model of NMDA receptor hypofunction. Schizophr Bull 45(1):138–147, 2019 29394409

Orhan F, Fatouros-Bergman H, Goiny M, et al; Karolinska Schizophrenia Project (KaSP) Consortium: CSF GABA is reduced in first-episode psychosis and associates to symptom severity. Mol Psychiatry 23(5):1244–1250, 2018 28289277

Plavén-Sigray P, Matheson GJ, Collste K, et al: Positron emission tomography studies of the glial cell marker translocator protein in patients with psychosis: a meta-analysis using individual participant data. Biol Psychiatry 84(6):433–442, 2018 29653835

Purcell SM, Moran JL, Fromer M, et al: A polygenic burden of rare disruptive mutations in schizophrenia. Nature 506(7487):185–190, 2014 24463508

Rabiner EA: Imaging of striatal dopamine release elicited with NMDA antagonists: is there anything there to be seen? J Psychopharmacol 21(3):253–258, 2007 17591653

Radua J, Ramella-Cravaro V, Ioannidis JPA, et al: What causes psychosis? An umbrella review of risk and protective factors. World Psychiatry 17(1):49–66, 2018 29352556

Ramirez S, Liu X, Lin PA, et al: Creating a false memory in the hippocampus. Science 341(6144):387–391, 2013 23888038

Ramsden HL, Sürmeli G, McDonagh SG, et al: Laminar and dorsoventral molecular organization of the medial entorhinal cortex revealed by large-scale anatomical analysis of gene expression. PLoS Comput Biol 11(1):e1004032, 2015 25615592

Recillas-Morales S, Sánchez-Vega L, Ochoa-Sánchez N, et al: L-type Ca2+ channel activity determines modulation of GABA release by dopamine in the substantia nigra reticulata and the globus pallidus of the rat. Neuroscience 256:292–301, 2014 24505607

Redondo RL, Kim J, Arons AL, et al: Bidirectional switch of the valence associated with a hippocampal contextual memory engram. Nature 513(7518):426–430, 2014 25162525

Reith J, Benkelfat C, Sherwin A, et al: Elevated dopa decarboxylase activity in living brain of patients with psychosis. Proc Natl Acad Sci USA 91(24):11651–11654, 1994 7972118

Ruggiero RN, Rossignoli MT, De Ross JB, et al: Cannabinoids and vanilloids in schizophrenia: neurophysiological evidence and directions for basic research. Front Pharmacol 8:399, 2017 28680405

Schizophrenia Working Group of the Psychiatric Genomics Consortium: Biological insights from 108 schizophrenia-associated genetic loci. Nature 511(7510):421–427, 2014 25056061

Schobel SA, Lewandowski NM, Corcoran CM, et al: Differential targeting of the CA1 subfield of the hippocampal formation by schizophrenia and related psychotic disorders. Arch Gen Psychiatry 66(9):938–946, 2009 19736350

Schobel SA, Chaudhury NH, Khan UA, et al: Imaging patients with psychosis and a mouse model establishes a spreading pattern of hippocampal dysfunction and implicates glutamate as a driver. Neuron 78(1):81–93, 2013 23583108

Schwarcz R, Stone TW: The kynurenine pathway and the brain: challenges, controversies and promises. Neuropharmacology 112 (Pt B):237–247, 2017 27511838

Schwarcz R, Rassoulpour A, Wu HQ, et al: Increased cortical kynurenate content in schizophrenia. Biol Psychiatry 50(7):521–530, 2001 11600105

Shergill SS, Samson G, Bays PM, et al: Evidence for sensory prediction deficits in schizophrenia. Am J Psychiatry 162(12):2384–2386, 2005 16330607

Sherman SM: Thalamus plays a central role in ongoing cortical functioning. Nat Neurosci 19(4):533–541, 2016 27021938

Sherva R, Wang Q, Kranzler H, et al: Genome-wide association study of cannabis dependence severity, novel risk variants, and shared genetic risks. JAMA Psychiatry 73(5):472–480, 2016 27028160

Sheth SA, Mian MK, Patel SR, et al: Human dorsal anterior cingulate cortex neurons mediate ongoing behavioural adaptation. Nature 488(7410):218–221, 2012 22722841

Slifstein M, van de Giessen E, Van Snellenberg J, et al: Deficits in prefrontal cortical and extrastriatal dopamine release in schizophrenia: a positron emission tomographic functional magnetic resonance imaging study. JAMA Psychiatry 72(4):316–324, 2015 25651194

Spellman TJ, Gordon JA: Synchrony in schizophrenia: a window into circuit-level pathophysiology. Curr Opin Neurobiol 30:17–23, 2015 25215626

Steullet P, Cabungcal JH, Monin A, et al: Redox dysregulation, neuroinflammation, and NMDA receptor hypofunction: a "central hub" in schizophrenia pathophysiology? Schizophr Res 176(1):41–51, 2016 25000913

Strauss GP, Cohen AS: A transdiagnostic review of negative symptom phenomenology and etiology. Schizophr Bull 43(4):712–719, 2017 28969356

Strauss GP, Waltz JA, Gold JM: A review of reward processing and motivational impairment in schizophrenia. Schizophr Bull 40 (suppl 2):S107–S116, 2014 24375459

Sullivan PF, Kendler KS, Neale MC: Schizophrenia as a complex trait: evidence from a meta-analysis of twin studies. Arch Gen Psychiatry 60(12):1187–1192, 2003 14662550

Taylor SF, Tso IF: GABA abnormalities in schizophrenia: a methodological review of in vivo studies. Schizophr Res 167(1–3):84–90, 2015 25458856

Tseng HH, Watts JJ, Kiang M, et al: Nigral stress-induced dopamine release in clinical high risk and antipsychotic-naïve schizophrenia. Schizophr Bull 44(3):542–551, 2018 29036383

Tseng KY, Chambers RA, Lipska BK: The neonatal ventral hippocampal lesion as a heuristic neurodevelopmental model of schizophrenia. Behav Brain Res 204(2):295–305, 2009 19100784

Ursini G, Punzi G, Chen Q, et al: Convergence of placenta biology and genetic risk for schizophrenia. Nat Med 24(6):792–801, 2018 29808008

van Haren NE, Schnack HG, Cahn W, et al: Changes in cortical thickness during the course of illness in schizophrenia. Arch Gen Psychiatry 68(9):871–880, 2011 21893656

Varese F, Smeets F, Drukker M, et al: Childhood adversities increase the risk of psychosis: a meta-analysis of patient-control, prospective- and cross-sectional cohort studies. Schizophr Bull 38(4):661–671, 2012 22461484

Verma A, Moghaddam B: NMDA receptor antagonists impair prefrontal cortex function as assessed via spatial delayed alternation performance in rats: modulation by dopamine. J Neurosci 16(1):373–379, 1996 8613804

Volk DW, Lewis DA: Early developmental disturbances of cortical inhibitory neurons: contribution to cognitive deficits in schizophrenia. Schizophr Bull 40(5):952–957, 2014 25053651

Wagatsuma A, Okuyama T, Sun C, et al: Locus coeruleus input to hippocampal CA3 drives single-trial learning of a novel context. Proc Natl Acad Sci USA 115(2):E310–E316, 2018 29279390

Walton E, Hass J, Liu J, et al: Correspondence of DNA methylation between blood and brain tissue and its application to schizophrenia research. Schizophr Bull 42(2):406–414, 2016 26056378

Walton E, Hibar DP, van Erp TGM, et al; Karolinska Schizophrenia Project Consortium (KaSP): Prefrontal cortical thinning links to negative symptoms in schizophrenia via the ENIGMA consortium. Psychol Med 48(1):82–94, 2018 28545597

Wamsley EJ, Tucker MA, Shinn AK, et al: Reduced sleep spindles and spindle coherence in schizophrenia: mechanisms of impaired memory consolidation? Biol Psychiatry 71(2):154–161, 2012 21967958

Wang M, Pei L, Fletcher PJ, et al: Schizophrenia, amphetamine-induced sensitized state and acute amphetamine exposure all show a common alteration: increased dopamine D2 receptor dimerization. Mol Brain 3:25, 2010 20813060

Xu MQ, Sun WS, Liu BX, et al: Prenatal malnutrition and adult schizophrenia: further evidence from the 1959–1961 Chinese famine. Schizophr Bull 35(3):568–576, 2009 19155344

Zeng B, Ardekani BA, Tang Y, et al: Abnormal white matter microstructure in drug-naive first episode schizophrenia patients before and after eight weeks of antipsychotic treatment. Schizophr Res 172(1–3):1–8, 2016 26852402

CHAPTER 7

Neurobiology

L. Fredrik Jarskog, M.D.
T. Wilson Woo, M.D., Ph.D.

Given its prominent clinical manifestations, the neuropathological phenotype of schizophrenia is remarkably subtle. Kraeplin (1919/1971) originally suggested that schizophrenia was characterized by a degenerative pathology. However, with the ascendance of psychoanalytic theory, the pathophysiological underpinnings remained largely unexplored until rigorous biological inquiry was again applied to schizophrenia in the last third of the twentieth century. Over the past 4–5 decades, researchers have begun to reveal the complex neurobiology of schizophrenia, demonstrating a brain disorder that appears to be fundamentally neurodevelopmental in origin and associated with subtle yet consistent deficits in synaptic connectivity and brain circuitry. The aim of this chapter is to review the research that has contributed to this neurobiological conceptualization, with a focus on postmortem studies of histopathology and neurochemistry, with selected neuroimaging and genetic findings that further illustrate the overarching themes. Given the scope of this chapter, the review is necessarily selective, and therefore some lines of research have been omitted or only briefly summarized.

Histopathology

Glia and Glial Markers

Although an early study found an increase in periventricular and subependymal gliosis in brains of individuals with schizophrenia (Stevens 1982), many subsequent studies have reported either no change in glial numbers (Arnold et al. 1998; Benes et al. 1991a; Roberts et al. 1986) or a decrease in cortical glial density (Cotter et al. 2001; Stark et al. 2004; Uranova et al. 2004). Consistent with these reports are studies that have found normal glial fibrillary acidic protein (GFAP) immunoreactivity (Arnold et al. 1998; Damadzic et al. 2001; Perrone-Bizzozero et al. 1996; Purohit et al. 1998; Roberts et al. 1987). GFAP is a structural protein that increases markedly in response to astrocytic infiltration following neuronal damage and is often elevated in classic neurodegenerative disorders such as Alzheimer's disease. However, reductions in GFAP-reactive astroglia have been reported in prefrontal cortex (PFC) in schizophrenia (Rajkowska et al. 2002). Furthermore, postmortem studies have revealed significant reductions in GFAP in frontal cortex and GFAP messenger RNA (mRNA) in cingulate cortex in schizophrenia compared with control subjects without schizophrenia (Johnston-Wilson et al. 2000; Webster et al. 2005). In a systematic review, of 33 studies that measured GFAP in postmortem brain in schizophrenia, 21 studies found no change compared with control subjects, 6 found reduced GFAP, and 6 found increased GFAP (Trépanier et al. 2016). The relatively consistent findings of either reduced or normal GFAP expression in diverse cortical brain regions suggest that classic neurodegenerative neuropathology is absent in schizophrenia.

Microglia, the primary immune cells of the central nervous system (CNS), have received increased attention in schizophrenia research as part of investigations into the potential pathophysiological role of inflammatory mechanisms. In a systematic review, Trépanier and colleagues (2016) identified 22 studies that reported on microglial markers in postmortem brain in patients with schizophrenia. Of these studies, 11 found increased microglial markers, 8 found no effect, and 3 found a decrease. Because increased numbers of reactive microglia typically occur in settings of CNS inflammation or injury and because such microgliosis subsequently resolves after the inflammatory process subsides, it becomes challenging to understand the postmortem microglial findings in a pathophysiological context, given that the onset of psychosis has usually predated postmortem examination by many decades. Also, most microglial studies in schizophrenia have had inadequate statistical power and include primarily elderly subjects, in whom incidental lesions are common; thus, it will be necessary to conduct larger studies that include adequate numbers of young subjects in order to more confidently relate the presence of reactive microglia to the pathophysiology of schizophrenia using postmortem brain tissue (Schnieder and Dwork 2011).

Microglial activation has also been studied in vivo using PET imaging to quantitate translocator protein 18kD (TSPO) expression. PET imaging can potentially probe for the presence of microglial activity at the time of psychosis onset. Early studies using first-generation TSPO radiotracers found elevated TSPO levels in patients with chronic schizophrenia (van Berckel et al. 2008), and a study of people at ultrahigh risk of psychosis using a second-generation tracer also found elevated levels (Bloomfield et al. 2016). However, other studies using second-generation tracers have found no change or reduced TSPO levels (Coughlin et al. 2016). A recent meta-analysis showed evidence for lower TSPO levels in frontal and temporal cortices and in the hippocampus in 75 patients with schizophrenia or first-episode psychosis compared with 77 healthy control subjects across five studies using second-generation TSPO ligands (Plaven-Sigray et al. 2018). Taken together with the postmortem findings, the PET data suggest the presence of an altered immune response in schizophrenia involving microglia, but additional research is needed to better understand the nature of these alterations.

Neurons and Neuronal Distribution

Classic neurodegenerative disorders are generally characterized by large-scale neuronal loss, but there is little evidence that schizophrenia is associated with significant cortical neuronal loss. Using unbiased stereology, one study found no change in total cortical neuronal number in patients with schizophrenia compared with control subjects (Pakkenberg 1993). Likewise, multiple studies found no evidence of neuronal loss in dorsal PFC (DPFC) in schizophrenia (Akbarian et al. 1995; Selemon et al. 1995, 1998; Thune et al. 2001). Several studies found small but significant increases in neuronal density in prefrontal and occipital cortex in patients with schizophrenia compared with control subjects, which the authors interpreted as representing reductions in neuropil rather than absolute changes in neuronal number (Selemon et al. 1995, 1998). However, other studies have reported reduced density of cortical neuronal subpopulations in patients with schizophrenia compared with control subjects, including interneurons in layer II of DPFC and in layers II–VI of the anterior cingulate cortex (ACC) (Benes et al. 1991a, 2001).

In contrast, reduced neuronal numbers have been reported in subcortical areas in patients with schizophrenia. An early stereological study reported about 30% fewer neurons in nucleus accumbens and mediodorsal thalamus in patients with schizophrenia (Pakkenberg 1990). The mediodorsal thalamus findings have been replicated in many (Byne et al. 2002; Popken et al. 2000; Young et al. 2000) but not all (Cullen et al. 2003; Dorph-Petersen et al. 2004) studies. A meta-analysis of neuroimaging studies found consistent volume reductions in the hippocampus (Nelson et al. 1998), but most postmortem studies have not demonstrated an overall loss of neurons (Heckers et al. 1991; Walker et al. 2002). Several studies, however, have identified reductions in hippocampal neuronal subpopulations, specifically in GABAergic interneurons (Benes et al. 1998; Zhang and Reynolds 2002). Thus, although overall cortical neuronal numbers in patients with schizophrenia appear mostly unchanged, discrete neuronal reductions may occur with laminar and regional specificity. Several studies have found reduced neuronal numbers in several subcortical regions, whereas other studies have found no differences, highlighting the variability for this outcome across postmortem studies in schizophrenia.

Another focus of postmortem research has involved neuronal distribution and organization in schizophrenia. Several studies have reported abnormal lamination as well as neuronal disorganization in the entorhinal cortex, consistent with potential migration deficits early in development (Arnold et al. 1991, 1997; Jakob and Beckmann 1986). In frontal and temporal cortices, abnormal distribution of nicotinamide adenine dinucleotide phosphate–diaphorase (NADPH-d)–containing neurons in gray and white matter has been reported and is thought to reflect deficits in neuronal migration or apoptosis (Akbarian et al. 1993a, 1993b, 1996a, 1996b). Although evidence of neuronal maldistribution has been interpreted as supporting the neurodevelopmental hypothesis of schizophrenia, other studies have failed to replicate these findings (Akil and Lewis 1997). Taken together, these data indicate a need for further research to better understand the potential role of neuronal disorganization in the neuropathology of schizophrenia.

Neuropil and Synaptic Markers

Evidence suggests that the cortical neuropathology of schizophrenia involves reduced cortical neuropil (Selemon and Goldman-Rakic 1999). Neuropil is composed primarily of axons, dendrites, and synaptic terminals. Consistent with the reduced neuropil hypothesis is evidence of reduced dendritic spine density and total dendritic length of pyramidal neurons in DPFC in patients with schizophrenia (Black et al. 2002; Garey et al. 1998; Glantz and Lewis 2000; Konopaske et al. 2014). Notably, reduced dendritic spine density appears to be layer specific, with reductions in DPFC layer III but not in layer V or VI (Glantz and Lewis 2000; Kolluri et al. 2005). Consistent with reduced spines and dendritic length, there is also evidence of fewer parvalbumin and γ-aminobutyric acid (GABA) membrane transporter GAT-1 cartridges (Lewis et al. 2001; Pierri et al. 1999) and reductions of the presynaptic marker protein synaptophysin across multiple brain regions (Eastwood et al. 1995; Glantz and Lewis 1997; Karson et al. 1999; Perrone-Bizzozero et al. 1996). In a recent meta-analysis, significant reductions in synaptophysin protein or mRNA emerged for frontal and cingulate cortices and in the hippocampus but not in temporal or occipital cortices (Osimo et al. 2019). Presynaptic vesicle docking protein synaptosomal nerve-associated protein 25 (SNAP-25) has also been reduced in DPFC in several studies (Gabriel et al. 1997; Karson et al. 1999), but this conclusion was not supported by meta-analysis (Osimo et al. 2019). Several studies have also found lower SNAP-25 levels in the hippocampus (Thompson et al. 2003; Young et al. 1998). Two other synaptic markers, complexin I and complexin II, are associated with inhibitory and excitatory neurons, respectively. Alterations in complexin I and II proteins and mRNA have been reported in the hippocampus and DPFC in patients with schizophrenia (Eastwood and Harrison 2000, 2005; Harrison and Eastwood 1998; Sawada et al. 2005). Neural cell adhesion molecule (NCAM), another protein increasingly appreciated for its diverse roles in neurodevelopment and synaptic stabilization, has also been implicated in the neuropathology of schizophrenia. In the hippocampus, NCAM has been reported as both reduced (Barbeau et al. 1995) and increased (Vawter et al. 1999). In DPFC, NCAM has been reported to be reduced in some (Gilabert-Juan et al. 2012) but not all (Barbeau et al. 1995) studies in subjects with schizophrenia compared with control subjects.

Research has begun to shed light on some of the molecular mechanisms that may underlie the reduction in dendritic spine density found in DPFC in patients with schizophrenia. Rho GTPase cell division cycle 42 (CDC42) is involved in spine morphogenesis, and its activity promotes spine formation (Nakayama et al. 2000; Scott et al. 2003; Stankiewicz and Linseman 2014). CDC42 mRNA was significantly reduced in DPFC in 15 matched pairs of subjects with schizophrenia and control subjects by in situ hybridization, and its expression also correlated with dendritic spine density in a subset of the same subjects (Hill et al. 2006). CDC42 interacts with CDC42 effector protein (CDC42EP). CDC42 is activated by glutamate stimulation, and in turn CDC42 inhibits CDC42EP, which then allows for movement of cytoskeletal proteins and other molecules between the dendrite and the spine across the spine neck (reviewed by Glausier and Lewis 2018). Interestingly, CDC42EP mRNA expression was increased in DPFC in schizophrenia compared with control subjects (Ide and Lewis 2010). This research group subsequently used laser microdissection to demonstrate increased CDC42EP mRNA specifically in DPFC deep layer III pyramidal neurons, the same neurons that have consistently demonstrated reduced density in schizophrenia (Datta et al. 2015). One possible consequence of reduced CDC42 and increased CDC42EP is impairment of glutamate-stimulated movement across the spine neck, thereby limiting synaptic plasticity and promoting dendritic spine loss (Glausier and Lewis 2018).

The postmortem data implicating synaptic and neuropil changes in the neuropathology of schizophrenia are also supported by gene array studies, including use of laser-captured pyramidal neurons showing altered RNA expression in cytoskeletal and synaptic plasticity pathways (Mirnics et al. 2000; Pietersen et al. 2014). Functional gene group analysis using genome-wide association study data has also identified variants associated with synaptic signaling in schizophrenia (Lips et al. 2012; Schijven et al. 2018). Genetic findings include identification of the association of complement component 4 gene variants in schizophrenia, providing support for schizophrenia as a disorder of excessive cortical synaptic pruning (Sekar et al. 2016). Furthermore, posttranscriptional gene expression is regulated in part by noncoding microRNAs. Variants of microRNA-137 (miR-137) have been associated with increased schizophrenia risk, and four specific miR-137 risk alleles have been found to impair synaptic vesicle trafficking and alter presynaptic plasticity (Siegert et al. 2015). Taken together, the postmortem and genetic evidence implicating neuropil and synaptic abnormalities in the pathophysiology of schizophrenia has grown increasingly strong.

Neuronal Soma

Neuronal somal size has been associated with the extent of dendritic and axonal arborization (Elston and Rosa 1997; Jacobs et al. 1997). Given evidence for reduced dendritic length and reduced dendritic spine density in schizophrenia, neuronal somal size has also been studied. In DPFC, small but significant reductions in pyramidal neuronal size have been reported in patients with schizophrenia compared with control subjects (Pierri et al. 2001, 2003; Rajkowska et al. 1998). Several studies have also reported smaller hippocampal pyramidal neurons in patients with schizophrenia (Arnold et al. 1995; Benes et al. 1991b; Zaidel et al. 1997). Other studies in DPFC and ACC did not find differences in neuronal somal size (Benes et al. 1986, 2000; Cotter et al. 2001). Although the etiology remains unclear, smaller somal volumes could stem from early developmental agenesis or subtle atrophy at a subsequent pathophysiological stage (Rajkowska et al. 1998).

Perineuronal Nets

Perineuronal nets (PNNs) are lattice-like structures comprising four major extracellular matrix components: hyaluronan; link proteins; the lectican family of proteins (i.e., chondroitin sulfate proteoglycans [CSPGs], including aggrecan, neurocan, versican, and brevican); and tenascin-R (Hynes and Yamada 2012; Wang and Fawcett 2012; Yamaguchi 2000). Chains of hyaluronan are directly attached to the cell membrane of neurons. Link proteins in turn bind CSPGs to hyaluronan chains. Finally, tenascin-R links together CSPGs. The precise functions of PNNs remain elusive, but they may play a role in neuroprotection, ion homeostasis, and synaptic plasticity, as well as in regulating the excitatory-inhibitory balance of neural circuits.

During the course of postnatal development, the density of PNNs progressively increases until it plateaus during late adolescence and early adulthood (Mauney et al. 2013). At the same time, parvalbumin (PV) neurons become increasingly encapsulated by PNNs, which may serve as a cation buffer in the extracellular matrix and hence facilitate fast-spiking firing of PV neurons (Härtig et al. 1999). The functional maturation of PV neurons also requires the presence of the homeoprotein orthodenticle homeobox 2 (OTX2), which is produced in the choroid plexus, secreted into the cerebrospinal fluid (CSF), and delivered to the cerebral cortex (Prochiantz et al. 2014). In the cerebral cortex, the transport of OTX2 into PV neurons is mediated by PNNs (Lee et al. 2017). Of note, in patients with schizophrenia, the densities of PNNs in the PFC and also in temporal structures, such as the amygdala, have been found to be significantly decreased (Mauney et al. 2013; Pantazopoulos et al. 2010). Hence, PNN deficits may contribute to the pathophysiology of schizophrenia, at least in part, by impairing the uptake of OTX2 into PV neurons and thus leading to their dysmaturation and dysfunction.

Neurochemistry

GABA System

Over the past few decades, multiple lines of evidence have strongly implicated inhibitory neurons in the cerebral cortex as functionally impaired in the pathophysiology of schizophrenia (Benes 2000; Costa et al. 2001; Lewis et al. 2005). Subsets of these neurons regulate distinct aspects of information processing (Gabbott and Bacon 1996; Wang et al. 2004). For example, inhibitory neurons that contain PV provide perisomatic (basket cells) and axoaxonic (chandelier cells) inhibition to pyramidal cells. In the PFC in patients with schizophrenia, the expression of the mRNA for the GABA-synthesizing enzyme glutamic acid decarboxylase 67 (GAD_{67}) is undetectable in about 45% of PV neurons (Hashimoto et al. 2003), suggesting that inhibition furnished by PV neurons is reduced. Furthermore, the number of axon terminals of chandelier cells, labeled with an antibody against GAT-1, is decreased by as much as 40% (Pierri et al. 1999; Woo et al. 1998). Also, the $GABA_A$ receptor α2 subunit, which is selectively localized to synapses formed by chandelier cells, has been found to be upregulated (Volk et al. 2002). This increase in density of postsynaptic $GABA_A$ receptor $α_2$ subunit on the pyramidal axon initial segment suggests a compensatory response to reduced GABAergic activity in the presynaptic chandelier cells. Unlike those of chandelier neurons, axon terminals of basket cells cannot be reliably identified under light microscopy. Hence, there is currently no definitive evidence directly indicating the involvement of basket cell terminals in the neuropathology of schizophrenia. However, because basket cells represent the majority—possibly 80%–90%—of all PV neurons in the cerebral cortex (Kawaguchi 1995; Krimer et al. 2005; Markram et al. 2004; Zaitsev et al. 2005), it is almost certain that at least a subset of basket cells must also be affected in order to account for the finding of Hashimoto and colleagues (2003).

PV neurons play a key role in the generation of neural circuitry oscillation in the gamma frequency band (Soltesz 2005), which is thought to represent the neurophysiological substrate of advanced cognitive and perceptive operations. Examining neuronal oscillations in schizophrenia represents an important in vivo approach to understanding the consequences of altered GABAergic signaling. In fact, many studies have implicated altered synchrony of neuronal oscillations in patients with schizophrenia (Uhlhaas and Singer 2010), and reduced GABA synthesis in PV neurons has been hypothesized as an important contributing factor (Gonzalez-Burgos and Lewis 2008). Altered neural oscillations in patients with schizophrenia are in turn thought to contribute to various clinical symptoms and deficits, including perceptual abnormalities, thought disorder, and working memory impairments (Ford et al. 2007; Gonzalez-Burgos and Lewis 2008; Spencer et al. 2004; Uhlhaas and Singer 2015).

The GABA system has also been studied in vivo in patients with schizophrenia using proton magnetic resonance spectroscopy (^{1}H-MRS). ^{1}H-MRS is useful for providing net tissue GABA levels in specific brain regions; however, because of the required size of the voxel, it cannot provide information in small areas such as synaptic or cellular compartments, cannot separate cortical gray versus white matter, and cannot provide cortical layer-specific data. A meta-analysis of available ^{1}H-MRS studies did not find significant differences in GABA levels when levels were analyzed by brain region in patients with schizophrenia compared with control subjects, although a small reduction in schizophrenia emerged after averaging GABA levels across multiple brain regions from the same study (Schür et al. 2016). Notably, in one of the few MRS studies to examine GABA levels in unmedicated patients with schizophrenia, GABA levels were increased by 30% in medial PFC, with no change in dorsolateral PFC, in patients with schizophrenia compared with control subjects (Kegeles et al. 2012). This elevation in medial PFC was not seen in patients treated with antipsychotics, suggesting a possible normalization of net GABA levels associated with treatment.

Glutamate System

It has long been known that treatment with antagonists of the N-methyl-D-aspartate (NMDA) class of glutamate receptors produces a syndrome with symptomatic, cognitive, and electrophysiological features very similar to those of schizophrenia (Javitt and Zukin 1991; Krystal et al. 1994). Such findings led to the NMDA receptor hypofunction model of the disorder (Olney and Farber 1995; Olney et al. 1999). NMDA receptors occur on both GABA and pyramidal neurons; thus, it is of interest that the NMDA receptors located on GABA neurons are approximately 10-fold more sensitive to NMDA receptor antagonists than those on pyramidal neurons (Greene et al. 2000; Grunze et al. 1996). In addition, in primary neuronal cultures, Kinney and colleagues (2006) showed that mRNA expression for the NR2A subunit of the NMDA receptor in PV neurons is fivefold greater than that in pyramidal cells. These findings support the idea that deficient glutamatergic neurotransmission via NMDA receptors on inhibitory neurons is involved in the pathophysiology of schizophrenia. Further support is provided by postmortem studies that have shown that in subjects with schizophrenia, NR2A subunit expression in GABA neurons appears to be decreased (Woo et al. 2004, 2008). Furthermore, NR2A- but not NR2B-selective antagonist downregulates GAD_{67} and PV expression in PV neurons (Kinney et al. 2006). Similarly, NMDA antagonism in vivo reduces PV expression (Abdul-Monim et al. 2007; Braun et al. 2007; Keilhoff et al. 2004; Reynolds et al. 2004; Rujescu et al. 2006) and the number of axoaxonic cartridges of chandelier cells (Morrow et al. 2007). Taken together, reduced glutamatergic inputs to PV neurons via NMDA receptors, possibly especially those that contain the NR2A subunit, may mediate the functional deficits of PV neurons. In fact, the number of PV cells that express a detectable level of NR2A mRNA is reduced by as much as 50% in subjects with schizophrenia (Bitanihirwe et al. 2009). Functionally, NMDA receptor blockade has been shown to disrupt gamma rhythms in the entorhinal cortex in animals, and this disruption is thought to be mediated by NMDA receptors on PV neurons (Cunningham et al. 2006). The available evidence appears, therefore, to suggest that deficient glutamatergic neurotransmission via NMDA receptors on PV neurons may contribute to the pathophysiology of schizophrenia by disrupting gamma network oscillations.

Glutamatergic abnormalities have also been identified in vivo with ^{1}H-MRS in patients with schizophrenia. Studies have consistently reported elevated Glx (glutamate+glutamine) levels in medial PFC in unmedicated patients with schizophrenia versus healthy control subjects, whereas no difference has been found between medicated patients and healthy control subjects (reviewed by Poels et al. 2014). Increased Glx levels have also been reported in medial PFC in people at ultrahigh risk for psychosis, supporting a pathophysiological role for hypoglutamatergia in the early stages of psychosis (de la Fuente-Sandoval et al. 2015), because increased glutamate levels may reflect a compensatory response to an underlying hypoglutamatergic state, consistent with the glutamate hypothesis of schizophrenia. Elevated glutamate and Glx levels have also been reported in basal ganglia in patients with first-episode psychosis, including in associative striatum (de la Fuente-Sandoval et al. 2011, 2013), further supporting the glutamate hypothesis.

Dopamine System

The dopamine hypothesis of schizophrenia suggests that subcortical hyperdopaminergia coexists with cortical hypodopaminergia and that this imbalance of subcortical-to-cortical dopamine contributes to positive, negative, and cognitive symptoms of schizophrenia (Abi-Dargham and Moore 2003). A more recent iteration specifically links risk factors for psychosis (e.g., early-life neurobiological stressors, drug use, genes) with increased presynaptic striatal dopaminergic function (Howes and Kapur 2009). Direct evidence of subcortical hyperdopaminergia was first provided by several single-photon emission computed tomography (SPECT) studies using the radiolabeled dopamine D_2 receptor antagonist ^{123}I-iodobenzamide ([^{123}I]IBZM); evidence of increased striatal dopamine transmission was found both in first-episode neuroleptic-naïve patients and in previously treated patients with chronic schizophrenia experiencing acute exacerbation (Abi-Dargham et al. 1998, 2000). PET imaging of striatal dopamine capacity using 3,4-dihydroxy-5-fluorophenylalanine (^{18}F-DOPA) has confirmed these findings, and they have been extended to people with prodromal symptoms of schizophrenia (Howes et al. 2009). Subsequent studies have also demonstrated that increased dopamine capacity is present not only in striatal nerve terminals but also in the substantia nigra, the site of dopamine neuron cell bodies (Howes et al. 2013). Notably, striatal synaptic dopamine levels have been correlated with the severity of positive symptoms and were also predictive of antipsychotic treatment response (Abi-Dargham et al. 2000; Howes et al. 2013). The hypothesis that positive symptoms of schizophrenia are in part mediated by increased subcortical dopamine activity is consistent with the mechanism of action of D_2 receptor antagonists, which are thought to act primarily in the striatum (including the nucleus accumbens) because of the greater density of D_2 receptors in the striatum than in DPFC (Lidow and Goldman-Rakic 1994).

A consistent postmortem finding has been increased dopamine striatal D_2 receptor density in patients with schizophrenia (Zakzanis and Hansen 1998). However, haloperidol treatment for 6–12 months in rats can produce substantial elevations in striatal D_2 receptor number (Joyce 2001; Laruelle et al. 1992), indicating that the increase in striatal D_2 receptor density in patients with schizophrenia most likely represents a compensatory upregulation in response to chronic antipsychotic treatment. Another marker of dopamine activity is tyrosine hydroxylase (TH), the rate-limiting enzyme of dopamine production. Consistent with ^{18}F-DOPA PET findings (Howes et al. 2013), postmortem studies in the substantia nigra have also found increased TH protein levels in subjects with schizophrenia compared with control subjects (Howes et al. 2013; Schoonover et al. 2017). TH mRNA in the substantia nigra was increased in one study (Mueller et al. 2004) but unchanged in another (Ichinose et al. 1994). Importantly, rodent studies have found no significant effect of chronic antipsychotic treatment on TH immunolabeling in the substantia nigra (Perez-Costas et al. 2012).

Although it has been studied less, evidence for cortical hypodopaminergia has also emerged. Decreased lengths of tyrosine hydroxylase–immunoreactive (TH-IR) axons and dopamine membrane transporter–positive axons in layer VI of DPFC and decreased density of TH-IR axons in the entorhinal cortex have been identified in schizophrenia (Akil et al. 1999, 2000). Research on monkeys treated chronically with haloperidol indicates that these findings were not secondary to antipsychotic medication (Akil et al. 1999). Another study found no changes in TH-IR varicosities in DPFC or ACC in schizophrenia compared with control subjects, although reductions in schizophrenia were found in several layers of ACC in antipsychotic-treated patients only (Benes et al. 1997). Consistent with these postmortem data is a PET study using the D_2/D_3 radiotracer [^{11}C]FLB457; this study found blunted capacity for dopamine release in DPFC in schizophrenia compared with control subjects (Slifstein et al. 2015). In another study using [^{11}C]NNC112, a PET ligand for the D_1 receptor, patients with schizophrenia had increased availability of D_1 receptors in the frontal cortex. This availability was strongly associated with impaired working memory function (Abi-Dargham et al. 2002). This finding was interpreted as reflecting evidence of compensatory D_1 receptor upregulation secondary to chronic hypodopaminergia in the frontal cortex.

Taken together, these imaging and postmortem studies interrogating the dopamine system in schizophrenia suggest a pattern of dopamine dysregulation that involves both cortical and subcortical areas. Although certain striatal dopamine D_2 receptor findings appear related to antipsychotic treatment, most dopamine-related abnormalities seem to represent treatment-independent, pathophysiological features of the illness.

Neurotrophins

Neurotrophins are a family of small target-derived proteins with pleiotropic functions that support normal neurodevelopment. Brain-derived neurotrophic factor (BDNF) is the most widely expressed neurotrophin in the CNS. It is of particular interest in schizophrenia given its important roles in GABAergic interneuron development (Woo and Lu 2006), synaptic plasticity, learning and memory (Poo 2001; von Bohlen Und Halbach and von Bohlen Und Halbach 2018), and maintenance of synaptic stability and neuronal integrity in the adult brain (Gorski et al. 2003).

In the frontal cortex, BDNF mRNA expression rises from infancy through adolescence and then plateaus through adulthood (Webster et al. 2002). In postmortem DPFC, mean BDNF protein level was 40% lower using Western blot analysis, and mean BDNF mRNA was 23% lower using RNase protection assay in subjects with schizophrenia compared with control subjects (Weickert et al. 2003). In addition, postmortem DPFC in 15 subjects with schizophrenia and 15 matched control subjects showed BDNF mRNA expression and its receptor tropomyosin receptor kinase B (TrkB) mRNA reduced by 28% and 27%, respectively, using in situ hybridization (Hashimoto et al. 2005). Testing the hypothesis that reduced BDNF and TrkB expression may contribute to altered GABA-related gene expression, these investigators also measured GAD_{67} mRNA and analyzed the correlation between GAD_{67} and the BDNF and TrkB expression. GAD_{67} mRNA was decreased by 28% in the schizophrenia cohort, and both BDNF mRNA and TrkB correlated with GAD_{67} mRNA in the same matched patient–control subject pairs (Hashimoto et al. 2005). The BDNF, TrkB, and GAD_{67} mRNA findings were replicated in an additional 12 matched patient–control subject pairs (Hashimoto et al. 2005). These data support a role for altered BDNF signaling in DPFC in schizophrenia, in particular contributing to the evidence for deficits in GABAergic interneurons. The findings show consistent reductions in cortical BDNF levels that correlate with GABAergic deficits and suggest a pathophysiological role underlying alterations in cortical circuitry and cognitive impairment in people with schizophrenia.

Peripheral BDNF has also been assessed in patients with schizophrenia as a potential marker of CNS expression. Although it remains unclear whether peripheral BDNF levels accurately reflect cortical BDNF, studies have measured BDNF protein in blood. A meta-analysis across 1,114 patients with schizophrenia and 970 age-matched healthy control subjects found significantly lower BDNF levels in patients with schizophrenia, with a moderate effect size (Hedges $g=-0.594$, $P=0.001$) and overall moderate quality of evidence (Green et al. 2011). Several small studies have also found concordant reductions of BDNF in CSF and plasma in drug-naïve patients with first-episode psychosis (Pillai et al. 2010) and significantly lower BDNF in PFC and CSF from the same subjects (Issa et al. 2010). Replication studies with larger numbers of subjects comparing plasma and CSF BDNF levels are needed to provide reliable evidence that peripheral BDNF levels accurately represent central BDNF.

Conclusion

The neuropathology of schizophrenia is subtle, and pathognomonic lesions are lacking. Usually, even when certain findings are generally well accepted, one or more studies have reported opposite or negative results. Nevertheless, converging lines of investigation increasingly identify schizophrenia as a disorder of synaptic dysconnectivity that in turn adversely impacts broad areas of brain circuitry. Most postmortem studies find no reduction in overall cortical neuronal numbers in patients with schizophrenia, and there is an absence of gliosis that might otherwise indicate a neurodegenerative process. However, numerous studies demonstrate reductions in presynaptic and postsynaptic marker proteins and mRNA together with significant reductions in dendritic arborization and dendritic spine density. Whether these findings indicate an entirely neurodevelopmental origin or the result, in part, of atrophy or degeneration remains uncertain. Emerging research implicates activated microglial functioning and changes in other immune-related processes, which may have important pathophysiological consequences. Several consistent neurochemical deficits have been identified, including dopaminergic and GABAergic changes. Although not as well defined, evidence of glutamatergic deficits that broadly supports the integrated glutamate-dopamine hypothesis of schizophrenia is also emerging. The genetic basis for schizophrenia is highly complex and appears related to numerous genes, each with small effect (Schizophrenia Working Group of the Psychiatric Genomics Consortium 2014). Although the neurobiological functions of most of these genes are not well understood, it is notable that genes related to glutamatergic and immune function appear overrepresented. Understanding how specific genetic polymorphisms may contribute to etiopathogenic mechanisms that can account for the regional, cellular, and molecular diversity of neuropathological findings in schizophrenia represents one of the major challenges that lie ahead for the field.

References

Abdul-Monim Z, Neill JC, Reynolds GP: Sub-chronic psychotomimetic phencyclidine induces deficits in reversal learning and alterations in parvalbumin-immunoreactive expression in the rat. J Psychopharmacol 21(2):198–205, 2007 17329300

Abi-Dargham A, Moore H: Prefrontal DA transmission at D1 receptors and the pathology of schizophrenia. Neuroscientist 9(5):404–416, 2003 14580124

Abi-Dargham A, Gil R, Krystal J, et al: Increased striatal dopamine transmission in schizophrenia: confirmation in a second cohort. Am J Psychiatry 155(6):761–767, 1998 9619147

Abi-Dargham A, Rodenhiser J, Printz D, et al: Increased baseline occupancy of D2 receptors by dopamine in schizophrenia. Proc Natl Acad Sci USA 97(14):8104–8109, 2000 10884434

Abi-Dargham A, Mawlawi O, Lombardo I, et al: Prefrontal dopamine D1 receptors and working memory in schizophrenia. J Neurosci 22(9):3708–3719, 2002 11978847

Akbarian S, Bunney WE Jr, Potkin SG, et al: Altered distribution of nicotinamide-adenine dinucleotide phosphate-diaphorase cells in frontal lobe of schizophrenics implies disturbances of cortical development. Arch Gen Psychiatry 50(3):169–177, 1993a 7679891

Akbarian S, Viñuela A, Kim JJ, et al: Distorted distribution of nicotinamide-adenine dinucleotide phosphate-diaphorase neurons in temporal lobe of schizophrenics implies anomalous cortical development. Arch Gen Psychiatry 50(3):178–187, 1993b 7679892

Akbarian S, Kim JJ, Potkin SG, et al: Gene expression for glutamic acid decarboxylase is reduced without loss of neurons in prefrontal cortex of schizophrenics. Arch Gen Psychiatry 52(4):258–266, 1995 7702443

Akbarian S, Kim JJ, Potkin SG, et al: Maldistribution of interstitial neurons in prefrontal white matter of the brains of schizophrenic patients. Arch Gen Psychiatry 53(5):425–436, 1996a 8624186

Akbarian S, Sucher NJ, Bradley D, et al: Selective alterations in gene expression for NMDA receptor subunits in prefrontal cortex of schizophrenics. J Neurosci 16(1):19–30, 1996b 8613785

Akil M, Lewis DA: Cytoarchitecture of the entorhinal cortex in schizophrenia. Am J Psychiatry 154(7):1010–1012, 1997 9210754

Akil M, Pierri JN, Whitehead RE, et al: Lamina-specific alterations in the dopamine innervation of the prefrontal cortex in schizophrenic subjects. Am J Psychiatry 156(10):1580–1589, 1999 10518170

Akil M, Edgar CL, Pierri JN, et al: Decreased density of tyrosine hydroxylase-immunoreactive axons in the entorhinal cortex of schizophrenic subjects. Biol Psychiatry 47(5):361–370, 2000 10704948

Arnold SE, Hyman BT, Van Hoesen GW, et al: Some cytoarchitectural abnormalities of the entorhinal cortex in schizophrenia. Arch Gen Psychiatry 48(7):625–632, 1991 2069493

Arnold SE, Franz BR, Gur RC, et al: Smaller neuron size in schizophrenia in hippocampal subfields that mediate cortical-hippocampal interactions. Am J Psychiatry 152(5):738–748, 1995 7726314

Arnold SE, Ruscheinsky DD, Han LY: Further evidence of abnormal cytoarchitecture of the entorhinal cortex in schizophrenia using spatial point pattern analyses. Biol Psychiatry 42(8):639–647, 1997 9325556

Arnold SE, Trojanowski JQ, Gur RE, et al: Absence of neurodegeneration and neural injury in the cerebral cortex in a sample of elderly patients with schizophrenia. Arch Gen Psychiatry 55(3):225–232, 1998 9510216

Barbeau D, Liang JJ, Robitalille Y, et al: Decreased expression of the embryonic form of the neural cell adhesion molecule in schizophrenic brains. Proc Natl Acad Sci USA 92(7):2785–2789, 1995 7708724

Benes FM: Emerging principles of altered neural circuitry in schizophrenia. Brain Res Brain Res Rev 31(2–3):251–269, 2000 10719152

Benes FM, Davidson J, Bird ED: Quantitative cytoarchitectural studies of the cerebral cortex of schizophrenics. Arch Gen Psychiatry 43(1):31–35, 1986 3942472

Benes FM, McSparren J, Bird ED, et al: Deficits in small interneurons in prefrontal and cingulate cortices of schizophrenic and schizoaffective patients. Arch Gen Psychiatry 48(11):996–1001, 1991a 1747023

Benes FM, Sorensen I, Bird ED: Reduced neuronal size in posterior hippocampus of schizophrenic patients. Schizophr Bull 17(4):597–608, 1991b 1805353

Benes FM, Todtenkopf MS, Taylor JB: Differential distribution of tyrosine hydroxylase fibers on small and large neurons in layer II of anterior cingulate cortex of schizophrenic brain. Synapse 25(1):80–92, 1997 8987151

Benes FM, Kwok EW, Vincent SL, et al: A reduction of nonpyramidal cells in sector CA2 of schizophrenics and manic depressives. Biol Psychiatry 44(2):88–97, 1998 9646890

Benes FM, Todtenkopf MS, Logiotatos P, et al: Glutamate decarboxylase(65)-immunoreactive terminals in cingulate and prefrontal cortices of schizophrenic and bipolar brain. J Chem Neuroanat 20(3–4):259–269, 2000 11207424

Benes FM, Vincent SL, Todtenkopf M: The density of pyramidal and nonpyramidal neurons in anterior cingulate cortex of schizophrenic and bipolar subjects. Biol Psychiatry 50(6):395–406, 2001 11566156

Bitanihirwe BK, Lim MP, Kelley JF, et al: Glutamatergic deficits and parvalbumin-containing inhibitory neurons in the prefrontal cortex in schizophrenia. BMC Psychiatry 9:71, 2009 19917116

Black JE, Klintsova AY, Kodish IM, et al: What is missing in the reduced neuropil of schizophrenic prefrontal cortex? A combined Golgi and electron microscopy study. Biol Psychiatry 51(8):54S, 2002

Bloomfield PS, Selvaraj S, Veronese M, et al: Microglial activity in people at ultra high risk of psychosis and in schizophrenia: an [(11)C]PBR28 PET brain imaging study. Am J Psychiatry 173(1):44–52, 2016 26472628

Braun I, Genius J, Grunze H, et al: Alterations of hippocampal and prefrontal GABAergic interneurons in an animal model of psychosis induced by NMDA receptor antagonism. Schizophr Res 97(1–3):254–263, 2007 17601703

Byne W, Buchsbaum MS, Mattiace LA, et al: Postmortem assessment of thalamic nuclear volumes in subjects with schizophrenia. Am J Psychiatry 159(1):59–65, 2002 11772691

Costa E, Davis J, Grayson DR, et al: Dendritic spine hypoplasticity and downregulation of reelin and GABAergic tone in schizophrenia vulnerability. Neurobiol Dis 8(5):723–742, 2001 11592844

Cotter DR, Pariante CM, Everall IP: Glial cell abnormalities in major psychiatric disorders: the evidence and implications. Brain Res Bull 55(5):585–595, 2001 11576755

Coughlin JM, Wang Y, Ambinder EB, et al: In vivo markers of inflammatory response in recent-onset schizophrenia: a combined study using [(11)C]DPA-713 PET and analysis of CSF and plasma. Transl Psychiatry 6:e777, 2016 27070405

Cullen TJ, Walker MA, Parkinson N, et al: A postmortem study of the mediodorsal nucleus of the thalamus in schizophrenia. Schizophr Res 60(2–3):157–166, 2003 12591579

Cunningham MO, Hunt J, Middleton S, et al: Region-specific reduction in entorhinal gamma oscillations and parvalbumin-immunoreactive neurons in animal models of psychiatric illness. J Neurosci 26(10):2767–2776, 2006 16525056

Damadzic R, Bigelow LB, Krimer LS, et al: A quantitative immunohistochemical study of astrocytes in the entorhinal cortex in schizophrenia, bipolar disorder and major depression: absence of significant astrocytosis. Brain Res Bull 55(5):611–618, 2001 11576757

Datta D, Arion D, Corradi JP, et al: Altered expression of CDC42 signaling pathway components in cortical layer 3 pyramidal cells in schizophrenia. Biol Psychiatry 78(11):775–785, 2015 25981171

de la Fuente-Sandoval C, León-Ortiz P, Favila R, et al: Higher levels of glutamate in the associative-striatum of subjects with prodromal symptoms of schizophrenia and patients with first-episode psychosis. Neuropsychopharmacology 36(9):1781–1791, 2011 21508933

de la Fuente-Sandoval C, León-Ortiz P, Azcárraga M, et al: Glutamate levels in the associative striatum before and after 4 weeks of antipsychotic treatment in first-episode psychosis: a longitudinal proton magnetic resonance spectroscopy study. JAMA Psychiatry 70(10):1057–1066, 2013 23966023

de la Fuente-Sandoval C, Reyes-Madrigal F, Mao X, et al: Cortico-striatal GABAergic and glutamatergic dysregulations in subjects at ultra-high risk for psychosis investigated with proton magnetic resonance spectroscopy. Int J Neuropsychopharmacol 19(3):pyv105, 2015 26364273

Dorph-Petersen KA, Pierri JN, Sun Z, et al: Stereological analysis of the mediodorsal thalamic nucleus in schizophrenia: volume, neuron number, and cell types. J Comp Neurol 472(4):449–462, 2004 15065119

Eastwood SL, Harrison PJ: Hippocampal synaptic pathology in schizophrenia, bipolar disorder and major depression: a study of complexin mRNAs. Mol Psychiatry 5(4):425–432, 2000 10889554

Eastwood SL, Harrison PJ: Decreased expression of vesicular glutamate transporter 1 and complexin II mRNAs in schizophrenia: further evidence for a synaptic pathology affecting glutamate neurons. Schizophr Res 73(2–3):159–172, 2005 15653259

Eastwood SL, Burnet PW, Harrison PJ: Altered synaptophysin expression as a marker of synaptic pathology in schizophrenia. Neuroscience 66(2):309–319, 1995 7477874

Elston GN, Rosa MG: The occipitoparietal pathway of the macaque monkey: comparison of pyramidal cell morphology in layer III of functionally related cortical visual areas. Cereb Cortex 7(5):432–452, 1997 9261573

Ford JM, Krystal JH, Mathalon DH: Neural synchrony in schizophrenia: from networks to new treatments. Schizophr Bull 33(4):848–852, 2007 17567628

Gabbott PL, Bacon SJ: Local circuit neurons in the medial prefrontal cortex (areas 24a,b,c, 25 and 32) in the monkey, I: cell morphology and morphometrics. J Comp Neurol 364(4):567–608, 1996 8821449

Gabriel SM, Haroutunian V, Powchik P, et al: Increased concentrations of presynaptic proteins in the cingulate cortex of subjects with schizophrenia. Arch Gen Psychiatry 54(6):559–566, 1997 9193197

Garey LJ, Ong WY, Patel TS, et al: Reduced dendritic spine density on cerebral cortical pyramidal neurons in schizophrenia. J Neurol Neurosurg Psychiatry 65(4):446–453, 1998 9771764

Gilabert-Juan J, Varea E, Guirado R, et al: Alterations in the expression of PSA-NCAM and synaptic proteins in the dorsolateral prefrontal cortex of psychiatric disorder patients. Neurosci Lett 530(1):97–102, 2012 23022470

Glantz LA, Lewis DA: Reduction of synaptophysin immunoreactivity in the prefrontal cortex of subjects with schizophrenia: regional and diagnostic specificity. Arch Gen Psychiatry 54(10):943–952, 1997 9337775

Glantz LA, Lewis DA: Decreased dendritic spine density on prefrontal cortical pyramidal neurons in schizophrenia. Arch Gen Psychiatry 57(1):65–73, 2000 10632234

Glausier JR, Lewis DA: Mapping pathologic circuitry in schizophrenia. Handb Clin Neurol 150:389–417, 2018 29496154

Gonzalez-Burgos G, Lewis DA: GABA neurons and the mechanisms of network oscillations: implications for understanding cortical dysfunction in schizophrenia. Schizophr Bull 34(5):944–961, 2008 18586694

Gorski JA, Zeiler SR, Tamowski S, et al: Brain-derived neurotrophic factor is required for the maintenance of cortical dendrites. J Neurosci 23(17):6856–6865, 2003 12890780

Green MJ, Matheson SL, Shepherd A, et al: Brain-derived neurotrophic factor levels in schizophrenia: a systematic review with meta-analysis. Mol Psychiatry 16(9):960–972, 2011 20733577

Greene R, Bergeron R, McCarley R, et al: Short-term and long-term effects of N-methyl-D-aspartate receptor hypofunction. Arch Gen Psychiatry 57(12):1180–1181, author reply 1182–1183, 2000 11115333

Grunze HC, Rainnie DG, Hasselmo ME, et al: NMDA-dependent modulation of CA1 local circuit inhibition. J Neurosci 16(6):2034–2043, 1996 8604048

Harrison PJ, Eastwood SL: Preferential involvement of excitatory neurons in medial temporal lobe in schizophrenia. Lancet 352(9141):1669–1673, 1998 9853440

Härtig W, Derouiche A, Welt K, et al: Cortical neurons immunoreactive for the potassium channel Kv3.1b subunit are predominantly surrounded by perineuronal nets presumed as a buffering system for cations. Brain Res 842(1):15–29, 1999 10526091

Hashimoto T, Volk DW, Eggan SM, et al: Gene expression deficits in a subclass of GABA neurons in the prefrontal cortex of subjects with schizophrenia. J Neurosci 23(15):6315–6326, 2003 12867516

Hashimoto T, Bergen SE, Nguyen QL, et al: Relationship of brain-derived neurotrophic factor and its receptor TrkB to altered inhibitory prefrontal circuitry in schizophrenia. J Neurosci 25(2):372–383, 2005 15647480

Heckers S, Heinsen H, Geiger B, et al: Hippocampal neuron number in schizophrenia: a stereological study. Arch Gen Psychiatry 48(11):1002–1008, 1991 1747014

Hill JJ, Hashimoto T, Lewis DA: Molecular mechanisms contributing to dendritic spine alterations in the prefrontal cortex of subjects with schizophrenia. Mol Psychiatry 11(6):557–566, 2006 16402129

Howes OD, Kapur S: The dopamine hypothesis of schizophrenia: version III—the final common pathway. Schizophr Bull 35(3):549–562, 2009 19325164

Howes OD, Montgomery AJ, Asselin MC, et al: Elevated striatal dopamine function linked to prodromal signs of schizophrenia. Arch Gen Psychiatry 66(1):13–20, 2009 19124684

Howes OD, Williams M, Ibrahim K, et al: Midbrain dopamine function in schizophrenia and depression: a post-mortem and positron emission tomographic imaging study. Brain 136 (Pt 11):3242–3251, 2013 24097339

Hynes RO, Yamada KM: Extracellular Matrix Biology. Cold Spring Harbor, NY, Cold Spring Harbor Laboratory Press, 2012

Ichinose H, Ohye T, Fujita K, et al: Quantification of mRNA of tyrosine hydroxylase and aromatic L-amino acid decarboxylase in the substantia nigra in Parkinson's disease and schizophrenia. J Neural Transm Park Dis Dement Sect 8(1–2):149–158, 1994 7893377

Ide M, Lewis DA: Altered cortical CDC42 signaling pathways in schizophrenia: implications for dendritic spine deficits. Biol Psychiatry 68(1):25–32, 2010 20385374

Issa G, Wilson C, Terry AV Jr, et al: An inverse relationship between cortisol and BDNF levels in schizophrenia: data from human postmortem and animal studies. Neurobiol Dis 39(3):327–333, 2010 20451611

Jacobs B, Driscoll L, Schall M: Life-span dendritic and spine changes in areas 10 and 18 of human cortex: a quantitative Golgi study. J Comp Neurol 386(4):661–680, 1997 9378859

Jakob H, Beckmann H: Prenatal developmental disturbances in the limbic allocortex in schizophrenics. J Neural Transm 65(3–4):303–326, 1986 3711886

Javitt DC, Zukin SR: Recent advances in the phencyclidine model of schizophrenia. Am J Psychiatry 148(10):1301–1308, 1991 1654746

Johnston-Wilson NL, Sims CD, Hofmann JP, et al; The Stanley Neuropathology Consortium: Disease-specific alterations in frontal cortex brain proteins in schizophrenia, bipolar disorder, and major depressive disorder. Mol Psychiatry 5(2):142–149, 2000 10822341

Joyce JN: D2 but not D3 receptors are elevated after 9 or 11 months chronic haloperidol treatment: influence of withdrawal period. Synapse 40(2):137–144, 2001 11252025

Karson CN, Mrak RE, Schluterman KO, et al: Alterations in synaptic proteins and their encoding mRNAs in prefrontal cortex in schizophrenia: a possible neurochemical basis for 'hypofrontality.' Mol Psychiatry 4(1):39–45, 1999 10089007

Kawaguchi Y: Physiological subgroups of nonpyramidal cells with specific morphological characteristics in layer II/III of rat frontal cortex. J Neurosci 15(4):2638–2655, 1995 7722619

Kegeles LS, Mao X, Stanford AD, et al: Elevated prefrontal cortex γ-aminobutyric acid and glu-
tamate-glutamine levels in schizophrenia measured in vivo with proton magnetic resonance spectroscopy. Arch Gen Psychiatry 69(5):449–459, 2012 22213769

Keilhoff G, Becker A, Grecksch G, et al: Repeated application of ketamine to rats induces
changes in the hippocampal expression of parvalbumin, neuronal nitric oxide synthase
and cFOS similar to those found in human schizophrenia. Neuroscience 126(3):591–598,
2004 15183509

Kinney JW, Davis CN, Tabarean I, et al: A specific role for NR2A-containing NMDA receptors
in the maintenance of parvalbumin and GAD67 immunoreactivity in cultured interneurons. J Neurosci 26(5):1604–1615, 2006 16452684

Kolluri N, Sun Z, Sampson AR, et al: Lamina-specific reductions in dendritic spine density in
the prefrontal cortex of subjects with schizophrenia. Am J Psychiatry 162(6):1200–1202,
2005 15930070

Konopaske GT, Lange N, Coyle JT, et al: Prefrontal cortical dendritic spine pathology in schizophrenia and bipolar disorder. JAMA Psychiatry 71(12):1323–1331, 2014 25271938

Kraeplin E: Dementia Praecox and Paraphrenia (1919). Translated by Barkley RM, Edited by
Robertson GM. Edinburgh, E. & S. Livingstone, 1971

Krimer LS, Zaitsev AV, Czanner G, et al: Cluster analysis-based physiological classification and
morphological properties of inhibitory neurons in layers 2–3 of monkey dorsolateral prefrontal cortex. J Neurophysiol 94(5):3009–3022, 2005 15987765

Krystal JH, Karper LP, Seibyl JP, et al: Subanesthetic effects of the noncompetitive NMDA antagonist, ketamine, in humans: psychotomimetic, perceptual, cognitive, and neuroendocrine responses. Arch Gen Psychiatry 51(3):199–214, 1994 8122957

Laruelle M, Jaskiw GE, Lipska BK, et al: D1 and D2 receptor modulation in rat striatum and
nucleus accumbens after subchronic and chronic haloperidol treatment. Brain Res
575(1):47–56, 1992 1387032

Lee HHC, Bernard C, Ye Z, et al: Genetic Otx2 mis-localization delays critical period plasticity
across brain regions. Mol Psychiatry 22(5):680–688, 2017 28194008

Lewis DA, Cruz DA, Melchitzky DS, et al: Lamina-specific deficits in parvalbumin-
immunoreactive varicosities in the prefrontal cortex of subjects with schizophrenia:
evidence for fewer projections from the thalamus. Am J Psychiatry 158(9):1411–1422, 2001
11532725

Lewis DA, Hashimoto T, Volk DW: Cortical inhibitory neurons and schizophrenia. Nat Rev
Neurosci 6(4):312–324, 2005 15803162

Lidow MS, Goldman-Rakic PS: A common action of clozapine, haloperidol, and remoxipride
on D1- and D2-dopaminergic receptors in the primate cerebral cortex. Proc Natl Acad Sci
USA 91(10):4353–4356, 1994 8183912

Lips ES, Cornelisse LN, Toonen RF, et al; International Schizophrenia Consortium: Functional
gene group analysis identifies synaptic gene groups as risk factor for schizophrenia. Mol
Psychiatry 17(10):996–1006, 2012 21931320

Markram H, Toledo-Rodriguez M, Wang Y, et al: Interneurons of the neocortical inhibitory system. Nat Rev Neurosci 5(10):793–807, 2004 15378039

Mauney SA, Athanas KM, Pantazopoulos H, et al: Developmental pattern of perineuronal nets
in the human prefrontal cortex and their deficit in schizophrenia. Biol Psychiatry
74(6):427–435, 2013 23790226

Mirnics K, Middleton FA, Marquez A, et al: Molecular characterization of schizophrenia
viewed by microarray analysis of gene expression in prefrontal cortex. Neuron 28(1):53–
67, 2000 11086983

Morrow BA, Elsworth JD, Roth RH: Repeated phencyclidine in monkeys results in loss of parvalbumin-containing axo-axonic projections in the prefrontal cortex. Psychopharmacology
(Berl) 192(2):283–290, 2007 17265073

Mueller HT, Haroutunian V, Davis KL, et al: Expression of the ionotropic glutamate receptor
subunits and NMDA receptor-associated intracellular proteins in the substantia nigra in
schizophrenia. Brain Res Mol Brain Res 121(1–2):60–69, 2004 14969737

Nakayama AY, Harms MB, Luo L: Small GTPases Rac and Rho in the maintenance of dendritic spines and branches in hippocampal pyramidal neurons. J Neurosci 20(14):5329–5338, 2000 10884317

Nelson MD, Saykin AJ, Flashman LA, et al: Hippocampal volume reduction in schizophrenia as assessed by magnetic resonance imaging: a meta-analytic study. Arch Gen Psychiatry 55(5):433–440, 1998 9596046

Olney JW, Farber NB: Glutamate receptor dysfunction and schizophrenia. Arch Gen Psychiatry 52(12):998–1007, 1995 7492260

Olney JW, Newcomer JW, Farber NB: NMDA receptor hypofunction model of schizophrenia. J Psychiatr Res 33(6):523–533, 1999 10628529

Osimo EF, Beck K, Reis Marques T, et al: Synaptic loss in schizophrenia: a meta-analysis and systematic review of synaptic protein and mRNA measures. Mol Psychiatry 24(4):549–561, 2019 29511299

Pakkenberg B: Pronounced reduction of total neuron number in mediodorsal thalamic nucleus and nucleus accumbens in schizophrenics. Arch Gen Psychiatry 47(11):1023–1028, 1990 2241504

Pakkenberg B: Total nerve cell number in neocortex in chronic schizophrenics and controls estimated using optical disectors. Biol Psychiatry 34(11):768–772, 1993 8292680

Pantazopoulos H, Woo T-UW, Lim MP, et al: Extracellular matrix-glial abnormalities in the amygdala and entorhinal cortex of subjects diagnosed with schizophrenia. Arch Gen Psychiatry 67(2):155–166, 2010 20124115

Perez-Costas E, Melendez-Ferro M, Rice MW, et al: Dopamine pathology in schizophrenia: analysis of total and phosphorylated tyrosine hydroxylase in the substantia nigra. Front Psychiatry 3:31, 2012 22509170

Perrone-Bizzozero NI, Sower AC, Bird ED, et al: Levels of the growth-associated protein GAP-43 are selectively increased in association cortices in schizophrenia. Proc Natl Acad Sci USA 93(24):14182–14187, 1996 8943081

Pierri JN, Chaudry AS, Woo TU, et al: Alterations in chandelier neuron axon terminals in the prefrontal cortex of schizophrenic subjects. Am J Psychiatry 156(11):1709–1719, 1999 10553733

Pierri JN, Volk CL, Auh S, et al: Decreased somal size of deep layer 3 pyramidal neurons in the prefrontal cortex of subjects with schizophrenia. Arch Gen Psychiatry 58(5):466–473, 2001 11343526

Pierri JN, Volk CL, Auh S, et al: Somal size of prefrontal cortical pyramidal neurons in schizophrenia: differential effects across neuronal subpopulations. Biol Psychiatry 54(2):111–120, 2003 12873800

Pietersen CY, Mauney SA, Kim SS, et al: Molecular profiles of pyramidal neurons in the superior temporal cortex in schizophrenia. J Neurogenet 28(1–2):53–69, 2014 24702465

Pillai A, Kale A, Joshi S, et al: Decreased BDNF levels in CSF of drug-naive first-episode psychotic subjects: correlation with plasma BDNF and psychopathology. Int J Neuropsychopharmacol 13(4):535–539, 2010 19941699

Plaven-Sigray P, Matheson GJ, Collste K, et al: Positron emission tomography studies of the glial cell marker translocator protein in patients with psychosis: a meta-analysis using individual participant data. Biol Psychiatry 84(6):433–442, 2018 29653835

Poels EM, Kegeles LS, Kantrowitz JT, et al: Glutamatergic abnormalities in schizophrenia: a review of proton MRS findings. Schizophr Res 152(2–3):325–332, 2014 24418122

Poo MM: Neurotrophins as synaptic modulators. Nat Rev Neurosci 2(1):24–32, 2001 11253356

Popken GJ, Bunney WE Jr, Potkin SG, et al: Subnucleus-specific loss of neurons in medial thalamus of schizophrenics. Proc Natl Acad Sci USA 97(16):9276–9280, 2000 10908653

Prochiantz A, Fuchs J, Di Nardo AA: Postnatal signalling with homeoprotein transcription factors. Philos Trans R Soc Lond B Biol Sci 369(1652):20130518, 2014 25135979

Purohit DP, Perl DP, Haroutunian V, et al: Alzheimer disease and related neurodegenerative diseases in elderly patients with schizophrenia: a postmortem neuropathologic study of 100 cases. Arch Gen Psychiatry 55(3):205–211, 1998 9510214

Rajkowska G, Selemon LD, Goldman-Rakic PS: Neuronal and glial somal size in the prefrontal cortex: a postmortem morphometric study of schizophrenia and Huntington disease. Arch Gen Psychiatry 55(3):215–224, 1998 9510215

Rajkowska G, Miguel-Hidalgo JJ, Makkos Z, et al: Layer-specific reductions in GFAP-reactive astroglia in the dorsolateral prefrontal cortex in schizophrenia. Schizophr Res 57(2–3):127–138, 2002 12223243

Reynolds GP, Abdul-Monim Z, Neill JC, et al: Calcium binding protein markers of GABA deficits in schizophrenia—postmortem studies and animal models. Neurotox Res 6(1):57–61, 2004 15184106

Roberts GW, Colter N, Lofthouse R, et al: Gliosis in schizophrenia: a survey. Biol Psychiatry 21(11):1043–1050, 1986 2943323

Roberts GW, Colter N, Lofthouse R, et al: Is there gliosis in schizophrenia? Investigation of the temporal lobe. Biol Psychiatry 22(12):1459–1468, 1987 3315013

Rujescu D, Bender A, Keck M, et al: A pharmacological model for psychosis based on N-methyl-D-aspartate receptor hypofunction: molecular, cellular, functional and behavioral abnormalities. Biol Psychiatry 59(8):721–729, 2006 16427029

Sawada K, Barr AM, Nakamura M, et al: Hippocampal complexin proteins and cognitive dysfunction in schizophrenia. Arch Gen Psychiatry 62(3):263–272, 2005 15753239

Schijven D, Kofink D, Tragante V, et al: Comprehensive pathway analyses of schizophrenia risk loci point to dysfunctional postsynaptic signaling. Schizophr Res 199:195–202, 2018 29653892

Schizophrenia Working Group of the Psychiatric Genomics Consortium: Biological insights from 108 schizophrenia-associated genetic loci. Nature 511(7510):421–427, 2014 25056061

Schnieder TP, Dwork AJ: Searching for neuropathology: gliosis in schizophrenia. Biol Psychiatry 69(2):134–139, 2011 21035789

Schoonover KE, McCollum LA, Roberts RC: Protein markers of neurotransmitter synthesis and release in postmortem schizophrenia substantia nigra. Neuropsychopharmacology 42(2):540–550, 2017 27550734

Schür RR, Draisma LW, Wijnen JP, et al: Brain GABA levels across psychiatric disorders: a systematic literature review and meta-analysis of (1) H-MRS studies. Hum Brain Mapp 37(9):3337–3352, 2016 27145016

Scott EK, Reuter JE, Luo L: Small GTPase Cdc42 is required for multiple aspects of dendritic morphogenesis. J Neurosci 23(8):3118–3123, 2003 12716918

Sekar A, Bialas AR, de Rivera H, et al; Schizophrenia Working Group of the Psychiatric Genomics Consortium: Schizophrenia risk from complex variation of complement component 4. Nature 530(7589):177–183, 2016 26814963

Selemon LD, Goldman-Rakic PS: The reduced neuropil hypothesis: a circuit based model of schizophrenia. Biol Psychiatry 45(1):17–25, 1999 9894571

Selemon LD, Rajkowska G, Goldman-Rakic PS: Abnormally high neuronal density in the schizophrenic cortex: a morphometric analysis of prefrontal area 9 and occipital area 17. Arch Gen Psychiatry 52(10):805–818, discussion 819–820, 1995 7575100

Selemon LD, Rajkowska G, Goldman-Rakic PS: Elevated neuronal density in prefrontal area 46 in brains from schizophrenic patients: application of a three-dimensional, stereologic counting method. J Comp Neurol 392(3):402–412, 1998 9511926

Siegert S, Seo J, Kwon EJ, et al: The schizophrenia risk gene product miR-137 alters presynaptic plasticity. Nat Neurosci 18(7):1008–1016, 2015 26005852

Slifstein M, van de Giessen E, Van Snellenberg J, et al: Deficits in prefrontal cortical and extrastriatal dopamine release in schizophrenia: a positron emission tomographic functional magnetic resonance imaging study. JAMA Psychiatry 72(4):316–324, 2015 25651194

Soltesz I: Diversity in the Neuronal Machine. New York, Oxford University Press, 2005

Spencer KM, Nestor PG, Perlmutter R, et al: Neural synchrony indexes disordered perception and cognition in schizophrenia. Proc Natl Acad Sci USA 101(49):17288–17293, 2004 15546988

Stankiewicz TR, Linseman DA: Rho family GTPases: key players in neuronal development, neuronal survival, and neurodegeneration. Front Cell Neurosci 8:314, 2014 25339865

Stark AK, Uylings HB, Sanz-Arigita E, et al: Glial cell loss in the anterior cingulate cortex, a sub-region of the prefrontal cortex, in subjects with schizophrenia. Am J Psychiatry 161(5):882–888, 2004 15121654

Stevens JR: Neuropathology of schizophrenia. Arch Gen Psychiatry 39(10):1131–1139, 1982 7125843

Thompson PM, Egbufoama S, Vawter MP: SNAP-25 reduction in the hippocampus of patients with schizophrenia. Prog Neuropsychopharmacol Biol Psychiatry 27(3):411–417, 2003 12691775

Thune JJ, Uylings HB, Pakkenberg B: No deficit in total number of neurons in the prefrontal cortex in schizophrenics. J Psychiatr Res 35(1):15–21, 2001 11287052

Trépanier MO, Hopperton KE, Mizrahi R, et al: Postmortem evidence of cerebral inflammation in schizophrenia: a systematic review. Mol Psychiatry 21(8):1009–1026, 2016 27271499

Uhlhaas PJ, Singer W: Abnormal neural oscillations and synchrony in schizophrenia. Nat Rev Neurosci 11(2):100–113, 2010 20087360

Uhlhaas PJ, Singer W: Oscillations and neuronal dynamics in schizophrenia: the search for basic symptoms and translational opportunities. Biol Psychiatry 77(12):1001–1009, 2015 25676489

Uranova NA, Vostrikov VM, Orlovskaya DD, et al: Oligodendroglial density in the prefrontal cortex in schizophrenia and mood disorders: a study from the Stanley Neuropathology Consortium. Schizophr Res 67(2–3):269–275, 2004 14984887

van Berckel BN, Bossong MG, Boellaard R, et al: Microglia activation in recent-onset schizo-phrenia: a quantitative (R)-[11C]PK11195 positron emission tomography study. Biol Psy-chiatry 64(9):820–822, 2008 18534557

Vawter MP, Howard AL, Hyde TM, et al: Alterations of hippocampal secreted N-CAM in bi-polar disorder and synaptophysin in schizophrenia. Mol Psychiatry 4(5):467–475, 1999 10523820

Volk DW, Pierri JN, Fritschy JM, et al: Reciprocal alterations in pre- and postsynaptic inhibitory markers at chandelier cell inputs to pyramidal neurons in schizophrenia. Cereb Cortex 12(10):1063–1070, 2002 12217970

von Bohlen Und Halbach O, von Bohlen Und Halbach V: BDNF effects on dendritic spine mor-phology and hippocampal function. Cell Tissue Res 373(3):729–741, 2018 29450725

Walker MA, Highley JR, Esiri MM, et al: Estimated neuronal populations and volumes of the hippocampus and its subfields in schizophrenia. Am J Psychiatry 159(5):821–828, 2002 11986137

Wang D, Fawcett J: The perineuronal net and the control of CNS plasticity. Cell Tissue Res 349(1):147–160, 2012 22437874

Wang XJ, Tegnér J, Constantinidis C, et al: Division of labor among distinct subtypes of inhibi-tory neurons in a cortical microcircuit of working memory. Proc Natl Acad Sci USA 101(5):1368–1373, 2004 14742867

Webster MJ, Weickert CS, Herman MM, et al: BDNF mRNA expression during postnatal devel-opment, maturation and aging of the human prefrontal cortex. Brain Res Dev Brain Res 139(2):139–150, 2002 12480128

Webster MJ, O'Grady J, Kleinman JE, et al: Glial fibrillary acidic protein mRNA levels in the cin-gulate cortex of individuals with depression, bipolar disorder and schizophrenia. Neuro-science 133(2):453–461, 2005 15885920

Weickert CS, Hyde TM, Lipska BK, et al: Reduced brain-derived neurotrophic factor in prefron-tal cortex of patients with schizophrenia. Mol Psychiatry 8(6):592–610, 2003 12851636

Woo NH, Lu B: Regulation of cortical interneurons by neurotrophins: from development to cognitive disorders. Neuroscientist 12(1):43–56, 2006 16394192

Woo TUW, Whitehead RE, Melchitzky DS, et al: A subclass of prefrontal gamma-aminobutyric acid axon terminals are selectively altered in schizophrenia. Proc Natl Acad Sci USA 95(9):5341–5346, 1998 9560277

Woo TUW, Walsh JP, Benes FM: Density of glutamic acid decarboxylase 67 messenger RNA-containing neurons that express the N-methyl-D-aspartate receptor subunit NR2A in the anterior cingulate cortex in schizophrenia and bipolar disorder. Arch Gen Psychiatry 61(7):649–657, 2004 15237077

Woo TUW, Kim AM, Viscidi E: Disease-specific alterations in glutamatergic neurotransmission on inhibitory interneurons in the prefrontal cortex in schizophrenia. Brain Res 1218:267–277, 2008 18534564

Yamaguchi Y: Lecticans: organizers of the brain extracellular matrix. Cell Mol Life Sci 57(2):276–289, 2000 10766023

Young CE, Arima K, Xie J, et al: SNAP-25 deficit and hippocampal connectivity in schizophrenia. Cereb Cortex 8(3):261–268, 1998 9617921

Young KA, Manaye KF, Liang C, et al: Reduced number of mediodorsal and anterior thalamic neurons in schizophrenia. Biol Psychiatry 47(11):944–953, 2000 10838062

Zaidel DW, Esiri MM, Harrison PJ: Size, shape, and orientation of neurons in the left and right hippocampus: investigation of normal asymmetries and alterations in schizophrenia. Am J Psychiatry 154(6):812–818, 1997 9167509

Zaitsev AV, Gonzalez-Burgos G, Povysheva NV, et al: Localization of calcium-binding proteins in physiologically and morphologically characterized interneurons of monkey dorsolateral prefrontal cortex. Cereb Cortex 15(8):1178–1186, 2005 15590911

Zakzanis KK, Hansen KT: Dopamine D2 densities and the schizophrenic brain. Schizophr Res 32(3):201–206, 1998 9720125

Zhang ZJ, Reynolds GP: A selective decrease in the relative density of parvalbumin-immunoreactive neurons in the hippocampus in schizophrenia. Schizophr Res 55(1–2):1–10, 2002 11955958

PART III

Treatment and
Rehabilitative Therapies

CHAPTER 8

Pharmacological and Somatic Therapies

T. Scott Stroup, M.D., M.P.H.

Diana O. Perkins, M.D., M.P.H.

Daniel C. Javitt, M.D.

Pharmacological treatments, especially antipsychotic medications, are an essential component of a comprehensive approach to the treatment of schizophrenia. Used judiciously, pharmacotherapies can greatly reduce symptoms and promote recovery. However, medications do not cure schizophrenia and can create significant burdens that may hinder personal and treatment goals. Guidelines strongly assert that treatment plans should be individualized and should integrate pharmacotherapies and psychosocial interventions (Buchanan et al. 2010; Dixon et al. 2010).

In this chapter, we discuss drugs commonly used in the treatment of schizophrenia and provide guidance for their use. The goal of pharmacological treatment of schizophrenia is to minimize symptoms and functional impairments to allow individuals to pursue personal goals. Antipsychotic drugs effectively treat positive symptoms, such as hallucinations, delusions, and disorganized speech and behavior. Antipsychotics are only partially effective for treating negative symptoms, including anhedonia, avolition, alogia, affective flattening, and social withdrawal. Antipsychotic drugs are also used to treat behavioral disturbances such as aggression and hostility and to reduce anxiety and suicidal behaviors. Anxiolytics, antidepressants, and mood stabilizers such as lithium and some antiepileptic drugs are often used as adjunctive treatments. Although cognitive impairments are common in schizophrenia and are related to functional outcomes, and are an important focus of research, there are neither drugs approved by the U.S. Food and Drug Administration (FDA) nor commonly used drugs to address this issue. After discussing antipsychotic medications and other pharmacological treatments for schizophrenia, the chapter ends with an examination of neuromodulation-based treatments that may have an increasing role in the treatment of schizophrenia.

Antipsychotic Medications

Modern drug treatment for schizophrenia dates to the early 1950s, when Deniker and Delay reported the antipsychotic effects of chlorpromazine (Healy 2002). Chlorpromazine was introduced in the United States in 1954, followed over the next three decades by several drugs, including haloperidol and perphenazine, which had similar therapeutic effects. These and all subsequent antipsychotics that are approved to treat schizophrenia block postsynaptic dopamine receptors in the brain, with the dopamine blockade in frontal cortical and limbic regions thought to account for the antipsychotic effect. Antipsychotics also interact with other neurotransmitter systems that may have therapeutic effects as well as adverse effects.

Antipsychotic medicines ameliorate psychotic symptoms such as hallucinations, delusions, and disorganized speech or behavior. The drugs reduce the intensity of the symptoms, shorten exacerbations of illness, and reduce the risk of relapse. An early landmark study led by the U.S. National Institute of Mental Health (NIMH) found that approximately 60% of the subjects who received antipsychotic drugs, as compared with 20% of placebo-treated subjects, had a nearly complete resolution of acute positive symptoms during a 6-week trial (Guttmacher 1964). Only 8% of the medication-treated subjects showed no improvement or worsened, whereas almost half of the placebo-treated subjects did not improve or worsened. Positive symptoms responded to a greater degree and more consistently than negative symptoms. The antipsychotics studied—fluphenazine, perphenazine, and thioridazine—did not differ in efficacy. Subsequent research showed that patients with schizophrenia who achieve remission and then consistently take antipsychotic drugs are about three times less likely to relapse than patients who do not take the medicines consistently (Hogarty et al. 1976).

Adverse effects were important considerations from the beginning of modern antipsychotic therapy. Rigidity, bradykinesia, and tremor resembling Parkinson's disease were particularly prominent, along with a sometimes severe restlessness known as akathisia and persistent, involuntary choreoathetoid (jerky and/or writhing) movements called tardive dyskinesia (TD). These adverse effects, together known as extrapyramidal side effects (EPS), were extremely problematic in the early decades of antipsychotic use, and TD was the source of several prominent lawsuits (Healy 2002).

In the late 1980s, clozapine, a drug first tested in the late 1950s, was shown to have greater efficacy than chlorpromazine in patients with refractory symptoms. In the critical study of clozapine in patients with treatment-resistant schizophrenia, 30% of clozapine-treated patients met response criteria compared with only 4% of chlorpromazine-treated patients (Kane et al. 1988). Clozapine was remarkable not only for its superior efficacy for patients with refractory symptoms but also for its very low risk of EPS and TD. However, clozapine had a significant risk of agranulocytosis and other life-threatening side effects that greatly limited its use.

Clozapine's unique clinical benefits and pharmacological profile led to the development of many drugs with pharmacological similarities. In particular, clozapine has prominent effects on neurotransmitter receptors other than dopamine and a different side-effect profile from that of the chlorpromazine-like drugs. The goal of drug developers was to achieve clozapine's efficacy advantages and very low risk of EPS and TD without the risk of agranulocytosis. The very low risk of EPS and TD was key to its influence on antipsychotic development in the wake of lawsuits over liability for TD (Healy 2002).

The antipsychotic drugs introduced before clozapine all block dopamine receptors and have side effects that tend to vary according to drug potency. High-potency drugs have a stronger affinity for dopamine receptors than low-potency drugs; lower dosages of the high-potency drugs achieve the same antipsychotic effect as higher dosages of low-potency drugs. Newer antipsychotics also block postsynaptic dopamine receptors. Antagonism of central serotonergic receptors and perhaps relatively loose binding to dopamine D_2 receptors are common features in their actions. The different effects of antipsychotics on dopamine receptors and on other neurotransmitter systems determine their pharmacological actions and side effects.

Although the drugs introduced after clozapine are often grouped as a class of "second-generation antipsychotics," they differ from each other in many ways (Leucht et al. 2009a, 2009c, 2009b). In general, these drugs cause fewer EPS than the drugs that came before clozapine, but there is considerable variation of this risk within both the newer and the older groups. Similarly, there is variation within and overlap between the older and newer groups in the propensity to cause sedation, anticholinergic effects, weight gain, and dyslipidemias. Therefore, when possible, we avoid the terms *first-* and *second-generation* when referring to antipsychotic medications. This decision is based on research questioning the validity and helpfulness of the distinction, as well as considerable heterogeneity within both of the groupings (Leucht et al. 2009a, 2009b). For these reasons, antipsychotics are best considered on their individual merits. Below we describe the key clinical features of selected antipsychotics that are of interest because they are in common use, represent a group of similar antipsychotics, or have been recently introduced. They are listed in the approximate order in which they were introduced for clinical use.

Low-Potency Antipsychotics

Low-potency drugs (e.g., chlorpromazine, thioridazine) have a relatively low risk of EPS, high risk of sedation, and high risk of anticholinergic (e.g., dry mouth, constipation, blurred vision) and antiadrenergic (e.g., orthostatic hypotension) side effects. Chlorpromazine, the first antipsychotic approved for use, has been available since 1954. It is effective in treating psychotic symptoms but is associated with substantial weight gain, sedation, orthostatic hypotension, anticholinergic side effects, and modest EPS when used at currently recommended dosages. The use of dosages above those recommended in Table 8–1 is not associated with better outcomes but has an increased risk of adverse effects, including TD.

Medium-Potency Antipsychotics

Medium-potency drugs (e.g., loxapine, perphenazine) tend to have a moderate risk of common side effects. For example, perphenazine, which has been available since 1958, is effective in treating psychotic symptoms but is associated with moderate hypotension and EPS when used at currently recommended dosages. The Clinical Antipsychotic Trials of Intervention Effectiveness (CATIE) study, a large clinical trial initiated by the NIMH, brought increased attention to perphenazine because it worked well and caused only moderate EPS and little or no weight gain (Lieberman

TABLE 8–1.   Selected information on commonly used antipsychotic medications

	Recommended dosage range (mg/day)	Weight/ metabolic side effects	EPS/TD	Prolactin elevation	Sedation	Anticholinergic side effects	Hypotension
Aripiprazole	10–30	–	+	–	+	–	–
Asenapine	10–20	++	++	++	++	–	+
Brexpiprazole	2–4	+	+	–	+	–	–
Cariprazine	1.5–6	+	++	–	+	–	–
Chlorpromazine	300–1,000	+++	+	++	+++	+++	+++
Clozapine	150–600	+++	–	–	+++	+++	+++
Fluphenazine	5–20	+	+++	+++	+	–	–
Haloperidol	5–20	+	+++	+++	++	–	–
Iloperidone	12–24	++	–	+	+	+	+++
Loxapine (oral)	30–100	++	++	++	++	+	+
Lurasidone	40–160	–	++	–	++	–	+
Olanzapine	10–30	+++	+	+	++	++	–
Paliperidone	6–12	++	++	+++	+	–	+
Perphenazine	12–48	++	++	++	++	–	–
Quetiapine	300–750	++	–	–	++	–	++
Risperidone	2–8	++	++	+++	+	–	++
Ziprasidone	120–160	–	+	+	+	–	+

Note.   EPS=extrapyramidal side effects; TD=tardive dyskinesia. Symbols are defined as follows: – indicates none or equivocal/occurs rarely; +indicatesmild/occurs sometimes; ++indicates moderate/occurs frequently; +++indicatessevere/occurs very frequently.

et al. 2005). The use of dosages above those recommended in Table 8–1 is not associated with better outcomes but has an increased risk of adverse effects, including TD.

High-Potency Antipsychotics

High-potency drugs (e.g., haloperidol, fluphenazine) have a high risk of EPS, moderate risk of sedation, and low risk of anticholinergic and antiadrenergic effects. Haloperidol, which has been widely used for decades, is effective in reducing schizophrenic psychopathology and in reducing acutely agitated behaviors. It is associated with a high risk of EPS but with little risk of sedation, orthostatic hypotension, weight gain, or anticholinergic side effects. Haloperidol's short-acting injections are commonly used in emergency situations when rapid effects are needed, whereas a long-acting haloperidol formulation that allows monthly injections is used when patients have trouble regularly taking oral antipsychotic medications (see Table 8–2). Because high-potency antipsychotics pose a relatively high, dose-related risk of TD, it is important to use the lowest dose that is effective in controlling symptoms (Buchanan et al. 2010).

Clozapine

Clozapine was approved for use in the United States in 1990, despite a significant risk of the potentially lethal side effect agranulocytosis, because of the medication's unique efficacy for treatment-resistant schizophrenia. The key study in clozapine's approval by the FDA found that among patients with rigorously defined treatment resistance (lack of response to at least three prior antipsychotics, with no period of good functioning in the past 5 years, then no response to haloperidol in a 6-week lead-in trial), 30% of the clozapine-treated group but only 4% of the chlorpromazine-treated group met a priori response criteria after 6 weeks. Clozapine is the most effective antipsychotic for treatment-resistant schizophrenia (Chakos et al. 2001). Additional meta-analyses comparing the effectiveness of antipsychotics have found that clozapine has the largest effect in reducing symptoms of schizophrenia (Leucht et al. 2009a, 2009c). A multiple-treatments meta-analysis of 15 antipsychotics in 212 clinical trials found clozapine to be the most efficacious (Leucht et al. 2013). The CATIE study provided additional evidence to support use of clozapine in patients with persistent symptoms (McEvoy et al. 2006). Furthermore, clozapine is effective in reducing suicidal behaviors in patients with schizophrenia or schizoaffective disorder at high risk for suicide (Meltzer et al. 2003) and in reducing hostility and aggression among patients with treatment-resistant symptoms (Chengappa et al. 2002; Citrome et al. 2001). Large observational studies of patients in real-world treatment settings have also found advantages of clozapine over other antipsychotics in reducing mortality (Tiihonen et al. 2009) and reducing hospitalization rates in patients with evidence of treatment resistance (Stroup et al. 2016).

Unfortunately, 0.5%–1% of patients taking clozapine develop agranulocytosis (Alvir et al. 1993). In the United States, this risk led to the establishment of the Clozapine Risk Evaluation and Mitigation Strategy (REMS) Program for clinicians, pharmacies, and patients. The Clozapine REMS Program provides online training that is required for clozapine prescribers and dispensing pharmacies; the program enforces requirements for monitoring of the patient's absolute neutrophil counts prior to dispensing the drug. Other serious medical risks of clozapine include seizures, which occur in up to 2% of patients, and myocarditis, which is rare but is life-threatening. Common side effects include sedation, hypotension, and tachycardia. Clozapine is associated with more weight gain and

TABLE 8–2. Long-acting antipsychotic drugs (all given intramuscularly)

	How supplied	Half-life (days)	Starting dose (mg)	Second dose (mg)	Maintenance dose (mg)
Aripiprazole (extended release)	Prefilled syringes of 300 or 400 mg		400	400 (4 weeks later)	300 or 400 every 4 weeks
Aripiprazole lauroxil	Prefilled syringes of 441, 662, 882, or 1,064 mg		441, 662, 882, or 1,064 based on prior oral dosage	After 4 weeks for 441, 662 After 4–6 weeks for 882 After 8 weeks for 1,064	Every 4 weeks for 441, 662 Every 4–6 weeks for 882 Every 8 weeks for 1,064
Fluphenazine decanoate	25 mg/mL		12.5	12.5–25 (6–14 days later)	12.5–50 every 2–3 weeks
Haloperidol decanoate	50 or 100 mg/mL	21	50	50–100 (3–28 days later)	50–200 every 3–4 weeks
Paliperidone palmitate (1-month version)	Prefilled syringes of 39, 78, 117, 156, or 234 mg	25–49	117	158 (7 days later)	39–234 every 4 weeks
Paliperidone palmitate (3-month version)	Prefilled syringes of 273 mg/0.875 mL, 410 mg/1.315 mL, 546 mg/1.75 mL, or 819 mg/2.625 mL	84–139	273–819	273–819 (12 weeks later)	273–819 every 12 weeks
Risperidone microspheres	Prepared packages of 12.5, 25, 37.5, or 50 mg	3–6	25	25–50 (2 weeks later)	25–50 every 2 weeks
Olanzapine pamoate	Prepared packages of 210, 300, or 405 mg	30	210–300	210–300 (2 weeks later)	150–300 every 2 weeks or 300–405 every 4 weeks

higher risk of glucose and lipid abnormalities than most other antipsychotic drugs (American Diabetes Association et al. 2004). Nevertheless, because of its efficacy in reducing refractory positive symptoms, with virtually no acute EPS or TD, clozapine represents a unique and important treatment option for severely ill patients for whom adequate medical supervision is available. Importantly, clozapine provided the impetus for the development of other antipsychotic drugs and hope for better outcomes.

Because clozapine is the only available medication for treatment-resistant schizophrenia, a trial should last at least 12 weeks at an effective dosage. Clinical benefits may continue to accrue for up to 12 months. Clozapine should be continued as a maintenance treatment if it is effective. However, because of its side effects and the need for continued white blood cell monitoring, if after a substantial trial of 6 months clozapine does not offer advantages over previous treatments, then it should be slowly discontinued and replaced with a new or previously helpful treatment.

Risperidone

Risperidone is a widely used antipsychotic that has been available in the United States since 1994. At typical dosages (2–6 mg/day), risperidone has a relatively low risk of EPS, but this risk increases at higher dosages. Risperidone frequently causes serum prolactin elevation and sometimes leads to weight gain, glucose abnormalities, and lipid abnormalities. Risperidone occasionally causes orthostatic hypotension. A long-acting, injectable microsphere formulation of risperidone for injection every 2 weeks is available to help enhance treatment adherence.

Paliperidone

Paliperidone, 9-hydroxy-risperidone, is an active metabolite of risperidone that is available in a once-daily oral preparation and injectable preparations that can be given monthly or every 3 months. Its pharmacological profile is similar to risperidone's, but paliperidone appears to cause somewhat more prolactin elevation at typical dosages. It is not extensively metabolized in the liver and thus may be suitable for individuals with hepatic impairment. The monthly long-acting injectable formulation is given every 4 weeks following two initial injections 1 week apart, without a need for supplementation by an oral antipsychotic medication. An every-3-months version of paliperidone is available for people who have been adequately treated on a stable dose of the monthly formulation.

Olanzapine

Olanzapine was approved by the FDA as a treatment for schizophrenia in 1996. Olanzapine frequently causes sedation and weight gain at therapeutic dosages and is thought to cause more glucose and lipid abnormalities than do all other antipsychotics except clozapine (American Diabetes Association et al. 2004). Olanzapine does not increase prolactin levels. Olanzapine has a low risk of causing EPS. The association of olanzapine with weight gain and adverse metabolic effects is so significant that the evidence-based Schizophrenia Patient Outcomes Research Team (PORT) treatment recommendations excluded olanzapine as a first-line choice for individuals experiencing a first episode of psychosis (Buchanan et al. 2010).

Olanzapine is also available as an extended-release intramuscular suspension (olanzapine pamoate) that can be administered every 2 or 4 weeks. Patients receiving this formulation are at risk for a postinjection delirium/sedation syndrome. As a result, patients must be observed in a registered health care facility for at least 3 hours after each injection.

Quetiapine

Quetiapine was approved for use as a treatment for schizophrenia in the United States in 1997. Because of a half-life of only 6 hours, doses of quetiapine should be given two or three times daily, although once-daily dosing may be feasible (Chengappa et al. 2003). A once-daily, sustained-release oral preparation is also available. At recommended dosages, quetiapine causes no elevation in prolactin levels and few or no EPS. It often causes sedation and sometimes leads to hypotension, weight gain, and lipid and glucose abnormalities. Because of its sedative properties, quetiapine is sometimes selected for patients with prominent insomnia.

Ziprasidone

Ziprasidone causes little or no weight gain, a feature that distinguishes it from most other antipsychotics. With a half-life of 7 hours, it is recommended as a twice-daily drug. Administration with food enhances absorption; because of the substantial food effects on absorption, ziprasidone should be taken with meals. Unlike other antipsychotics, it very rarely causes sedation. Ziprasidone rarely causes EPS (except possibly akathisia). It is rarely associated with glucose or lipid abnormalities but sometimes causes prolactin elevations.

Initial FDA approval of ziprasidone was delayed because clinical trial data showed that it delayed cardiac repolarization, as measured by the QT interval on electrocardiograms (ECGs). The FDA issued a warning about QT prolongation and instructed prescribers to avoid coadministration with other QT-prolonging drugs and to avoid prescribing ziprasidone to patients with histories of, or at significant risk for, cardiac arrhythmias. The FDA did not, however, require pretreatment ECGs. Clinical use over several years now indicates that ziprasidone can be safely used with attention to current labeling related to QT prolongation.

Lurasidone

Lurasidone has demonstrated efficacy for positive and negative symptoms of schizophrenia (Loebel et al. 2013; Nasrallah et al. 2013). Lurasidone has low risk of weight gain, lipid abnormalities, and hence metabolic syndrome. However, lurasidone is associated with akathisia, especially at higher dosages, as well as nausea.

The absorption of lurasidone is reduced by 50% if the medication is not taken with at least 350 kilocalories of fat (Preskorn et al. 2013). Therefore, to avoid rapid changes in blood levels and the consequential impact on efficacy and side effects, patients should be instructed either to always take lurasidone with a meal or to always take lurasidone on an empty stomach. Because strong cytochrome P450 3A inhibitors or inducers alter the metabolism of lurasidone, their concomitant use is not recommended (Chiu et al. 2014).

Aripiprazole

Unlike antipsychotics that preceded it, aripiprazole has partial agonist activity at D_2 receptors. This has the theoretical advantage of agonist activity when dopamine levels are relatively low and antagonist activity when dopamine levels are high (Lieberman 2004).

Of the common antipsychotic side effects, only occasional or mild sedation results from use of aripiprazole. The medication is very rarely associated with weight gain, glucose or lipid abnormalities, or hypotension. Aripiprazole sometimes causes akathisia or an akathisia-like syndrome, and other forms of EPS, including TD, may occur but are not common. Headache, insomnia, and nausea early in treatment are relatively more common for aripiprazole than for other antipsychotics.

Two different long-acting injectable versions of aripiprazole are available. One is for use every 4 weeks and the other for every 4–8 weeks depending on dosage.

Brexpiprazole

Brexpiprazole, like aripiprazole, has partial agonist activity at D_2 receptors. It is also a partial agonist at the serotonin 5-HT_{1A} receptor. Brexpiprazole sometimes causes sedation and EPS but rarely causes prolactin elevation, anticholinergic effects, or hypotension.

Cariprazine

Cariprazine also has partial agonist activity at D_2 receptors. In addition, cariprazine has partial agonist activity at D_3 and 5-HT_{1A} receptors. Side effects include EPS and somnolence. Cariprazine rarely causes prolactin elevation, anticholinergic effects, or hypotension. One study found that compared with risperidone, cariprazine had more benefit for negative symptoms (Németh et al. 2017).

Iloperidone

Iloperidone has low risk of EPS and prolactin elevation but significant risk of orthostatic hypotension. Because of the risk of orthostatic hypotension during the initial treatment period, a slow titration schedule is recommended to achieve the recommended target dose after 1 week. Iloperidone is associated with QT prolongation similar in magnitude to that of ziprasidone and therefore should not be prescribed to patients also taking other QT-prolonging drugs or to those at significant risk for cardiac arrhythmias or with electrolyte disturbances.

Asenapine

Asenapine is only available as sublingual dissolvable tablets because it has very poor bioavailability if swallowed. The recommended starting dose (5 mg twice daily) is the same as the target dose for treating schizophrenia. In clinical trials, asenapine was associated with weight gain, EPS (particularly akathisia), oral hypoesthesia, and dizziness (presumed to be orthostatic hypotension).

Pimavanserin

Pimavanserin is approved for the treatment of psychosis associated with Parkinson's disease. Pimavanserin is a selective serotonin inverse agonist of serotonin 5-HT_{2A} receptors. (Inverse agonists induce the opposite effect of agonists.) It is not approved for treatment of schizophrenia but is under study as an adjunctive treatment of schizophrenia.

Drugs in Development

Additional investigational new drugs that use other putative therapeutic mechanisms are in various stages of clinical development. Such novel treatments are needed and offer considerable hope for greater treatment effects and chances for recovery, but an accounting of the relative benefits and risks of all of the possible treatments in the pipeline would be premature. Currently, all available information is from studies designed and reported by the drugs' developers.

Common Antipsychotic Side Effects and Management Recommendations

The benefits of antipsychotic medications must be weighed against their risks; realizing the benefits of antipsychotics requires working with patients to minimize the risks. Key prescribing principles to minimize problems due to side effects include soliciting patient preferences in treatment selection and using the lowest effective dose of medication. If an adverse effect is medically dangerous or life-threatening (e.g., myocarditis or neuroleptic malignant syndrome [NMS]), then the medication should be stopped while the medical condition is assessed and managed. Subsequent resumption of treatment with the same antipsychotic or a different one requires careful consideration and monitoring.

For routine management of adverse effects, we recommend the following series of approaches: 1) lower the dose or adjust the dosing schedule; 2) change to an antipsychotic with a different side-effect profile; 3) consider behavioral interventions; and, finally, 4) use concomitant medications to treat the adverse effect. Because side effects and individual responses vary, not all of these options are available for all situations. In addition, the preferred order of response may vary according to the specific side effect and an individual's preference (Stroup and Gray 2018).

Extrapyramidal Side Effects

Each type of extrapyramidal side effect has a characteristic time of onset. Akathisia typically occurs a few hours to days after medication administration, dystonia within the first few days, and parkinsonism within a few days to weeks after starting a new drug or after a dosage increase (Casey 1993). TD and tardive dystonia by definition occur only after prolonged exposure to antipsychotic medications. The risk of EPS varies considerably across drugs (see Table 8–1), but high-potency antipsychotics (e.g., haloperidol, fluphenazine) are more likely than other antipsychotics to cause EPS when the drugs are used at usual therapeutic dosages.

Akathisia.   Akathisia refers to a subjective feeling of restlessness often accompanied by almost constant movements, usually in the legs or feet. Severe akathisia can be diagnosed when a patient paces frequently, has restless foot movements, or is unable to sit still. Akathisia must be differentiated from psychotic agitation, which is often a response to disturbing hallucinations or delusions, but also may represent hostility related to acute psychosis or increased motor activity associated with excited catatonia. Patients who experience milder akathisia may not have any evidence of increased motor activity but may experience an unpleasant sensation of restlessness. Patients should be monitored for akathisia when starting a new antipsychotic drug or when the dosage is increased. Severe akathisia has been associated with an increased risk of suicidal behaviors. If symptoms of schizophrenia are adequately treated, lowering the antipsychotic dosage is a feasible first approach to reducing akathisia. Another common approach is to change to an antipsychotic less likely to cause akathisia. Drug treatments for akathisia include β-blockers, anticholinergic agents, and benzodiazepines, and vitamin B_6 is also used (Pringsheim et al. 2018). The comparative effectiveness of the various medication treatments for akathisia is unknown, but benzodiazepines are not the first choice because of an association with increased mortality among people with schizophrenia.

Drug-induced parkinsonism.   Drug-induced parkinsonism typically includes the classic Parkinson's disease symptoms of tremor, muscular rigidity, and a decrease in spontaneous movements (bradykinesia). It may include cognitive slowing, decreased facial expressiveness, and diminished arm swing. Recognition and management of parkinsonism are important because it is frequently associated with poor adherence to antipsychotic medication regimens (Perkins 2002; Robinson et al. 2002). The initial approach to parkinsonian side effects is to lower the dosage of antipsychotic, especially with the newer antipsychotics because the optimally effective dosage is typically lower than the dosage that induces parkinsonism. Another option is to change to an antipsychotic less likely to cause parkinsonism. Anticholinergic medications such as benztropine or trihexyphenidyl effectively treat parkinsonism but have their own adverse effects, including dry mouth, constipation, and cognitive impairment.

Dystonias.   Dystonias are intermittent or sustained muscular spasms and abnormal postures. Common forms of dystonia include abnormal positioning of the neck (torticollis), impaired swallowing (dysphagia), hypertonic or enlarged tongue, and deviations of the eyes (oculogyric crisis). These reactions usually appear within the first few days of treatment with antipsychotic drugs and sometimes occur within minutes to hours. Dystonic reactions can be painful and dramatic. They occur most commonly with high-potency antipsychotics, particularly when the medications are given in substantial doses (e.g., haloperidol 5–10 mg) to drug-naïve patients. For this reason, prophylactic treatment with benztropine 1–2 mg is recommended when a patient starts taking high-potency antipsychotics at these substantial doses, as may be required in emergency situations. The antihistamine antiemetic promethazine provided at a dose of 50 mg intramuscularly has also been shown to prevent acute dystonic reactions when given with intramuscular haloperidol, although use of promethazine in this way is not common practice in the United States (Huff et al. 2007; Raveendran et al. 2007). Acute dystonic reactions are treated with diphenhydramine 25–50 mg or benztropine 1–2 mg. Usually, these treatments are given intramuscularly to provide rapid relief from the considerable discomfort of dystonias.

Neuroleptic malignant syndrome.   NMS, another neurological side effect, is characterized by rigidity, hyperthermia, mental status changes, and autonomic instability. NMS has a lifetime incidence of approximately 0.2% among antipsychotic users (Caroff 2003). Hyperthermia and severe muscle rigidity may lead to rhabdomyolysis and renal failure. Serum levels of creatine kinase may rise dramatically. Risk factors for NMS include rapid dose escalation of high-potency antipsychotics, parenteral administration, and underlying neurological impairment. NMS is thought to be less common with drugs that have decreased risk of EPS, but the incidence with older antipsychotics may also be decreasing because doses now commonly used are lower than in the past.

NMS can be fatal if untreated. Treatment includes discontinuation of the antipsychotic and provision of supportive care. Temperature reduction by cooling blankets if necessary and correction of fluid imbalances are crucial. Data on the effectiveness of pharmacological interventions are limited, but the dopamine agonist bromocriptine

(2.5 mg every 8 hours) and the muscle relaxant dantrolene (1–2.5 mg/kg intravenously every 6 hours) are commonly used. Benzodiazepines (e.g., lorazepam, clonazepam) may also be beneficial (Pileggi and Cook 2016). Electroconvulsive therapy (ECT) is indicated if catatonia related to NMS persists or response is otherwise inadequate with drugs and supportive care. If NMS occurs, need for an antipsychotic medication should be carefully assessed before antipsychotic treatment is resumed. When another trial of an antipsychotic drug is attempted, drugs with low risk of EPS (in particular, clozapine) are preferred. A rechallenge should begin with a low dosage of a different antipsychotic, slow titration, and careful monitoring (Pileggi and Cook 2016).

Tardive dyskinesia and other tardive syndromes.   TD is characterized by involuntary, repetitive, purposeless, hyperkinetic, abnormal movements of the mouth, face and tongue, trunk, and extremities that occur during or following the cessation of long-term antipsychotic drug therapy. According to DSM-5 (American Psychiatric Association 2013) diagnostic criteria, the abnormal movements develop after use of an antipsychotic for at least a few months. Sometimes dyskinesias occur after an antipsychotic is discontinued or the dosage is reduced; withdrawal dyskinesias are usually time-limited. Oral-facial movements occur in about three-fourths of TD patients and can include lip smacking, sucking, puckering, and grimacing. Other movements include irregular movements of the limbs, particularly choreoathetoid (jerky and/or writhing) movements of the fingers, toes, or trunk. Other late-onset syndromes include tardive dystonia and tardive akathisia.

The incidence of TD was estimated to be 4%–5% per year in nonelderly adults taking older antipsychotics, using data collected when these medications were used at relatively high dosages and before drugs with lower risk of EPS were developed (Glazer et al. 1993; Kane et al. 1985; Morgenstern and Glazer 1993). The risk may be five to six times higher in older adults, with some data suggesting that up to 29% of elderly patients who take antipsychotics will develop TD each year (Jeste et al. 1999). A systematic review of 1-year studies that grouped amisulpride, olanzapine, quetiapine, risperidone, and ziprasidone as "second-generation antipsychotics" found a lower risk of TD in patients taking these antipsychotics (annual risk=2.1%) than in patients taking the high-potency antipsychotic haloperidol at relatively high dosages (annual risk=5.2%) (Correll et al. 2004). Low- and medium-potency antipsychotics cause fewer acute EPS compared with haloperidol and may have a lower risk of TD. Clozapine-induced TD is thought to be extremely rare. Risk factors for TD include increased age, female sex, higher dosages of antipsychotics, and longer periods of treatment.

For many decades, treatment of TD has been largely unsuccessful, although patients' symptoms sometimes diminish over time. In 2017, the FDA approved valbenazine and deutetrabenazine to treat TD. These new medications have the same mechanism as tetrabenazine—vesicular monoamine transporter 2 (VMAT2) inhibition—which was approved in 2008 to treat the chorea associated with Huntington's disease (Fernandez et al. 2017; Hauser et al. 2017). Clozapine has been used to treat TD, but there have been no methodologically rigorous trials to support this practice. Even with the availability of efficacious treatments, the recommended clinical approach is to use the lowest possible dose of antipsychotic that is effective and to consider changing to a medication with lower risk of TD (i.e., an antipsychotic with low risk of EPS) if TD is present or is an important concern.

TABLE 8–3.   **Recommended monitoring schedule for individuals taking antipsychotics**

	Baseline	4 weeks	8 weeks	12 weeks	Quarterly	Annually
Personal or family history	✔					✔
Weight (body mass index)	✔	✔	✔	✔	✔	
Blood pressure	✔	✔	✔	✔	✔	
Fasting plasma glucose or hemoglobin A_{1c}	✔			✔		✔
Fasting lipid profile	✔			✔		✔

Monitoring for EPS.   Signs and symptoms of EPS should be assessed prior to starting an antipsychotic and at weekly intervals until the dose has been stabilized for at least 2 weeks (Marder et al. 2004). Although the risk of EPS varies, all antipsychotics—with the possible exception of clozapine—may cause akathisia or rigidity.

The examination for EPS includes observing patients for restlessness and inquiring whether the patient feels restless. Asking patients if they are having difficulty sitting still can be helpful. Parkinsonism is evaluated by observing the patient's gait and examining for rigidity in the elbow and wrist. Dystonias usually manifest as urgent, painful events reported by patients.

All antipsychotic treatment should include regular monitoring for TD. We recommend examining patients for TD before starting an antipsychotic and at 6-month intervals. Patients who are at high risk, including the elderly and those who are sensitive to EPS, should be examined more frequently. The Abnormal Involuntary Movement Scale (AIMS) (1988) provides instructions for examining patients as well as means for recording the results of the examination.

Metabolic Effects

Physicians prescribing antipsychotics should screen carefully and monitor patients who take antipsychotic drugs for signs of rapid weight gain or other problems that could lead to diabetes, obesity, and heart disease. Although the risk of weight gain and metabolic problems varies among medications, the importance of this problem is such that all patients taking antipsychotics should be monitored. Table 8–3 is adapted from the recommendations of experts from multiple disciplines (American Diabetes Association et al. 2004; Marder et al. 2004).

Weight gain.   Individuals with schizophrenia are more likely than the population at large to be overweight or obese (Allison et al. 1999). Antipsychotics vary widely in their association with weight gain (Leucht et al. 2013). Mental health providers should monitor and chart the body mass index (BMI: weight in kilograms divided by height in meters squared) of every patient with schizophrenia, regardless of the antipsychotic medication prescribed (Marder et al. 2004). Patients should be weighed at every visit for the first 6 months following a medication change. The relative risk of weight gain for the different antipsychotic medications should be a consideration in drug selection for patients who have a BMI >25. Interventions for patients who gain weight may include closer monitoring of weight, engagement in a weight management program, or a change in antipsychotic medication. If a patient is taking an antipsychotic medication that is associated with a high risk for weight gain, switching to a medication with less weight gain liability is an option, although it is important to consider the impact of such a change on the patient's overall clinical status (Stroup et al. 2011). Another approach is to add metformin, which appears to prevent further weight gain and may facilitate loss of antipsychotic-induced weight gain in patients with schizophrenia (Jarskog et al. 2013; Wu et al. 2008). The risks of adjunctive metformin are low, with gastrointestinal upset the most common problem. Vitamin B_{12} malabsorption is a rare consequence of metformin; thus, annual monitoring of B_{12} levels is recommended. In addition, there is some clinical trial evidence supporting the use of topiramate to counteract antipsychotic-induced weight gain (Mizuno et al. 2014).

Diabetes.   All newer (second-generation) antipsychotics are labeled with a warning that they are associated with an increased risk of hyperglycemia and diabetes. However, it is likely that all antipsychotic drugs that are associated with weight gain are also associated to some extent with an increased risk of diabetes.

Mental health practitioners should be aware of risk factors for diabetes and the symptoms of new-onset diabetes (including weight change, polyuria, and polydipsia) and should inform patients about these symptoms and monitor for their presence at regular intervals. Furthermore, a baseline measure of glucose—either a fasting glucose level or a hemoglobin A_{1c} level—should be collected for all patients before starting a new antipsychotic. This measure should be repeated after 3 months and then annually (American Diabetes Association et al. 2004; Marder et al. 2004). Patients who are gaining weight should have fasting glucose or hemoglobin A_{1c} levels monitored more frequently.

Mental health providers should ensure that patients who are diagnosed with diabetes receive follow-up with an appropriate medical provider. The patient's psychiatrist and medical care provider should communicate when medication changes are instituted that may affect the control of the patient's diabetes. If symptoms of diabetes are reported, a random blood glucose level should be collected, and if the level is elevated (≥126 if fasting or ≥200 if nonfasting), then the patient should be referred to a medical care provider.

Dyslipidemia.   Elevated levels of total cholesterol, low-density lipoprotein (LDL) cholesterol, and triglycerides may, in part, account for the high risk of coronary heart disease in schizophrenia. Prescribers should be aware of the lipid profiles of all patients with schizophrenia. If a lipid panel is not available, one should be obtained and reviewed. As noted in Table 8–3, lipid levels should be checked before medication changes, after 12 weeks, and then annually. Patients with significant abnormalities should be evaluated and then monitored by a medical care provider. The American College of Cardiology/American Heart Association Task Force on Clinical Practice Guidelines provide recommendations for management of blood cholesterol (Gundy et al. 2019).

Other Side Effects

Cardiac changes.   Antipsychotics can also cause varying amounts of sedation and postural hypotension, as noted in Table 8–1. Patients should be asked about these side effects at each visit after starting an antipsychotic until tolerance develops. If the side effects do not resolve, a dose reduction or change to an antipsychotic with a lower risk of sedation or hypotension is indicated.

Tachycardia may be a side effect of certain agents, particularly clozapine. β-Blockers are commonly used to control the heart rate of individuals with clozapine-associated tachycardia.

A patient's blood pressure and pulse should be monitored at least monthly after starting an antipsychotic until the dosage is stable. Thereafter, pulse and blood pressure should be measured quarterly.

Seizures.   Seizures are a rare side effect of antipsychotics; their occurrence with clozapine has gotten a great deal of attention. Because the risk is thought to be associated with rapid increases in clozapine blood levels, slow titration is recommended and care is needed with other changes that might affect clozapine metabolism (e.g., starting a drug that inhibits clozapine's metabolism, stopping smoking).

Prolactin changes.   Many antipsychotics, particularly high-potency antipsychotics, risperidone, paliperidone, sulpiride, and amisulpride, elevate serum prolactin levels through blockade of dopamine receptors in the anterior pituitary. Consequences may include decreased libido, anorgasmia, amenorrhea, galactorrhea, and gynecomastia. One large observational study found that dopamine receptor antagonists were associated with an increased risk of breast cancer, possibly related to elevated prolactin (Wang et al. 2002). High levels of prolactin associated with antipsychotic use may increase the risk of osteoporosis, but the precise nature of this relationship is uncertain (De Hert et al. 2016). Aripiprazole, which has agonist effects on pituitary dopamine receptors, is associated with decreases in serum prolactin levels, although the clinical significance of this effect is uncertain.

Guidelines recommend yearly monitoring of patients taking antipsychotics for symptoms of prolactin elevation, including galactorrhea, decreased libido or menstrual disturbances in women, and decreased libido or erectile or ejaculatory disturbances in men (Marder et al. 2004). Patients who are receiving an agent that is associated with prolactin elevation should be asked about symptoms of prolactin elevation at each visit after starting the agent until they are receiving a stable dose. If any symptoms of prolactin elevation are present, prolactin should be measured and, if possible, other medical causes ruled out. Antipsychotic dose reduction is one approach to prolactin elevation; consideration should also be given to switching to a non-prolactin-raising antipsychotic. The addition of aripiprazole is another approach to reducing elevated prolactin levels (Kane et al. 2009). If one of the interventions above leads to reduced signs and symptoms and the prolactin level declines to normal, an endocrine workup is not necessary. For patients with symptomatic antipsychotic-induced hyperprolactinemia, hormone replacement therapy (estrogen/progestogen for amenorrhea in women and testosterone for symptoms of testosterone deficiency in men) is an option if it is deemed important not to discontinue an antipsychotic that has been effective (Miller 2004).

Maintenance Antipsychotic Treatment and Relapse Prevention

Many studies have reported that maintenance antipsychotic treatment for schizophrenia that has responded to antipsychotic medication reduces symptom relapse and rehospitalization (Davis 1975; Kane and Lieberman 1987). A systematic review and meta-analysis of antipsychotic drugs versus placebo that examined relapse rates at 1 year in 65 randomized trials found relapse rates of 27% for antipsychotics and 64% for placebo—a risk ratio of 0.40 (Leucht et al. 2013). Hogarty and colleagues (1976) found a relapse rate of 66% within 1 year of treatment discontinuation, even among patients who had been successfully maintained in the community for 2–3 years with antipsychotic drugs. First-episode patients who meet symptom response criteria may have lower relapse rates. During the year following initial recovery, the relapse rate was 40% for patients taking placebo compared with 0% for patients taking medication (Kane et al. 1982). Furthermore, Robinson and colleagues (1999a) showed that discontinuing drug therapy increased the risk of relapse almost five times in a sample of patients with first-episode schizophrenia or schizoaffective disorder over several years of follow-up.

The benefits of maintenance antipsychotic drug treatment are tempered by the risk of long-term side effects, such as the development of TD as well as obesity, diabetes, hyperlipidemias, and other factors associated with heart disease. Targeted, intermittent antipsychotic medication strategies that involve slow titration off medication for stabilized patients and reintroduction of medication when signs or symptoms of imminent relapse occur have not been found to reduce the risk of TD and are associated with risks of symptom exacerbation and relapse (Carpenter et al. 1990; Gaebel et al. 1993; Herz et al. 1991; Jolley et al. 1990; Schooler 1993). The Schizophrenia PORT (Buchanan et al. 2010) and the American Psychiatric Association's "Practice Guideline for the Treatment of Patients With Schizophrenia" (Lehman et al. 2004b) recommend continuous maintenance treatment for all patients with chronic schizophrenia. Targeted, intermittent therapy is acceptable only for patients who cannot tolerate or will not accept continuous antipsychotic treatment.

Since the first long-term observational studies by Emil Kraepelin at the turn of the twentieth century, it has been known that even without antipsychotics, about 5% of persons with schizophrenia fully recover after a single episode of psychosis (for further details, see Chapter 2, "Natural History"). Maintenance treatment with antipsychotics has become more controversial with the publication of observational studies that similarly report that some patients with schizophrenia may not need long-term antipsychotic treatment (Harrow et al. 2012; Wunderink et al. 2013). Because it is currently impossible to predict who will be in the small subgroup of patients who do not need long-term treatment, treatment guidelines still recommend continuous treatment. If antipsychotics are, nevertheless, stopped, continued monitoring and follow-up are indicated to help identify early signs of relapse so that antipsychotic treatment can be restarted and adverse consequences of relapse can be avoided.

Choice of Antipsychotics

The antipsychotics introduced after clozapine were developed with the hope that they would lead to improved outcomes for individuals with schizophrenia, in part by reducing negative symptoms and the burden of EPS. Although advantages for clozapine have been shown in many studies, only some of the drugs that have followed have advantages in efficacy over the older antipsychotics when the older drugs are prescribed at appropriate dosages. Meta-analyses of randomized clinical trials consistently show modest advantages for clozapine and small advantages for amisulpride, olanzapine, and risperidone over other antipsychotics in reducing psychotic symptoms (Leucht et al. 2009c, 2013). Side effects vary considerably among the medications and have an impact on overall effectiveness by affecting patients' willingness to continue taking them. The most recent Schizophrenia PORT recommendations, based on exhaustive reviews of the literature, suggest that any antipsychotic other than clozapine is an appropriate treatment for people with multi-episode schizophrenia (Buchanan et al. 2010). For patients experiencing a first episode of psychosis, the Schizophrenia PORT recommendation is for any antipsychotic other than clozapine or olanzapine. Clozapine is excluded in both instances because of its risk of agranulocytosis; olanzapine is not recommended in first-episode psychosis because of its association with weight gain and other metabolic risk factors for cardiovascular disease (Buchanan et al. 2010). Beyond these recommendations in specific situations, the current recommendation is to select antipsychotics based on side-effect profiles (Goff 2014).

Antipsychotic Polypharmacy

Combining antipsychotics (polypharmacy) for schizophrenia is a common treatment strategy that has limited evidence of effectiveness (Fleischhacker and Uchida 2014; Freudenreich and Goff 2002). In the most recent systematic review of randomized clinical trials from the Cochrane Collaboration, Ortiz-Orendain et al. (2017) found that evidence regarding combining antipsychotics for schizophrenia is of very low quality but concluded that there is limited support for using combinations of antipsychotics in reducing the risk of no clinical response, particularly if clozapine is the monotherapy and is compared with clozapine plus another antipsychotic. The authors found no difference between combinations of antipsychotics and antipsychotic monotherapy in reducing hospitalizations, leaving the study early, or serious adverse events.

In general, clozapine monotherapy is preferable to antipsychotic polypharmacy for the treatment of schizophrenia that does not respond to standard antipsychotic monotherapy. Limited data are available to guide the use of specific antipsychotic combinations. However, in a large observational study from Finland, the combination of clozapine and aripiprazole was associated with lower rehospitalization rates than all other combinations of antipsychotics and all monotherapies studied (Tiihonen et al. 2019). This finding will need confirmation in other studies, preferably randomized clinical trials (Goff 2019).

Implementing and Monitoring Antipsychotic Drug Treatment

Dosing

Recommended dosage ranges for commonly used oral antipsychotics are shown in Table 8–1, earlier in this chapter. Few data support the usefulness of dosages beyond these recommendations, and a greater incidence of side effects is likely with higher dosages. During treatment of an acute episode of schizophrenia, antipsychotic drugs usually have a therapeutic effect within 1–3 weeks, with the greatest gains in the first 6–8 weeks (Davis et al. 1989). To minimize side effects, a gradual titration to the lowest antipsychotic dosage that achieves therapeutic aims is recommended. Unfortunately, the lowest effective dosage varies among individuals and must be determined empirically. The administration of large parenteral doses of antipsychotics within a 24-hour period ("rapid neuroleptization") has not shown any gains in efficacy over standard treatment and therefore is not a recommended strategy (Lehman et al. 2004a).

Evidence suggests that antipsychotic effects may begin within the first week of treatment (Agid et al. 2003). Some patients, however, may require several months to achieve a full clinical response. This also applies to first-episode patients, whose symptoms typically respond relatively rapidly to modest dosages of antipsychotic medications (Lieberman 1993). When patients' symptoms do not respond to a standard course of treatment, clinicians generally increase the dosage, switch to another antipsychotic drug, or maintain the initial treatment for an extended period. Little evidence from randomized clinical trials supports the efficacy of any of these strategies (Kinon et al. 1993; Levinson et al. 1990; Rifkin et al. 1991; Van Putten et al. 1990; Volavka et al. 1992), although an individual patient may show a better response to one particular drug than to another (Gardos 1974).

Route of Administration

Pills are the most commonly used form of antipsychotic medication and are suitable for most patients in most situations. Liquids and dissolvable tablets are useful for patients who cannot or will not swallow pills or who prefer this form. One antipsychotic is available for inhalation; inhaled loxapine is delivered by activation of an aerosol powder and must be monitored by a health care professional. Short-acting injections that are rapidly active are available for emergency treatment of agitated, psychotic patients or others in need of rapid decreases in symptoms or dangerous behavior.

Long-Acting Injectable Antipsychotic Medications

Long-acting injectable antipsychotics, also known as *depot antipsychotics*, are commonly thought to have important advantages over oral medications in some situations, although the evidence to support such advantages is limited (Buchanan et al. 2010). The primary indication for long-acting formulations is to improve adherence to antipsychotic regimens; thus, they are recommended for individuals who do not regularly take medications or who are expected not to do so. However, most persons have difficulty adhering to maintenance medication regimens, and even brief episodes of intermittent antipsychotic nonadherence are associated with increased risk of psychotic relapse (Kozma and Weiden 2009). Therefore, clinicians should consider routinely discussing the option of long-acting injectable formulations with patients and their family members, mentioning the advantage of consistent dosing as well as potential disadvantages (e.g., patient dislike of injections, injection pain, inconvenience). Table 8–2, presented earlier in this chapter, contains summary information on the long-acting injectable antipsychotics available in the United States.

Treatment Targets

The primary benefit of antipsychotics is reduction of positive psychotic symptoms, such as delusions, hallucinations, and disorganization. Antipsychotic drugs that have been approved by regulatory agencies are all superior to placebo in reducing positive symptoms. Antipsychotic drugs also reduce negative symptoms (e.g., affective flattening, alogia, avolition), but the magnitude of the effect is smaller than the effect on positive symptoms (Leucht et al. 1999), and any effect on residual negative symptoms or the deficit syndrome is small (Carpenter 1996; Kirkpatrick et al. 2000). The clearest types of negative symptoms that can be reduced with antipsychotic medicines are those secondary to positive symptoms, such as social withdrawal due to delusions or paranoia (Carpenter et al. 1988). As positive symptoms decrease in response to antipsychotic drugs, secondary negative symptoms also diminish.

Because cognitive impairments are common in schizophrenia and are strongly associated with functional outcomes, cognitive functioning is now an important focus of research and a target for drug development (Buchanan et al. 2011; Green et al. 2004). The cognitive domains under study include learning and secondary memory, motor function, verbal fluency, attention, and executive functioning. Studies of antipsychotic drugs have failed to demonstrate significant cognitive-enhancing effects of these medications, and there is no evidence to support the use of any adjunctive treatment for this purpose (Buchanan et al. 2011).

Factors Influencing Antipsychotic Response

Significant efforts are under way to identify factors associated with treatment-resistant schizophrenia because preventive measures may offer more hope than new drugs. For example, a delay in treatment of the first episode of schizophrenia (Addington et al. 2004; Kane et al. 2016; Loebel et al. 1992), known as the duration of untreated psychosis, and a delay in the treatment of acute exacerbations (May et al. 1976; Wyatt 1995) are associated with poorer clinical outcomes. Robinson and colleagues (1999b) reported that 87% of their sample of first-episode patients with schizophrenia or schizoaffective disorder responded to treatment within 1 year. Male sex, a history of obstetric complications, poorer attention at baseline, more severe hallucinations and delusions, and the development of EPS during antipsychotic treatment were associated with a significantly lower likelihood of response.

Antipsychotics in Special Populations

First-Episode Psychosis

A priority in first-episode psychosis is to reduce the duration of untreated psychosis by initiating treatment early. Another priority is to minimize adverse effects so that an individual's first exposure to potentially lifetime antipsychotic treatment is as favorable as possible. Because there is little known advantage of any specific antipsychotic medication for individuals experiencing a first psychotic episode, the recommendation is to choose an antipsychotic that is expected to minimize side effects. The Schizophrenia PORT recommends avoiding olanzapine because of potential weight gain and clozapine because of the risk of agranulocytosis (Buchanan et al. 2010). Others suggest avoiding haloperidol in this population because of its relatively high risk of neurological side effects. The recommendation to use the lowest effective dose applies to first-episode psychosis; this dose is expected to be lower in first-episode psychosis than in multi-episode schizophrenia.

Treatment-Resistant Schizophrenia

Clozapine is the treatment of choice for treatment-resistant schizophrenia and can provide enormous benefits for people who have not responded to other treatments. Because only a minority of patients with treatment-resistant schizophrenia have a good response to clozapine (Kane et al. 1988; Siskind et al. 2017), much attention has been paid to what to do when clozapine does not help sufficiently. The results of a recent observational study suggest that combining a second antipsychotic with clozapine may be helpful in this situation (Tiihonen et al. 2019), but this needs to be confirmed in prospective studies. Evidence from randomized clinical trials supports the use of adjunctive ECT for people with treatment-resistant schizophrenia who do not respond to clozapine (Lally et al. 2016).

Women of Reproductive Age

Women of reproductive age who take antipsychotic medications and wish to become pregnant should avoid medications that raise prolactin levels because elevated prolactin levels reduce the chances of conception (National Institute for Health and Care Excellence 2014). Several non-prolactin-raising antipsychotics to choose from are listed earlier in Table 8–1. An individualized risk-benefit assessment regarding the use of antipsychotic medications is recommended for women with schizophrenia who are or wish to become pregnant (Jones et al. 2014). For most of these women, the risk-benefit ratio favors continuing antipsychotics because of the risk of relapse and possible consequences of relapse for mother and child (Howard et al. 2004). Little evidence is available to guide choice of antipsychotics during pregnancy, but many experts recommend haloperidol because of decades of experience with its use. Pregnant women who are stable on an antipsychotic should continue with that treatment; switching during pregnancy is not recommended. Antipsychotics cross the placenta, but any teratogenicity is uncertain; children born to mothers with schizophrenia have an increased risk of congenital malformations, but it is unclear if any of this increased risk is due to antipsychotic medications (Hasan et al. 2015). Because antipsychotics may increase the risks of excessive weight gain and gestational diabetes, it is particularly important to monitor for these conditions in women taking an antipsychotic. In 2011, the FDA issued a safety communication about an association of antipsychotic use in pregnancy with newborn withdrawal syndromes and EPS (U.S. Food and Drug Administration 2011). Long-term effects of maternal use of antipsychotics on offspring are unknown.

For women with schizophrenia who have a newborn baby, the decision about breast-feeding should also be individualized. Because antipsychotics are present in breast milk, the possible risks of antipsychotic exposure to the newborn should be weighed against the benefits of breast-feeding to the baby and mother.

Other Pharmacological Treatments

Because antipsychotic medications often fail to resolve the full range of schizophrenic psychopathology and other common symptoms (e.g., anxiety, depression, mood instability, motor unrest), adjunctive treatments are commonly tried. Adjunctive pharmacological treatments in patients with schizophrenia have been the subject of numerous reviews (Ballon and Stroup 2013; Christison et al. 1991; Correll et al. 2017; Donaldson et al. 1983; Farmer and Blewett 1993; Johns and Thompson 1995; Lehman et al. 2004b; Lindenmayer 1995; Meltzer 1992; Rifkin 1993; Siris 1993). In this section, we summarize information on the use of benzodiazepines, antidepressants, mood stabilizers, and over-the-counter supplements to treat either symptoms of schizophrenia or common comorbid conditions.

Benzodiazepines

Although benzodiazepines have long been prescribed for patients with schizophrenia to treat anxiety, depression, or hostility, little systematic research supports their use for this purpose. The systematic review conducted by the Schizophrenia PORT and a meta-analysis conducted for the Cochrane Collaboration each determined that there is insufficient evidence to reach a conclusion about the usefulness of benzodiazepines for schizophrenia (Buchanan et al. 2010; Volz et al. 2007). More recently, evidence that adjunctive benzodiazepines may have adverse effects on mortality strongly suggests that caution is needed if benzodiazepines are considered for use in this population (Fontanella et al. 2016; Tiihonen et al. 2016).

Antidepressants

There appears to be an important role for antidepressants in the treatment of schizophrenia. Antidepressants are widely used to treat depression in individuals with schizophrenia, and there is now evidence from clinical trials that adjunctive antidepressants have benefits in reducing depressive symptoms in this population (Helfer et al. 2016). In addition, there is evidence that antidepressants may reduce negative symptoms (Galling et al. 2018). Previous concerns that antidepressants may worsen psychotic symptoms in people experiencing an acute episode (Plasky 1991) do not appear warranted. In addition, there is evidence from patient registry data in Scandinavia that antidepressants are associated with decreased risk of mortality (Tiihonen et al. 2016). A large observational study in the United States found that adjunctive antidepressants were associated with lower hospitalization rates compared with other augmentation strategies (Stroup et al. 2019).

Important practical issues must be considered when antidepressants are used in combination with clozapine. Some selective serotonin reuptake inhibitors (SSRIs)—especially fluvoxamine—inhibit the metabolism of clozapine and can cause large increases in clozapine levels that are potentially toxic. Serum clozapine levels and side effects, particularly anticholinergic side effects, should be monitored when using the combination of SSRIs and clozapine. Because bupropion and clozapine both increase the risk of seizures, this combination is not recommended.

Lithium and Antiepileptic Drugs

Lithium

Lithium is not an effective monotherapy for people with schizophrenia (Leucht et al. 2015), and there is inadequate evidence to support its use as an adjunct to antipsychotics for people with residual positive symptoms (Buchanan et al. 2010). In the Cochrane Collaboration's most current meta-analysis, lithium augmentation was associated with a higher response rate than augmentation with placebo, but this effect was nonsignificant when patients with schizoaffective disorder were excluded (Leucht et al. 2015). It remains unclear if lithium has beneficial effects on the core symptoms of schizophrenia or if any benefit is restricted to those patients with affective symptoms (Leucht et al. 2015).

Carbamazepine

Leucht and colleagues (2014) reviewed randomized clinical trials of carbamazepine as a sole treatment for schizophrenia and as an adjunct to treatment with an antipsychotic. They found no evidence to support its use as a sole treatment. They also reviewed studies that compared carbamazepine plus antipsychotics with placebo plus antipsychotics and concluded that carbamazepine should not be recommended for routine clinical use for treatment of schizophrenia or augmentation of antipsychotic treatment of schizophrenia. In clinical practice, carbamazepine is sometimes used as an adjunct to antipsychotics to treat aggressive, agitated patients, but strong evidence supporting this use is lacking.

Because of carbamazepine's ability to upregulate hepatic enzymes, plasma antipsychotic levels may be lowered when carbamazepine is used. Because of carbamazepine's risk of bone marrow toxicity, including agranulocytosis, it should not be used in combination with clozapine.

Valproate

Valproate (the active component of valproic acid and divalproex) is widely used as an adjunctive treatment for schizophrenia, but the Schizophrenia PORT concluded that there is inadequate evidence to support its use (Buchanan et al. 2010). The most recent Cochrane review of valproate for schizophrenia found evidence that adjunctive valproate may have benefits for overall clinical response and in reducing excitement and aggression but concluded that this evidence was weak and needs confirmation in randomized clinical trials that are blinded (Wang et al. 2016).

Over-the-Counter Adjunctive Pharmaceuticals

Over-the-counter supplements have undergone randomized placebo-controlled clinical trials as adjuncts to antipsychotics, motivated by molecular theories of the etiopathology of schizophrenia and interest in addressing residual symptoms. Several agents theoretically target *N*-methyl-D-aspartate (NMDA) receptor function, because dysregulation of this glutamate receptor is hypothesized to have a causal role in schizophrenia. Similarly, other agents target abnormalities observed in schizophrenia, such as oxidative stress, inflammation, and levels of certain vitamins. These etiopathological theories are discussed in further detail in Chapter 5, "Causes"; Chapter 6, "Pathophysiological Theories"; and Chapter 7, "Neurobiology." In this section, we provide a brief summary of the clinical trial literature, emphasizing evidence for safety as well as for efficacy.

NMDA Receptor Coagonists

To be activated, the NMDA receptor requires occupancy by glutamate and a co-neurotransmitter, such as D-serine or glycine. In fact, one hypothesized mechanism to explain clozapine's superiority to other antipsychotics is that clozapine inhibits the cellular reuptake of glycine, increasing glycine availability at the NMDA receptor (Javitt et al. 2005). The results of numerous clinical trials of several agents, including glycine, D-serine, D-cycloserine, sarcosine (a glycine reuptake inhibitor), and sodium benzoate (a food additive that enhances production of D-isomers), are mixed (Girgis et al. 2019). Safety concerns, especially prostate cancer risk from sarcosine (de Vogel et al. 2014; Heger et al. 2016), renal toxicity from D-serine (Iwakawa et al. 2019; Kaltenbach et al. 1979), and the difficulties posed to patients in consuming the large amount of glycine (several tablespoons) required to impact NMDA receptor function, limit adjunctive use of these agents.

N-Acetylcysteine

Oxidative damage and impaired redox status, especially involving the intracellular antioxidant glutathione, are consistent findings in schizophrenia (Do et al. 2009; Koga et al. 2016). Glutathione regulates NMDA receptor function at redox modulatory sites on the NMDA receptor as well as via regulation of glutamate levels. *N*-acetylcysteine (NAC), an orally bioavailable formulation of cysteine, is the rate-limiting amino acid in the synthesis of glutathione. These findings prompted several small NAC clinical trials with dosages ranging from 1,800 to 3,600 mg/day. The results of NAC trials are mixed, with some studies finding that NAC improves overall symptoms and negative symptoms, and perhaps cognition, especially in early-course schizophrenia patients (Berk et al. 2008; Carmeli et al. 2012; Conus et al. 2018; Farokhnia et al. 2013; Rapado-Castro et al. 2017). NAC has FDA approval to treat acetaminophen overdose and has a benign side-effect profile. Thus, although the potential benefits of adjunctive NAC to patients with schizophrenia are uncertain, there are no known health risks.

L-Theanine

L-Theanine is a natural constituent of green tea (~20–50 mg/cup). The traditional use of L-theanine is to reduce anxiety without causing sedation. Small placebo-controlled clinical trials in healthy humans similarly find that L-theanine reduces anxiety and also report improvements in attention, information processing speed, and working memory (Camfield et al. 2014; Dodd et al. 2015; White et al. 2016). L-Theanine impacts the glutamatergic system and regulates NMDA receptor function, facts that prompted investigation in schizophrenia. Two small double-blind, placebo-controlled adjunctive clinical trials of L-theanine alone (250 mg/day and 400 mg/day) (Ota et al. 2015; Ritsner et al. 2011) and a third in combination with pregnenolone (Kardashev et al. 2018) in persons with schizophrenia reported improvements in positive, activation, and anxiety symptoms; one of these trials also demonstrated improvements in sleep quality (Ota et al. 2015). Although confirmation in larger clinical trials is needed to determine efficacy in schizophrenia, it is possible that L-theanine may address residual sleep disturbances, anxiety, and positive symptoms in schizophrenia.

Folate

Several findings point toward disruptions in one-carbon metabolism (i.e., transfer of methyl groups) in schizophrenia, including results from genetic studies as well as observational studies reporting elevated homocysteine levels (Muntjewerff et al. 2006). That B vitamin folate serves as a methyl-donor in one-carbon metabolism prompted examination of the effects of folic acid supplementation in schizophrenia. A large double-blind randomized clinical trial found that folate supplementation plus vitamin B_{12} improved negative symptoms in patients with a genetic variant related to folate absorption (*FOLH1*) (Roffman et al. 2013), whereas a meta-analysis of seven studies found that addition of folate or methylfolate improved negative symptoms without genetic subtyping (Sakuma et al. 2018). A more recent trial found that benefits of L-methylfolate for negative symptoms were associated with an increase in ventromedial prefrontal cortical thickness (Roffman et al. 2018). Further studies are needed to establish benefits; however, folate supplementation to target negative symptoms in persons with schizophrenia carries no known risks.

Niacin

Symptoms of niacin (vitamin B_3) deficiency (pellagra) include psychosis, and there are consistent findings of abnormal skin flush response to niacin in patients with schizophrenia (Messamore 2018). However, randomized double-blind clinical trials with niacin failed to indicate benefit for patients with schizophrenia (Hoffer 1971).

Vitamin D

A critical step in the synthesis of vitamin D takes place in the skin and requires exposure to sunlight. For various reasons (e.g., sunscreen use, limited sun exposure), vitamin D insufficiency or deficiency is extremely common (Holick 2017). In the general population, the lower the vitamin D level, the greater the risk for a variety of health problems, including inflammation, metabolic syndrome, cardiovascular disease, diabetes, and bone demineralization; randomized placebo-controlled trials show that normalizing vitamin D levels improves these disorders (Mirhosseini et al. 2018; Tabrizi et al. 2018a, 2018b). Studies involving subjects with schizophrenia show that vitamin D levels are correlated with negative symptom severity and cognitive impairments (Doğan Bulut et al. 2016; Graham et al. 2015). One small randomized, double-blind, placebo-controlled clinical trial of vitamin D augmentation in clozapine-treated patients found that vitamin D improved cognitive function at a trend level (Krivoy et al. 2017). At present, there is insufficient evidence regarding the clinical consequences of low vitamin D levels or the benefits of vitamin D supplementation for persons with schizophrenia. Clinicians may consider screening vitamin D levels and recommending vitamin D supplementation for patients with demonstrated insufficiency, given that vitamin D has a low risk of adverse outcomes and the potential for overall health benefits.

Omega-3 Fatty Acids

Western diets are typically low in omega-3 fatty acids, which are key constituents of cell membranes influencing multiple aspects of brain function. A variety of health problems, including metabolic syndrome, are associated with low omega-3 levels; however, a meta-analysis of clinical trials of omega-3 supplementation failed to show reductions in cardiovascular disease risk (Aung et al. 2018). Clinical trials of omega-3 supplementation in persons with schizophrenia show mixed results, although there is more consistent evidence of potential benefits in general psychopathology and mood symptoms for persons with early-course schizophrenia (Chen et al. 2015; Firth et al. 2018). One study reported that omega-3 supplementation decreased the risk of psychosis in persons with clinical high-risk (prodromal) symptoms (Amminger et al. 2010), but a second study had negative results (McGorry et al. 2017). At present, there is no evidence to support fish oil or other omega-3 supplementation in treating schizophrenia, although there are also no health concerns.

Anti-inflammatory Drugs

Schizophrenia is associated with elevations in inflammatory biomarkers, and immune dysregulation is hypothesized to contribute to etiopathology. One randomized placebo-controlled trial with adjunctive aspirin found significant improvements in general, positive, and negative symptoms (Laan et al. 2010). In addition, several adjunctive randomized placebo-controlled trials with the prescription drug celecoxib had consistent findings of improvements in general, positive, and negative symptoms (Akhondzadeh et al. 2007; Müller et al. 2002, 2010; Rapaport et al. 2005; Zheng et al. 2017). In addition, randomized placebo-controlled trials of the prescription drug minocycline (an antibiotic with anti-inflammatory effects) have shown improved negative symptoms but mixed results for positive and cognitive symptoms (Chaudhry et al. 2012; Kelly et al. 2011; Khodaie-Ardakani et al. 2014; Levkovitz et al. 2010). Although the available evidence indicates that nonspecific anti-inflammatory drugs may benefit patients with schizophrenia, there are substantial risks associated with long-term use of these drugs (e.g., gastrointestinal bleeding, cardiovascular events). Further research is needed to support use in patients with schizophrenia, especially to identify biomarkers for persons most likely to benefit and to better delineate the risk-benefit ratio.

Neuromodulation

Neuromodulation-based treatments may be divided into invasive treatments such as ECT, which requires anesthesia, and more recently developed noninvasive brain stimulation approaches, such as transcranial magnetic stimulation (TMS) and transcranial electrical stimulation (tES).

Electroconvulsive Therapy

ECT was originally developed as a treatment for catatonia, which (at the time) was viewed as a subtype of schizophrenia, but currently, it is used mostly for the treatment of depression. A 2005 Cochrane review showed significant beneficial effects of ECT compared with placebo or sham treatment for psychosis, with a number needed to treat of 6. However, there was no advantage of ECT over antipsychotic treatment (Tharyan and Adams 2005).

The use of ECT in subjects with clozapine-refractory schizophrenia was recently reviewed (Lally et al. 2016). Although only two randomized trials were included (Masoudzadeh and Khalilian 2007; Petrides et al. 2015), a meta-analysis across all available open and blinded studies found a response rate of 62%, with relatively few adverse events (Lally et al. 2016). A longer course of treatments (up to 16), however, may be needed for treatment-resistant schizophrenia than for depression. Relatively high relapse rates were also observed post-ECT, suggesting the potential need for maintenance treatment.

In DSM-5, the diagnosis of catatonia has been divorced from schizophrenia, although it may be seen in the context of schizophrenia treatment. About 20% of individuals with catatonia do not respond to treatment with benzodiazepines (Fink et al. 2016). In such individuals, especially those with life-threatening illness, ECT may be viewed as the treatment of choice.

Transcranial Magnetic Stimulation

In TMS, electrical fields are induced in the brain by a rapidly alternating magnetic field administered over the scalp. Because magnetic pulses are not attenuated by the scalp, use of magnetic stimulation permits generation of much more focal currents inside the head than is possible with ECT. Because subconvulsive stimulation levels are used, no anesthesia is required. In general, low-frequency (≤1 Hz) repetitive TMS (rTMS) is considered inhibitory, whereas high-frequency (≥5 Hz) "theta-burst" stimulation is considered excitatory. High-frequency rTMS targeting dorsolateral prefrontal cortex has FDA approval for the treatment of refractory depression.

TMS has been used most extensively in schizophrenia for treatment of persistent auditory verbal hallucinations. For this indication, low-frequency rTMS is most commonly targeted at left temporoparietal language regions. Although results have been variable, a quantitative review of studies found significant but moderate benefits, supporting potential clinical use (Slotema et al. 2014). Studies have also investigated the use of high-frequency rTMS over left dorsolateral prefrontal cortex for the treatment of persistent negative symptoms, with inconsistent but encouraging results (Lefaucheur et al. 2014). A current limitation of clinical rTMS is that it is presently guided by surface landmarks rather than underlying brain structure and function.

Transcranial Electrical Stimulation

tES incorporates both transcranial direct current stimulation (tDCS) and transcranial alternating current stimulation (tACS). In tES, low-level currents (generally 1–2 mA) are applied across the scalp and configured to target specific brain regions. The currents are thought to modulate excitability within underlying brain regions.

As with TMS, tDCS has been studied most extensively in connection to persistent auditory verbal hallucinations, for which inhibitory (cathodal) current is applied over the left temporoparietal junction. A twice-per-day, 5-day treatment course has been found to produce beneficial effects across multiple studies, although issues related to optimal populations and concurrent antipsychotic use are still being investigated (Kantrowitz et al. 2019). As with TMS, tDCS studies targeting prefrontal cortex for persistent negative symptoms are also ongoing (Brunoni et al. 2014). To date, the majority of tDCS studies have used only single cathodal and anodal electrodes (1×montage), which produce relatively widespread electrical fields. Newer approaches that use higher-density arrays to more specifically target the electrical energy may be associated with superior results.

Conclusion

There is an urgent need for better treatments for schizophrenia, a need that has gained the attention of numerous researchers and pharmaceutical companies. Many people diagnosed with schizophrenia experience substantial reductions in psychotic symptoms with currently available antipsychotics, but some patients receive little benefit. There are no established drug treatments that address negative and cognitive symptoms associated with schizophrenia. Clozapine remains the only antipsychotic known to have advantages when other antipsychotics do not work; improved access to and wider use of clozapine are public health priorities that would improve outcomes for people with schizophrenia. A growing evidence base suggests that there is a role for adjunctive antidepressant medications in patients with schizophrenia to treat symptoms of depression and negative symptoms. There are a handful of over-the-counter supplements, particularly N-acetylcysteine, L-theanine, folate, and vitamin D, with well-established safety profiles and evidence of possible efficacy as adjunctive treatments for schizophrenia from clinical trials. Although the role of other adjunctive psychotropic medications is mostly unclear, benzodiazepines are best avoided because of an increased risk of adverse outcomes, including death. Neuromodulatory treatments are under active study and remain promising. Current and ongoing research offers tremendous hope for progress that will lead to better treatments and outcomes for people with schizophrenia.

References

Abnormal Involuntary Movement Scale (AIMS). Psychopharmacol Bull 24(4):781–783, 1988 3249784

Addington J, Van Mastrigt S, Addington D: Duration of untreated psychosis: impact on 2-year outcome. Psychol Med 34(2):277–284, 2004 14982133

Agid O, Kapur S, Arenovich T, Zipursky RB: Delayed-onset hypothesis of antipsychotic action: a hypothesis tested and rejected. Arch Gen Psychiatry 60(12):1228–1235, 2003 14662555

Akhondzadeh S, Tabatabaee M, Amini H, et al: Celecoxib as adjunctive therapy in schizophrenia: a double-blind, randomized and placebo-controlled trial. Schizophr Res 90(1–3):179–185, 2007 17208413

Allison DB, Fontaine KR, Heo M, et al: The distribution of body mass index among individuals with and without schizophrenia. J Clin Psychiatry 60(4):215–220, 1999 10221280

Alvir JM, Lieberman JA, Safferman AZ, et al: Clozapine-induced agranulocytosis: incidence and risk factors in the United States. N Engl J Med 329(3):162–167, 1993 8515788

American Diabetes Association; American Psychiatric Association; American Association of Clinical Endocrinologists; et al: Consensus Development Conference on Antipsychotic Drugs and Obesity and Diabetes. J Clin Psychiatry 65(2):267–272, 2004 15003083

American Psychiatric Association: Diagnostic and Statistical Manual of Mental Disorders, 5th Edition. Arlington, VA, American Psychiatric Association, 2013

Amminger GP, Schäfer MR, Papageorgiou K, et al: Long-chain omega-3 fatty acids for indicated prevention of psychotic disorders: a randomized, placebo-controlled trial. Arch Gen Psychiatry 67(2):146–154, 2010 20124114

Aung T, Halsey J, Kromhout D, et al; Omega-3 Treatment Trialists' Collaboration: Associations of omega-3 fatty acid supplement use with cardiovascular disease risks: meta-analysis of 10 trials involving 77,917 individuals. JAMA Cardiol 3(3):225–234, 2018 29387889

Ballon J, Stroup TS: Polypharmacy for schizophrenia. Curr Opin Psychiatry 26(2):208–213, 2013 23318662

Berk M, Copolov D, Dean O, et al: N-acetyl cysteine as a glutathione precursor for schizophrenia—a double-blind, randomized, placebo-controlled trial. Biol Psychiatry 64(5):361–368, 2008 18436195

Brunoni AR, Shiozawa P, Truong D, et al: Understanding tDCS effects in schizophrenia: a systematic review of clinical data and an integrated computation modeling analysis. Expert Rev Med Devices 11(4):383–394, 2014 24754366

Buchanan RW, Kreyenbuhl J, Kelly DL, et al; Schizophrenia Patient Outcomes Research Team (PORT): The 2009 Schizophrenia PORT psychopharmacological treatment recommendations and summary statements. Schizophr Bull 36(1):71–93, 2010 19955390

Buchanan RW, Keefe RS, Umbricht D, et al: The FDA-NIMH-MATRICS guidelines for clinical trial design of cognitive-enhancing drugs: What do we know 5 years later? Schizophre Bull 37(6):1209–1217, 2011 20410237

Camfield DA, Stough C, Farrimond J, et al: Acute effects of tea constituents L-theanine, caffeine, and epigallocatechin gallate on cognitive function and mood: a systematic review and meta-analysis. Nutr Rev 72(8):507–522, 2014 24946991

Carmeli C, Knyazeva MG, Cuénod M, et al: Glutathione precursor N-acetyl-cysteine modulates EEG synchronization in schizophrenia patients: a double-blind, randomized, placebo-controlled trial. PLoS One 7(2):e29341, 2012 22383949

Caroff S: Neuroleptic malignant syndrome: still a risk, but which patients may be in danger? Curr Psychiatry 2(12):36–42, 2003

Carpenter WT Jr: The treatment of negative symptoms: pharmacological and methodological issues. Br J Psychiatry Suppl (29):17–22, 1996 8733819

Carpenter WT Jr, Heinrichs DW, Wagman AM: Deficit and nondeficit forms of schizophrenia: the concept. Am J Psychiatry 145(5):578–583, 1988 3358462

Carpenter WT Jr, Hanlon TE, Heinrichs DW, et al: Continuous versus targeted medication in schizophrenic outpatients: outcome results. Am J Psychiatry 147(9):1138–1148, 1990 1974743

Casey DE: Neuroleptic-induced acute extrapyramidal syndromes and tardive dyskinesia. Psychiatr Clin North Am 16(3):589–610, 1993 8105453

Chakos M, Lieberman J, Hoffman E, et al: Effectiveness of second-generation antipsychotics in patients with treatment-resistant schizophrenia: a review and meta-analysis of randomized trials. Am J Psychiatry 158(4):518–526, 2001 11282684

Chaudhry IB, Hallak J, Husain N, et al: Minocycline benefits negative symptoms in early schizophrenia: a randomised double-blind placebo-controlled clinical trial in patients on standard treatment. J Psychopharmacol 26(9):1185–1193, 2012 22526685

Chen AT, Chibnall JT, Nasrallah HA: A meta-analysis of placebo-controlled trials of omega-3 fatty acid augmentation in schizophrenia: possible stage-specific effects. Ann Clin Psychiatry 27(4):289–296, 2015 26554370

Chengappa KN, Vasile J, Levine J, et al: Clozapine: its impact on aggressive behavior among patients in a state psychiatric hospital. Schizophr Res 53(1–2):1–6, 2002 11728832

Chengappa KN, Parepally H, Brar JS, et al: A random-assignment, double-blind, clinical trial of once- vs twice-daily administration of quetiapine fumarate in patients with schizophrenia or schizoaffective disorder: a pilot study. Can J Psychiatry 48(3):187–194, 2003 12728743

Chiu YY, Ereshefsky L, Preskorn SH, et al: Lurasidone drug-drug interaction studies: a comprehensive review. Drug Metabol Drug Interact 29(3):191–202, 2014 24825095

Christison GW, Kirch DG, Wyatt RJ: When symptoms persist: choosing among alternative somatic treatments for schizophrenia. Schizophr Bull 17(2):217–245, 1991 1679252

Citrome L, Volavka J, Czobor P, et al: Effects of clozapine, olanzapine, risperidone, and haloperidol on hostility among patients with schizophrenia. Psychiatr Serv 52(11):1510–1514, 2001 11684748

Conus P, Seidman LJ, Fournier M, et al: N-acetylcysteine in a double-blind randomized placebo-controlled trial: toward biomarker-guided treatment in early psychosis. Schizophr Bull 44(2):317–327, 2018 29462456

Correll CU, Leucht S, Kane JM: Lower risk for tardive dyskinesia associated with second-generation antipsychotics: a systematic review of 1-year studies. Am J Psychiatry 161(3):414–425, 2004 14992963

Correll CU, Rubio JM, Inczedy-Farkas G, et al: Efficacy of 42 pharmacologic cotreatment strategies added to antipsychotic monotherapy in schizophrenia: systematic overview and quality appraisal of the meta-analytic evidence. JAMA Psychiatry 74(7):675–684, 2017 28514486

Davis JM: Overview: maintenance therapy in psychiatry, I: schizophrenia. Am J Psychiatry 132(12):1237–1245, 1975 914

Davis JM, Barter JT, Kane JM (eds): Antipsychotic Drugs. Baltimore, MD, Williams & Wilkins, 1989

De Hert M, Detraux J, Stubbs B: Relationship between antipsychotic medication, serum prolactin levels and osteoporosis/osteoporotic fractures in patients with schizophrenia: a critical literature review. Expert Opin Drug Saf 15(6):809–823, 2016 26986209

de Vogel S, Ulvik A, Meyer K, et al: Sarcosine and other metabolites along the choline oxidation pathway in relation to prostate cancer—a large nested case-control study within the JANUS cohort in Norway. Int J Cancer 134(1):197–206, 2014 23797698

Dixon LB, Dickerson F, Bellack AS, et al; Schizophrenia Patient Outcomes Research Team (PORT): The 2009 Schizophrenia PORT psychosocial treatment recommendations and summary statements. Schizophr Bull 36(1):48–70, 2010 19955389

Do KQ, Cabungcal JH, Frank A, et al: Redox dysregulation, neurodevelopment, and schizophrenia. Curr Opin Neurobiol 19(2):220–230, 2009 19481443

Dodd FL, Kennedy DO, Riby LM, et al: A double-blind, placebo-controlled study evaluating the effects of caffeine and L-theanine both alone and in combination on cerebral blood flow, cognition and mood. Psychopharmacology (Berl) 232(14):2563–2576, 2015 25761837

Doğan Bulut S, Bulut S, Görkem Atalan D, et al: The relationship between symptom severity and low vitamin D levels in patients with schizophrenia. PLoS One 11(10):e0165284, 2016 27788194

Donaldson SR, Gelenberg AJ, Baldessarini RJ: The pharmacologic treatment of schizophrenia: a progress report. Schizophr Bull 9(4):504–527, 1983 6140750

Farmer AE, Blewett A: Drug treatment of resistant schizophrenia: limitations and recommendations. Drugs 45(3):374–383, 1993 7682908

Farokhnia M, Azarkolah A, Adinehfar F, et al: N-acetylcysteine as an adjunct to risperidone for treatment of negative symptoms in patients with chronic schizophrenia: a randomized, double-blind, placebo-controlled study. Clin Neuropharmacol 36(6):185–192, 2013 24201233

Fernandez HH, Factor SA, Hauser RA, et al: Randomized controlled trial of deutetrabenazine for tardive dyskinesia: the ARM-TD study. Neurology 88(21):2003–2010, 2017 28446646

Fink M, Kellner CH, McCall WV: Optimizing ECT technique in treating catatonia. J ECT 32(3):149–150, 2016 27428478

Firth J, Rosenbaum S, Ward PB, et al: Adjunctive nutrients in first-episode psychosis: a systematic review of efficacy, tolerability and neurobiological mechanisms. Early Interv Psychiatry 12(5):774–783, 2018 29561067

Fleischhacker WW, Uchida H: Critical review of antipsychotic polypharmacy in the treatment of schizophrenia. Int J Neuropsychopharmacol 17(7):1083–1093, 2014 22717078

Fontanella CA, Campo JV, Phillips GS, et al: Benzodiazepine use and risk of mortality among patients with schizophrenia: a retrospective longitudinal study. J Clin Psychiatry 77(5):661–667, 2016 27249075

Freudenreich O, Goff DC: Antipsychotic combination therapy in schizophrenia: a review of efficacy and risks of current combinations. Acta Psychiatr Scand 106(5):323–330, 2002 12366465

Gaebel W, Frick U, Kopcke W, et al: Early neuroleptic intervention in schizophrenia: are prodromal symptoms valid predictors of relapse? Br J Psychiatry Suppl (21):8–12, 1993 8105814

Galling B, Vernon JA, Pagsberg AK, et al: Efficacy and safety of antidepressant augmentation of continued antipsychotic treatment in patients with schizophrenia. Acta Psychiatr Scand 137(3):187–205, 2018 29431197

Gardos G: Are antipsychotic drugs interchangeable? J Nerv Ment Dis 159(5):343–348, 1974 4612111

Girgis RR, Zoghbi AW, Javitt DC, et al: The past and future of novel, non-dopamine-2 receptor therapeutics for schizophrenia: a critical and comprehensive review. J Psychiatr Res 108:57–83, 2019 30055853

Glazer WM, Morgenstern H, Doucette JT: Predicting the long-term risk of tardive dyskinesia in outpatients maintained on neuroleptic medications. J Clin Psychiatry 54(4):133–139, 1993 8098030

Goff DC: Maintenance treatment with long-acting injectable antipsychotics: comparing old with new. JAMA 311(19):1973–1974, 2014 24846032

Goff DC: Can adjunctive pharmacotherapy reduce hospitalization in schizophrenia? Insights from administrative databases. JAMA Psychiatry Feb 20, 2019 [Epub ahead of print] 30785617

Graham KA, Keefe RS, Lieberman JA, et al: Relationship of low vitamin D status with positive, negative and cognitive symptom domains in people with first-episode schizophrenia. Early Interv Psychiatry 9(5):397–405, 2015 24612563

Green MF, Nuechterlein KH, Gold JM, et al: Approaching a consensus cognitive battery for clinical trials in schizophrenia: the NIMH-MATRICS conference to select cognitive domains and test criteria. Biol Psychiatry 56(5):301–307, 2004 15336511

Grundy SM, Stone NJ, Bailey AL, et al: 2018 AHA/ACC/AACVPR/AAPA/ABC/ACPM/ADA/AGS/APhA/ASPC/NLA/PCNA Guideline on the Management of Blood Cholesterol: Executive Summary: a report of the American College of Cardiology/American Heart Association Task Force on Clinical Practice Guidelines. J Am Coll Cardiol 73(24):3168–3209, 2019 30423391

Guttmacher MS: Phenothiazine treatment in acute schizophrenia; effectiveness: the National Institute of Mental Health Psychopharmacology Service Center Collaborative Study Group. Arch Gen Psychiatry 10:246–261, 1964 14089354

Harrow M, Jobe TH, Faull RN: Do all schizophrenia patients need antipsychotic treatment continuously throughout their lifetime? A 20-year longitudinal study. Psychol Med 42(10):2145–2155, 2012 22340278

Hasan A, Falkai P, Wobrock T; WFSBP Task Force on Treatment Guidelines for Schizophrenia: World Federation of Societies of Biological Psychiatry (WFSBP) Guidelines for Biological Treatment of Schizophrenia, Part 3: Update 2015 Management of special circumstances: depression, suicidality, substance use disorders and pregnancy and lactation. World J Biol Psychiatry 16(3):142–170, 2015 25822804

Hauser RA, Factor SA, Marder SR, et al: KINECT 3: a phase 3 randomized, double-blind, placebo-controlled trial of valbenazine for tardive dyskinesia. Am J Psychiatry 174(5):476–484, 2017 28320223

Healy D: The Creation of Psychopharmacology. Cambridge, MA, Harvard University Press, 2002

Heger Z, Merlos Rodrigo MA, Michalek P, et al: Sarcosine up-regulates expression of genes involved in cell cycle progression of metastatic models of prostate cancer. PLoS One 11(11):e0165830, 2016 27824899

Helfer B, Samara MT, Huhn M, et al: Efficacy and safety of antidepressants added to antipsychotics for schizophrenia: a systematic review and meta-analysis. Am J Psychiatry 173(9):876–886, 2016 27282362

Herz MI, Glazer WM, Mostert MA, et al: Intermittent vs maintenance medication in schizophrenia: two-year results. Arch Gen Psychiatry 48(4):333–339, 1991 1672588

Hoffer A: Megavitamin B-3 therapy for schizophrenia. Can Psychiatr Assoc J 16(6):499–504, 1971 4947171

Hogarty GE, Ulrich RF, Mussare F, et al: Drug discontinuation among long term, successfully maintained schizophrenic outpatients. Dis Nerv Syst 37(9):494–500, 1976 971653

Holick MF: The vitamin D deficiency pandemic: approaches for diagnosis, treatment and prevention. Rev Endocr Metab Disord 18(2):153–165, 2017 28516265

Howard LM, Thornicroft G, Salmon M, Appleby L: Predictors of parenting outcome in women with psychotic disorders discharged from mother and baby units. Acta Psychiatr Scand 110(5):347–355, 2004 15458558

Huff G, Coutinho ES, Adams CE; TREC Collaborative Group: Rapid tranquillisation in psychiatric emergency settings in Brazil: pragmatic randomised controlled trial of intramuscular haloperidol versus intramuscular haloperidol plus promethazine. BMJ 335(7625):869, 2007 17954515

Iwakawa H, Makabe S, Ito T, et al: Urinary D-serine level as a predictive biomarker for deterioration of renal function in patients with atherosclerotic risk factors. Biomarkers 24(2):159–165, 2019 30252501

Jarskog LF, Hamer RM, Catellier DJ, et al; METS Investigators: Metformin for weight loss and metabolic control in overweight outpatients with schizophrenia and schizoaffective disorder. Am J Psychiatry 170(9):1032–1040, 2013 23846733

Javitt DC, Duncan L, Balla A, et al: Inhibition of system A-mediated glycine transport in cortical synaptosomes by therapeutic concentrations of clozapine: implications for mechanisms of action. Mol Psychiatry 10(3):275–287, 2005 15278098

Jeste DV, Rockwell E, Harris MJ, et al: Conventional vs. newer antipsychotics in elderly patients. Am J Geriatr Psychiatry 7(1):70–76, 1999 9919323

Johns CA, Thompson JW: Adjunctive treatments in schizophrenia: pharmacotherapies and electroconvulsive therapy. Schizophr Bull 21(4):607–619, 1995 8749888

Jolley AG, Hirsch SR, Morrison E, et al: Trial of brief intermittent neuroleptic prophylaxis for selected schizophrenic outpatients: clinical and social outcome at two years. BMJ 301(6756):837–842, 1990 2282421

Jones I, Chandra PS, Dazzan P, Howard LM: Bipolar disorder, affective psychosis, and schizophrenia in pregnancy and the post-partum period. Lancet 384(9956):1789–1799, 2014 25455249

Kaltenbach JP, Ganote CE, Carone FA: Renal tubular necrosis induced by compounds structurally related to D-serine. Exp Mol Pathol 30(2):209–214, 1979 421867

Kane J, Lieberman J (eds): Maintenance Pharmacotherapy in Schizophrenia. New York, Raven, 1987

Kane JM, Rifkin A, Quitkin F, et al: Fluphenazine vs placebo in patients with remitted, acute first-episode schizophrenia. Arch Gen Psychiatry 39(1):70–73, 1982 6275811

Kane JM, Woerner M, Lieberman J: Tardive dyskinesia: prevalence, incidence, and risk factors. Psychopharmacology Suppl 2:72–78, 1985 2860662

Kane J, Honigfeld G, Singer J, et al: Clozapine for the treatment-resistant schizophrenic: a double-blind comparison with chlorpromazine. Arch Gen Psychiatry 45(9):789–796, 1988 3046553

Kane JM, Correll CU, Goff DC, et al: A multicenter, randomized, double-blind, placebo-controlled, 16-week study of adjunctive aripiprazole for schizophrenia or schizoaffective disorder inadequately treated with quetiapine or risperidone monotherapy. J Clin Psychiatry 70(10):1348–1357, 2009 19906340

Kane JM, Robinson DG, Schooler NR, et al: Comprehensive versus usual community care for first-episode psychosis: 2-year outcomes from the NIMH RAISE Early Treatment Program. Am J Psychiatry 173(4):362–372, 2016 26481174

Kantrowitz JT, Sehatpour P, Avissar M, et al: Significant improvement in treatment resistant auditory verbal hallucinations after 5 days of double-blind, sham controlled, fronto-temporal, transcranial direct current stimulation (tDCS): a replication/extension study. Brain Stimul Mar 5, 2019 [Epub ahead of print] 30922713

Kardashev A, Ratner Y, Ritsner MS: Add-on pregnenolone with L-theanine to antipsychotic therapy relieves negative and anxiety symptoms of schizophrenia: an 8-week, randomized, double-blind, placebo-controlled trial. Clin Schizophr Relat Psychoses 12(1):31–41, 2018 26218236

Kelly DL, Vyas G, Richardson CM, et al: Adjunct minocycline to clozapine treated patients with persistent schizophrenia symptoms. Schizophr Res 133(1–3):257–258, 2011 21872445

Khodaie-Ardakani MR, Mirshafiee O, Farokhnia M, et al: Minocycline add-on to risperidone for treatment of negative symptoms in patients with stable schizophrenia: randomized double-blind placebo-controlled study. Psychiatry Res 215(3):540–546, 2014 24480077

Kinon BJ, Kane JM, Johns C, et al: Treatment of neuroleptic-resistant schizophrenic relapse. Psychopharmacol Bull 29(2):309–314, 1993 7904762

Kirkpatrick B, Kopelowicz A, Buchanan RW, et al: Assessing the efficacy of treatments for the deficit syndrome of schizophrenia. Neuropsychopharmacology 22(3):303–310, 2000 10693158

Koga M, Serritella AV, Sawa A, et al: Implications for reactive oxygen species in schizophrenia pathogenesis. Schizophr Res 176(1):52–71, 2016 26589391

Kozma CM, Weiden PJ: Partial compliance with antipsychotics increases mental health hospitalizations in schizophrenic patients: analysis of a national managed care database. Am Health Drug Benefits 2(1):31–38, 2009 25126270

Krivoy A, Onn R, Vilner Y, et al: Vitamin D supplementation in chronic schizophrenia patients treated with clozapine: a randomized, double-blind, placebo-controlled clinical trial. EBioMedicine 26:138–145, 2017 29226809

Laan W, Grobbee DE, Selten JP, et al: Adjuvant aspirin therapy reduces symptoms of schizophrenia spectrum disorders: results from a randomized, double-blind, placebo-controlled trial. J Clin Psychiatry 71(5):520–527, 2010 20492850

Lally J, Tully J, Robertson D, et al: Augmentation of clozapine with electroconvulsive therapy in treatment resistant schizophrenia: a systematic review and meta-analysis. Schizophr Res 171(1–3):215–224, 2016 26827129

Lefaucheur JP, André-Obadia N, Antal A, et al: Evidence-based guidelines on the therapeutic use of repetitive transcranial magnetic stimulation (rTMS). Clin Neurophysiol 125(11):2150–2206, 2014 25034472

Lehman AF, Kreyenbuhl J, Buchanan RW, et al: The Schizophrenia Patient Outcomes Research Team (PORT): updated treatment recommendations 2003. Schizophr Bull 30(2):193–217, 2004a 15279040

Lehman AF, Lieberman JA, Dixon LB, et al: Practice guideline for the treatment of patients with schizophrenia (second edition). Am J Psychiatry 161(2 suppl):1–56, 2004b 15000267

Leucht S, Pitschel-Walz G, Abraham D, et al: Efficacy and extrapyramidal side-effects of the new antipsychotics olanzapine, quetiapine, risperidone, and sertindole compared to conventional antipsychotics and placebo: a meta-analysis of randomized controlled trials. Schizophr Res 35(1):51–68, 1999 9988841

Leucht S, Corves C, Arbter D, et al: Second-generation versus first-generation antipsychotic drugs for schizophrenia: a meta-analysis. Lancet 373(9657):31–41, 2009a 19058842

Leucht S, Kissling W, Davis JM: Second-generation antipsychotics for schizophrenia: can we resolve the conflict? Psychol Med 39(10):1591–602, 2009b 19335931

Leucht S, Komossa K, Rummel-Kluge C, et al: A meta-analysis of head-to-head comparisons of second-generation antipsychotics in the treatment of schizophrenia. Am J Psychiatry 166(2):152–163, 2009c 19015230

Leucht S, Cipriani A, Spineli L, et al: Comparative efficacy and tolerability of 15 antipsychotic drugs in schizophrenia: a multiple-treatments meta-analysis. Lancet 382(9896):951–962, 2013 23810019

Leucht S, Helfer B, Dold M, et al: Carbamazepine for schizophrenia. Cochrane Database Syst Rev (5):CD001258, 2014 24789267

Leucht S, Helfer B, Dold M, et al: Lithium for schizophrenia. Cochrane Database Syst Rev (10):CD003834, 2015 26509923

Levinson DF, Simpson GM, Singh H, et al: Fluphenazine dose, clinical response, and extrapyramidal symptoms during acute treatment. Arch Gen Psychiatry 47(8):761–768, 1990 2378547

Levkovitz Y, Mendlovich S, Riwkes S, et al: A double-blind, randomized study of minocycline for the treatment of negative and cognitive symptoms in early phase schizophrenia. J Clin Psychiatry 71(2):138–149, 2010 19895780

Lieberman JA: Prediction of outcome in first-episode schizophrenia. J Clin Psychiatry 54(suppl):13–17, 1993 8097192

Lieberman JA: Dopamine partial agonists: a new class of antipsychotic. CNS Drugs 18(4):251–267, 2004 15015905

Lieberman JA, Stroup TS, McEvoy JP, et al; Clinical Antipsychotic Trials of Intervention Effectiveness (CATIE) Investigators: Effectiveness of antipsychotic drugs in patients with chronic schizophrenia. N Engl J Med 353(12):1209–1223, 2005 16172203

Lindenmayer JP: New pharmacotherapeutic modalities for negative symptoms in psychosis. Acta Psychiatr Scand Suppl 388:15–19, 1995 7541598

Loebel AD, Lieberman JA, Alvir JM, et al: Duration of psychosis and outcome in first-episode schizophrenia. Am J Psychiatry 149(9):1183–1188, 1992 1503130

Loebel A, Cucchiaro J, Sarma K, et al: Efficacy and safety of lurasidone 80 mg/day and 160 mg/day in the treatment of schizophrenia: a randomized, double-blind, placebo- and active-controlled trial. Schizophr Res 145(1–3):101–109, 2013 23415311

Marder SR, Essock SM, Miller AL, et al: Physical health monitoring of patients with schizophrenia. Am J Psychiatry 161(8):1334–1349, 2004 15285957

Masoudzadeh A, Khalilian AR: Comparative study of clozapine, electroshock and the combination of ECT with clozapine in treatment-resistant schizophrenic patients. Pak J Biol Sci 10(23):4287–4290, 2007 19086588

May PR, Tuma AH, Yale C, et al: Schizophrenia—a follow-up study of results of treatment. Arch Gen Psychiatry 33(4):481–486, 1976 938185

McEvoy JP, Lieberman JA, Stroup TS, et al; CATIE Investigators: Effectiveness of clozapine versus olanzapine, quetiapine, and risperidone in patients with chronic schizophrenia who did not respond to prior atypical antipsychotic treatment. Am J Psychiatry 163(4):600–610, 2006 16585434

McGorry PD, Nelson B, Markulev C, et al: Effect of ω-3 polyunsaturated fatty acids in young people at ultrahigh risk for psychotic disorders: the NEURAPRO randomized clinical trial. JAMA Psychiatry 74(1):19–27, 2017 27893018

Meltzer HY: Treatment of the neuroleptic-nonresponsive schizophrenic patient. Schizophr Bull 18(3):515–542, 1992 1357741

Meltzer HY, Alphs L, Green AI, et al; International Suicide Prevention Trial Study Group: Clozapine treatment for suicidality in schizophrenia: International Suicide Prevention Trial (InterSePT). Arch Gen Psychiatry 60(1):82–91, 2003 12511175

Messamore E: The niacin response biomarker as a schizophrenia endophenotype: a status update. Prostaglandins Leukot Essent Fatty Acids 136:95–97, 2018 28688777

Miller KK: Management of hyperprolactinemia in patients receiving antipsychotics. CNS Spectr 9(8) (suppl 7):28–32, 2004 15303078

Mirhosseini N, Vatanparast H, Mazidi M, et al: Vitamin D supplementation, glycemic control, and insulin resistance in prediabetics: a meta-analysis. J Endocr Soc 2(7):687–709, 2018 29951596

Mizuno Y, Suzuki T, Nakagawa A, et al: Pharmacological strategies to counteract antipsychotic-induced weight gain and metabolic adverse effects in schizophrenia: a systematic review and meta-analysis. Schizophr Bull 40(6):1385–1403, 2014 24636967

Morgenstern H, Glazer WM: Identifying risk factors for tardive dyskinesia among long-term outpatients maintained with neuroleptic medications: results of the Yale Tardive Dyskinesia Study. Arch Gen Psychiatry 50(9):723–733, 1993 8102845

Müller N, Riedel M, Scheppach C, et al: Beneficial antipsychotic effects of celecoxib add-on therapy compared to risperidone alone in schizophrenia. Am J Psychiatry 159(6):1029–1034, 2002 12042193

Müller N, Krause D, Dehning S, et al: Celecoxib treatment in an early stage of schizophrenia: results of a randomized, double-blind, placebo-controlled trial of celecoxib augmentation of amisulpride treatment. Schizophr Res 121(1–3):118–124, 2010 20570110

Muntjewerff JW, Kahn RS, Blom HJ, den Heijer M: Homocysteine, methylenetetrahydrofolate reductase and risk of schizophrenia: a meta-analysis. Mol Psychiatry 11(2):143–149, 2006 16172608

Nasrallah HA, Silva R, Phillips D, et al: Lurasidone for the treatment of acutely psychotic patients with schizophrenia: a 6-week, randomized, placebo-controlled study. J Psychiatr Res 47(5):670–677, 2013 23421963

National Institute for Health and Care Excellence: Antenatal and Postnatal Mental Health: Clinical Management and Service Guidance (NICE Clinical Guideline 192), December 17, 2014. Available at: https://www.nice.org.uk/guidance/cg192/resources/antenatal-and-postnatal-mental-health-clinical-management-and-service-guidance-pdf-35109869806789. Accessed July 25, 2019.

Németh G, Laszlovszky I, Czobor P, et al: Cariprazine versus risperidone monotherapy for treatment of predominant negative symptoms in patients with schizophrenia: a randomised, double-blind, controlled trial. Lancet 389(10074):1103–1113, 2017 28185672

Ortiz-Orendain J, Castiello-de Obeso S, Colunga-Lozano LE, et al: Antipsychotic combinations for schizophrenia. Cochrane Database Syst Rev 6:CD009005, 2017 28658515

Ota M, Wakabayashi C, Sato N, et al: Effect of L-theanine on glutamatergic function in patients with schizophrenia. Acta Neuropsychiatr 27(5):291–296, 2015 25896423

Perkins DO: Predictors of noncompliance in patients with schizophrenia. J Clin Psychiatry 63(12):1121–1128, 2002 12523871

Petrides G, Malur C, Braga RJ, et al: Electroconvulsive therapy augmentation in clozapine-resistant schizophrenia: a prospective, randomized study. Am J Psychiatry 172(1):52–58, 2015 25157964

Pileggi DJ, Cook AM: Neuroleptic malignant syndrome. Ann Pharmacother 50(11):973–981, 2016 27423483

Plasky P: Antidepressant usage in schizophrenia. Schizophr Bull 17(4):649–657, 1991 1687176

Preskorn S, Ereshefsky L, Chiu YY, et al: Effect of food on the pharmacokinetics of lurasidone: results of two randomized, open-label, crossover studies. Hum Psychopharmacol 28(5):495–505, 2013 24014143

Pringsheim T, Gardner D, Addington D, et al: The assessment and treatment of antipsychotic-induced akathisia. Can J Psychiatry Jan 1, 2018 [Epub ahead of print] 29685069

Rapado-Castro M, Dodd S, Bush AI, et al: Cognitive effects of adjunctive N-acetyl cysteine in psychosis. Psychol Med 47(5):866–876, 2017 27894373

Rapaport MH, Delrahim KK, Bresee CJ, et al: Celecoxib augmentation of continuously ill patients with schizophrenia. Biol Psychiatry 57(12):1594–1596, 2005 15953498

Raveendran NS, Tharyan P, Alexander J, Adams CE; TREC-India II Collaborative Group: Rapid tranquillisation in psychiatric emergency settings in India: pragmatic randomised controlled trial of intramuscular olanzapine versus intramuscular haloperidol plus promethazine. BMJ 335(7625):865, 2007 17954514

Rifkin A: Pharmacologic strategies in the treatment of schizophrenia. Psychiatr Clin North Am 16(2):351–363, 1993 8101372

Rifkin A, Doddi S, Karajgi B, et al: Dosage of haloperidol for schizophrenia. Arch Gen Psychiatry 48(2):166–170, 1991 1989572

Ritsner MS, Miodownik C, Ratner Y, et al: L-theanine relieves positive, activation, and anxiety symptoms in patients with schizophrenia and schizoaffective disorder: an 8-week, randomized, double-blind, placebo-controlled, 2-center study. J Clin Psychiatry 72(1):34–42, 2011 21208586

Robinson D, Woerner MG, Alvir JM, et al: Predictors of relapse following response from a first episode of schizophrenia or schizoaffective disorder. Arch Gen Psychiatry 56(3):241–247, 1999a 10078501

Robinson DG, Woerner MG, Alvir JM, et al: Predictors of treatment response from a first episode of schizophrenia or schizoaffective disorder. Am J Psychiatry 156(4):544–549, 1999b 10200732

Robinson DG, Woerner MG, Alvir JM, et al: Predictors of medication discontinuation by patients with first-episode schizophrenia and schizoaffective disorder. Schizophr Res 57(2–3):209–219, 2002 12223252

Roffman JL, Lamberti JS, Achtyes E, et al: Randomized multicenter investigation of folate plus vitamin B12 supplementation in schizophrenia. JAMA Psychiatry 70(5):481–489, 2013 23467813

Roffman JL, Petruzzi LJ, Tanner AS, et al: Biochemical, physiological and clinical effects of l-methylfolate in schizophrenia: a randomized controlled trial. Mol Psychiatry 23(2):316–322, 2018 28289280

Sakuma K, Matsunaga S, Nomura I, et al: Folic acid/methylfolate for the treatment of psychopathology in schizophrenia: a systematic review and meta-analysis. Psychopharmacology (Berl) 235(8):2303–2314, 2018 29785555

Schooler NR: Reducing dosage in maintenance treatment of schizophrenia: review and prognosis. Br J Psychiatry Suppl (22):58–65, 1993 7906525

Siris SG: Adjunctive medication in the maintenance treatment of schizophrenia and its conceptual implications. Br J Psychiatry Suppl (22):66–78, 1993 7906526

Siskind D, Siskind V, Kisely S: Clozapine response rates among people with treatment-resistant schizophrenia: data from a systematic review and meta-analysis. Can J Psychiatry 62(11):772–777, 2017 28655284

Slotema CW, Blom JD, van Lutterveld R, et al: Review of the efficacy of transcranial magnetic stimulation for auditory verbal hallucinations. Biol Psychiatry 76(2):101–110, 2014 24315551

Stroup TS, Gray N: Management of common adverse effects of antipsychotic medications. World Psychiatry 17(3):341–356, 2018 30192094

Stroup TS, McEvoy JP, Ring KD, et al; Schizophrenia Trials Network: A randomized trial examining the effectiveness of switching from olanzapine, quetiapine, or risperidone to aripiprazole to reduce metabolic risk: comparison of antipsychotics for metabolic problems (CAMP). Am J Psychiatry 168(9):947–956, 2011 21768610

Stroup TS, Gerhard T, Crystal S, et al: Comparative effectiveness of clozapine and standard antipsychotic treatment in adults with schizophrenia. Am J Psychiatry 173(2):166–173, 2016 26541815

Stroup TS, Gerhard T, Crystal S, et al: Comparative effectiveness of adjunctive psychotropic medications in patients with schizophrenia. JAMA Psychiatry 76(5):508–515, 2019 30785609

Tabrizi R, Akbari M, Lankarani KB, et al: The effects of vitamin D supplementation on endothelial activation among patients with metabolic syndrome and related disorders: a systematic review and meta-analysis of randomized controlled trials. Nutr Metab (Lond) 15:85, 2018a 30519274

Tabrizi R, Vakili S, Lankarani KB, et al: The effects of vitamin D supplementation on markers related to endothelial function among patients with metabolic syndrome and related disorders: a systematic review and meta-analysis of clinical trials. Horm Metab Res 50(8):587–596, 2018b 30081406

Tharyan P, Adams CE: Electroconvulsive therapy for schizophrenia. Cochrane Database Syst Rev (2):CD000076, 2005 15846598

Tiihonen J, Lönnqvist J, Wahlbeck K, et al: 11-year follow-up of mortality in patients with schizophrenia: a population-based cohort study (FIN11 study). Lancet 374(9690):620–627, 2009 19595447

Tiihonen J, Mittendorfer-Rutz E, Torniainen M, et al: Mortality and cumulative exposure to antipsychotics, antidepressants, and benzodiazepines in patients with schizophrenia: an observational follow-up study. Am J Psychiatry 173(6):600–606, 2016 26651392

Tiihonen J, Taipale H, Mehtälä J, et al: Association of antipsychotic polypharmacy vs monotherapy with psychiatric rehospitalization among adults with schizophrenia. JAMA Psychiatry Feb 20, 2019 [Epub ahead of print] 30785608

U.S. Food and Drug Administration: FDA Drug Safety Communication: Antipsychotic Drug Labels Updated on Use During Pregnancy and Risk of Abnormal Muscle Movements and Withdrawal Symptoms in Newborns, February 22, 2011. Available at: https://www.fda.gov/drugs/drug-safety-and-availability/fda-drug-safety-communication-antipsychotic-drug-labels-updated-use-during-pregnancy-and-risk. Accessed July 25, 2019.

Van Putten T, Marder SR, Mintz J: A controlled dose comparison of haloperidol in newly admitted schizophrenic patients. Arch Gen Psychiatry 47(8):754–758, 1990 2378546

Volavka J, Cooper T, Czobor P, et al: Haloperidol blood levels and clinical effects. Arch Gen Psychiatry 49(5):354–361, 1992 1586270

Volz A, Khorsand V, Gillies D, Leucht S: Benzodiazepines for schizophrenia. Cochrane Database Syst Rev Jan 24;(1):CD006391 2007 17253592

Wang PS, Walker AM, Tsuang MT, et al: Dopamine antagonists and the development of breast cancer. Arch Gen Psychiatry 59(12):1147–1154, 2002 12470131

Wang Y, Xia J, Helfer B, et al: Valproate for schizophrenia. Cochrane Database Syst Rev (11):CD001258, 2016 27884042

White DJ, de Klerk S, Woods W, et al: Anti-stress, behavioural and magnetoencephalography effects of an L-theanine-based nutrient drink: a randomised, double-blind, placebo-controlled, crossover trial. Nutrients 8(1):E53, 2016 26797633

Wu RR, Zhao JP, Jin H, et al: Lifestyle intervention and metformin for treatment of antipsychotic-induced weight gain: a randomized controlled trial. JAMA 299(2):185–193, 2008 18182600

Wunderink L, Nieboer RM, Wiersma D, et al: Recovery in remitted first-episode psychosis at 7 years of follow-up of an early dose reduction/discontinuation or maintenance treatment strategy: long-term follow-up of a 2-year randomized clinical trial. JAMA Psychiatry 70(9):913–920, 2013 23824214

Wyatt RJ: Early intervention for schizophrenia: can the course of the illness be altered? Biol Psychiatry 38(1):1–3, 1995 7548467

Zheng W, Cai DB, Yang XH, et al: Adjunctive celecoxib for schizophrenia: a meta-analysis of randomized, double-blind, placebo-controlled trials. J Psychiatr Res 92:139–146, 2017 28445800

CHAPTER 9

Psychosocial and Rehabilitative Therapies

Alice Medalia, Ph.D.

Alice Saperstein, Ph.D.

Paul Grant, Ph.D.

Treatment for schizophrenia focuses on symptom remission and helping the individual attain a meaningful and valued life in the community, with maximal independence. Even when pharmacological intervention is beneficial for symptom reduction, patients often continue to struggle with successful community functioning. This phenomenon is operationalized as the low rate of good functional outcome for people with schizophrenia. Considerable research has been devoted to extricating the factors that predict functional outcome. Models indicate that cognitive impairment, motivation, and social skills all account for more of the variance in real-world functioning than do positive symptoms, yet none of these predictors are particularly responsive to medication. Recognition of the need to supplement psychopharmacological treatment has led to the development of interventions aimed at addressing the factors that contribute to poor community functioning.

The main approaches to psychosocial intervention that are used for the treatment of schizophrenia include therapies that focus on cognition (cognitive-behavioral and cognitive remediation therapies), social skills training (SST), supported employment (SE), illness management and recovery (IMR), and psychoeducation. These treatments differ in the skills and components of functional recovery that they target; the focus might be on symptom stability, independent living, work or school functioning, or social functioning. Treatments may have obvious functional targets. For example, SST is expected to impact social functioning. There may also be indirect functional benefit, such as when SST facilitates better functioning at work. For each of the approaches to psychosocial intervention, we discuss the rationale, describe the intervention, present the goals and treatment principles, summarize research supporting it as an evidence-based treatment, and consider implementation issues.

Cognitive-Behavioral Therapy

Intervention Rationale

Cognitive-behavioral therapy (CBT) is a time-limited, structured, talking therapy that focuses on the interaction between an individual's thoughts, emotions, and behavior. Cognitive-behavioral therapy for psychosis (CBTp) provides adjunctive treatment for residual psychotic symptoms, using the same principles and intervention strategies developed for depression and anxiety. Residual positive and negative symptoms are experienced by the majority of patients who adhere to pharmacological treatment (Bustillo et al. 2001). Psychotic symptoms cause distress and contribute to feeling alienated, demoralized, and stigmatized. Since the 1990s, CBTp has evolved and been tested with numerous randomized controlled trials (RCTs) with acutely and chronically ill patients in all phases of the illness. Clinical guideline development groups in Europe and North America recognize CBTp as an effective intervention for schizophrenia and a key component of a treatment approach that integrates pharmacotherapy with psychosocial services.

Description of the Intervention

CBTp is done individually or in groups, in a collaborative and accepting atmosphere, with a CBT-trained therapist who establishes links between thoughts, feelings, and actions. Although the duration and pace of therapy may vary according to each individual's need, the treatment typically consists of 16–20 weekly sessions with an option for booster sessions. CBTp entails a modification of the CBT techniques used for depression and anxiety disorders. To address primary (e.g., cognitive dysfunction, lack of insight) and secondary (e.g., stigma) effects of the illness, clinicians already versed in CBT require specialized training to provide CBTp.

CBTp proceeds in phases that typically include assessment, engagement, introduction to a cognitive conceptualization of psychotic symptoms, goal setting, normalization, critical collaborative analysis, and development of alternative explanations. The various CBTp approaches share a goal of educating patients to understand and manage their psychotic symptoms by focusing on how their thoughts and behaviors impact their emotions. For example, the ABC model developed by Ellis and Harper (1975) teaches a patient to identify *a*ctivating events, modify distorted *b*eliefs about these events, and thereby change the emotional and behavioral *c*onsequences. Socratic questioning clarifies links between the patient's emotional distress and beliefs and gently challenges illogical conclusions. In CBTp, psychotic experiences are framed within the continuum of normal experience in order to decatastrophize them and help the patient feel less stigmatized and alone. Goal setting, respect for the recovery process, and caring promote engagement and collaboration.

Goals of Cognitive-Behavioral Therapy for Psychosis and Treatment Principles

CBTp aims to reduce psychotic symptoms and the associated distress, modify negative emotions, correct dysfunctional beliefs, and ultimately improve functioning. It is

TABLE 9–1.   **Key elements of cognitive-behavioral therapy for psychosis**

Formulation of the psychotic experience using the cognitive-behavioral therapy
conceptualization of an interaction between thoughts, feelings, and behavior

Establishment of a shared goal

Education about psychosis

Normalization of psychotic experiences

Collaborative work toward goals

Practice recognizing and changing appraisals

Development and practice of different responses to activating events in and out of sessions

Time-limited treatment

used to treat residual symptoms in those individuals considered to be adequately treated with antipsychotics, to treat those with medication-resistant positive symptoms, and to treat unmedicated patients. Whereas cognitive remediation (CR), discussed in the next section, targets basic cognitive functions such as attention and processing speed, CBTp targets higher-level cognition, as manifested in beliefs and thinking patterns. Table 9–1 lists the key elements of CBTp.

Research Support

CBTp has been studied in high-risk, first-episode, and chronically ill patient samples in RCTs that used active comparators or treatment as usual. Numerous meta-analyses and systematic reviews support the therapeutic benefit of CBTp for overall symptoms; greater reduction is seen in positive than in negative symptoms. An effect size (ES) measures the magnitude of difference between a treatment group and control group. When study quality is taken into account, a small to medium therapeutic benefit emerges for a wide range of CBTp approaches and indications, with an ES of –0.33 for overall symptoms (Jauhar et al. 2014). Most studies include patients who are taking medication; CBTp has been found to reduce positive and general symptoms in outpatients with incomplete medication response (Burns et al. 2014).

Acceptability of CBTp is indicated by low dropout rates across a broad range of CBTp approaches and durations (median 14.5%; range 0%–45%) (Wykes et al. 2008). CBTp is a cost-effective treatment for people with psychotic disorders, with reduced service use offsetting CBT costs. In a study reported by Myhr and Payne (2006), greater hospital admissions in the routine care cohort were the main driver of the cost difference. Additional research is needed to explore the longer-term impact of CBTp as well as the additive effects of combining CBTp with other psychological or pharmacological interventions to delay, if not prevent, a first episode of psychosis (van der Gaag et al. 2013).

The durability of effect after treatment ends has been the subject of study and controversy. Compared with treatment as usual and other psychological therapies, CBTp administered by well-trained clinicians resulted in improvements in positive symptoms, with medium effect sizes sustained at follow-up periods, lasting on average 6 months (Burns et al. 2014). Another meta-analysis of randomized controlled CBTp trials that included follow-up assessment found delayed beneficial effects on clinical symptoms that may not always be seen immediately following intervention (Sarin et al. 2011).

Not surprisingly, response to CBTp is variable (Wykes et al. 2008). An ongoing area of investigation is the expansion of the number of patients who benefit from treatment. Understanding the factors that are predictive of positive outcome can facilitate optimization of CBTp provision. Factors identified as contributing to a better response to CBTp include female gender, older age, higher clinical insight at baseline, shorter duration of the illness, and higher educational attainment (O'Keeffe et al. 2017).

Implications for Clinical Practice

Despite national guidelines from the Schizophrenia Patient Outcomes Research Team (PORT) in the United States (Dixon et al. 2010), the National Institute for Health and Care Excellence (NICE) in the United Kingdom (National Institute for Health and Care Excellence 2014), and the Canadian Psychiatric Association (Canadian Psychiatric Association Working Group 2005), widespread availability of CBTp is still lacking. One of the greatest challenges to availability is the lack of therapists trained to provide CBTp. The use of cognitive-behavioral techniques is within the scope of practicing clinical psychiatrists, psychologists, and community mental health professionals and can be feasibly integrated into a team approach of integrated care. At least four treatment manuals for CBTp have been empirically validated in RCTs. Publications and Web-based and live learning systems are expanding the opportunities for clinicians to learn how to provide CBTp.

Cognitive Remediation

Intervention Rationale

Cognitive impairment is a core symptom of schizophrenia that is evident already at first episode and persists throughout the course of illness, independent of positive symptoms. Deficits in cognitive skills such as working memory, attention, and declarative memory are also robustly characteristic of people at clinical high risk for schizophrenia. Cognitive deficits add to illness burden by imposing significant functional limitations, such as on the ability to adequately manage symptoms, to participate in and benefit from psychosocial rehabilitation programs, and to acquire social, vocational, and educational skills integral to community integration (Bowie et al. 2006). Although medication is the mainstay of treatment for schizophrenia symptoms, there are presently no pharmacological approaches that effectively treat the cognitive impairments of schizophrenia. In contrast, CR is moderately effective at improving both cognition and functional outcomes for people with schizophrenia (Best and Bowie 2017; Wykes et al. 2011).

Description of the Intervention

The Cognitive Remediation Expert Working Group (CREW), a group of international CR investigators, initially established a definition for *cognitive remediation* in 2005 and updated it in 2012: "Cognitive remediation is an intervention targeting cognitive deficit (attention, memory, executive function, social cognition, or meta-cognition) using scientific principles of learning with the ultimate goal of improving functional outcomes. Its effectiveness is enhanced when provided in a context (formal or informal) that provides support and opportunity for improving everyday functioning" (Cognitive Remediation Expert Working Group 2012). CR can be provided individually or in groups, as well as in inpatient and outpatient, residential, and other community settings. Delivery of CR may also vary by amount of in-person clinician contact, by whether it is embedded in a rehabilitation service, and by degree of time spent on computer-based cognitive exercises. Average dosing across efficacy studies is 32 sessions, held twice weekly (Wykes et al. 2011). The variations in CR delivery are associated with different outcomes for different populations and allow for tailoring treatment to the specific needs of the individual.

When conducted in a psychiatric rehabilitation setting, CR may be provided in groups of six to eight clients that meet for an hour. In each CR session, the bulk of time involves working on computer-based cognitive activities that are typically accessed through Web-based portals. There is also a group discussion about the use of cognitive skills and strategies in real-world situations. Because the treatment is personalized, each individual works at his or her own pace on computer tasks chosen to address that person's particular needs. Trained mental health clinicians provide individual guidance and support on the computer-based exercises, as well as facilitate the group discussion.

Goals of Cognitive Rehabilitation and Treatment Principles

CR is intended to improve neurocognitive and social-cognitive skills so that it will be easier for the person to meet recovery goals and function better in the community. Improvement on the cognitive training tasks is not a goal unto itself but rather a means to achieve gains on separate measures of the trained and untrained cognitive functions. Functional outcomes are measured as the capacity to perform everyday tasks (simulations) and actual everyday functioning (ratings, self-reports, objective data). Broader goals of CR may include promoting independent learning skills, a positive attitude about learning, self-confidence in one's ability to learn, and self-awareness about oneself as a learner (Medalia et al. 2019).

CR is a learning activity; participants learn to have better skills in areas such as attention, processing speed, or facial affect recognition. Therefore, the basic principles of learning and teaching apply to this intervention. Participants in CR make the most gains when they are motivated to learn, feel supported and empowered as a partner in the treatment process, feel understood, are appropriately challenged, and are afforded opportunities to practice their newfound skills in a safe environment that provides constructive feedback (Cella and Wykes 2019; Medalia et al. 2017). Table 9–2 lists the key elements of CR programs.

Learning in CR is predicated on the capacity for *neuroplasticity*, the process by which neurons in the brain adjust their activity in response to new situations or changes in the environment. There is evidence that people of all ages, even when they have psychiatric illnesses that affect brain functioning, are capable of learning, and this ability is reflected behaviorally and in neuroplasticity.

Research Support

CR for Neurocognitive Deficits

The efficacy and effectiveness of CR have been established in numerous RCTs. A 2011 meta-analysis of 40 independent studies of CR in over 2,100 people with schizophre-

TABLE 9–2.   **Key elements of cognitive remediation for psychosis**

Clinicians work collaboratively with individual participants to set cognitive goals that are relevant to their recovery goals (e.g., improve memory to help job/school performance).

Participants engage in training that is sufficiently intensive to produce meaningful effects.

The difficulty level of cognitive exercises adjusts to keep training tasks challenging and engaging; performance parameters (e.g., accuracy, speed) are tracked.

Participants learn strategies to improve cognitive performance.

Participant receives feedback on cognitive task performance and strategy use during the training session.

Session includes or is paired with activities that promote better use of cognition in daily life (e.g., discussion, role plays, other psychosocial interventions).

Clinicians help participants track progress toward cognitive and related functional goals, identify barriers, and adjust short- and long-term goals as needed.

nia (Wykes et al. 2011) indicated a medium ES for improving overall cognition (ES=0.45) and for daily functioning (ES=0.42), with an additional significant but small effect on improving psychiatric symptoms (ES=0.18). Gains persisted after CR ended, with effect sizes remaining moderate for global cognition (ES=0.43) and functional improvement (ES=0.37). Methodological quality of the studies was not a significant factor in the observed effect size differences; effect size did not diminish with better-quality studies. Despite the positive group findings, there are individual differences in response, with evidence that at least 25% of CR participants do not improve (Wykes et al. 2011). Therefore, key challenges for the field are to identify the therapeutic techniques that maximally impact neurocognition, to facilitate the generalization (transfer) of cognitive change to functional change, and to identify whether particular groups of patients differentially benefit from certain types of CR interventions. In this regard, research on moderators of treatment benefit is informative. Data indicate that gains are greater for functional outcome when CR includes provision of strategy coaching and is paired with other psychosocial interventions. An example of the functional and economic benefits of CR for people with schizophrenia is seen in the enhanced rates and maintenance of competitive employment, when CR is coupled with psychosocial rehabilitation (McGurk et al. 2016). Nonspecific benefits of CR include enhanced self-efficacy and self-confidence (Soumet-Leman et al. 2018).

CR for Social-Cognitive Deficits

A meta-analysis of 19 RCTs with 692 subjects (Kurtz and Richardson 2012) found moderate to large effects of social cognitive training on facial affect recognition (ES=0.71–1.01), moderate effects on theory of mind (ES=0.46), and moderate to large effects on total symptoms (ES=0.78) and observer-rated community and institutional functioning (ES=0.78). Moderator analyses indicated that CR training was more likely to generalize to total symptoms and community functioning in younger samples, but longer duration of illness predicted greater improvement in facial affect recognition and theory of mind.

Implications for Clinical Practice

CR is generally well accepted by participants, as indicated by high satisfaction rates and relatively low dropout rates (Medalia et al. 2019). CR initiatives exist at a national public health level in Europe and Asia, but public health initiatives that address cognitive symptoms associated with psychiatric illness are rare in the United States. Contributing factors may include the following: 1) cognitive health and its treatment are insufficiently addressed in behavioral health professional programs, and 2) there are inadequate funding streams to support cognitive interventions. Recent large-scale initiatives to disseminate CR are providing a precedent and road map to facilitate future efforts (e.g., www.teachrecovery.com; Medalia et al. 2019).

Social Skills Training

Intervention Rationale

Antipsychotic medications alone do not restore pre-illness levels of functioning, lead to normative role performance, or produce an acceptable quality of life for the majority of people living with schizophrenia. Owing to onset typically during late adolescence or young adulthood, schizophrenia disrupts a critical period of socialization and development of adult life skills, resulting in increasing social isolation, anxiety, maladaptive ways of coping, and frustration or even failure in attempts to fulfill desired social roles. As a result, skills deficits may accumulate, become more fixed, and worsen as the duration of illness increases. Systematic research over the past several decades has sought to use SST to reduce functional impairments in schizophrenia and to improve role functioning and quality of life. Social skills are the building blocks of social competence, including but not limited to verbal, nonverbal, and paralinguistic behaviors. Accurate social perception and social information processing underlie contextually appropriate responses, conversational skills, assertiveness skills, and skills related to illness self-management.

Description of the Intervention

SST is a psychosocial intervention that aims to enable individuals with schizophrenia to develop and strengthen a repertoire of instrumental and affiliative skills for improved functioning in their communities. SST can be flexibly implemented—conducted in hospitals, outpatient clinics, and residential settings, with individuals, families, or groups. Group-based training, usually involving 4–12 participants and 1–2 facilitators, is the principal modality because it is more cost-effective than individual training. Groups also provide opportunities for peer modeling, self-help, and peer support. Sessions last between 45 and 90 minutes, depending on participants' level of sustained attention, and make frequent use of visual aids, handouts, and repetition to compensate for cognitive problems (poor attention, working memory) that would otherwise hinder learning. Curricula and manuals are widely available in print and on the internet.

Goals of Social Skills Training and Treatment Principles

The primary goal of SST is to promote more adaptive interactions within social contexts. Meeting personal needs and eliciting positive responses from others will reinforce skill use, enhance personal efficacy, and open up further opportunities for real-world success. SST is predicated on social learning theory and principles of behavior therapy. Techniques include goal setting, behavioral rehearsal (role-playing), social modeling, coaching, prompting and corrective feedback, positive reinforcement, and homework assignments to facilitate generalization to the community. A standardized curriculum may teach knowledge and skills that the majority of persons with schizophrenia need for improved functioning and attainment of recovery goals such as social perception (i.e., accurate evaluation and interpretation of emotional expression), receptive and expressive skills (e.g., verbal and nonverbal communication), affiliative skills (e.g., appropriate expression of affection), instrumental role skills (e.g., scheduling a doctor's appointment), basic conversation skills (i.e., starting, maintaining, and ending a conversation), and social normative behavior (e.g., addressing a boss). SST is adaptable to specific content areas such as work or school (Mueser et al. 2005) and can address skill building for specific goals—for example, avoidance of substance use (Bellack et al. 2006), independent living, or relapse prevention (Liberman et al. 1993). In these ways, SST is often instrumental in other psychosocial interventions such as family interventions, vocational rehabilitation, and substance use treatment.

Research Support

SST, when delivered with sufficient intensity and duration, has been shown to improve social knowledge and behavior. Meta-analytic results (Kurtz and Mueser 2008) indicate large effect sizes for mastery of training content assessed via direct measures of knowledge (ES=1.20) and large effect size outcomes on performance-based measures of social and daily living skills (ES=0.52). Also encouraging are the moderate effect sizes for more intermediate outcome measures of community functioning (ES=0.52) and negative symptoms (ES=0.40). Improved social skills are hypothesized to reduce symptoms and relapses through improved coping and social support; however, the effects of SST are weakest for these outcome measures, with small and nonsignificant effects. Studies have reported on the retention of trained skills over periods of 1–2 years (Liberman et al. 1998; Wallace et al. 1992); however, additional research is needed to draw confident conclusions regarding the durability of training effects.

Although substantial evidence indicates that people with schizophrenia can learn a variety of interpersonal and everyday living skills, improving the generalization of newly learned behavioral skills for everyday life is an ongoing pursuit. A number of SST-based interventions have been developed to facilitate generalization. In comparison with skills training alone, the addition of community-based practice facilitated by a specialized case manager enhances improvements in interpersonal problem-solving skills and social adjustment (Glynn et al. 2002; Liberman et al. 2002). Another approach that adds family support persons to promote generalization has shown significant positive effects on skill acquisition and level of functioning, with better utilization of disease management skills linked to decreased rates of rehospitalization (Kopelowicz et al. 2003).

It is recognized that the disability associated with schizophrenia cannot be addressed with a single focused intervention. SST has been effectively paired with complementary interventions such as attention shaping (Silverstein et al. 2009) and computer-based CR (e.g., Bowie et al. 2012). Other comprehensive approaches to rehabilitation (Brenner et al. 1994; Hogarty and Flesher 1999; Roder et al. 2006) combine, either sequentially or concomitantly, training in social and problem-solving skills and training in specific cognitive functions. The results of several RCTs suggest that providing cognitive training is instrumental in improving social and vocational functioning (Medalia and Saperstein 2013; Spaulding and Sullivan 2016) and that SST is critically important for CR to generalize to improvement in social and vocational roles (Kurtz et al. 2015; Peña et al. 2016).

Implications for Clinical Practice

Combining SST with other skills-based and recovery-focused interventions in clinical practice is more likely than SST alone to enhance functioning in a range of goal-oriented contexts. Also, its integration with other evidence-based psychological treatments, such as CBTp, may more effectively target the residual symptoms of schizophrenia and comorbid conditions to improve quality of life.

Supported Employment

Intervention Rationale

The proportion of persons with schizophrenia who are competitively employed is low, between 10% and 20% (Marwaha and Johnson 2004). Their lack of sustainable living wages increases dependence on families and public assistance programs, contributes to low self-esteem and stigma, and often leads to an absence of daily structure and sense of purpose. However, employment is a common functional goal among individuals with schizophrenia. Factors that have been hypothesized to contribute to poor employment outcomes include symptomatology, poor premorbid functioning, employment history, and skills deficits. Vocational rehabilitation programs attempt to mitigate such factors to improve work outcomes. Traditional vocational services, including sheltered workshops, job clubs, and transitional employment programs, focus on the development of work interests, motivation, and skills. Although moderately effective at improving work activity, workshop-based and sheltered employment skills were not generalizable to competitive employment settings, and job tenure was not sustained as work services were discontinued upon job attainment (Bond et al. 2001). Other approaches have sought to overcome these shortcomings; however, among the programs described in the literature, only SE has a systematic body of research showing effectiveness in helping individuals with schizophrenia achieve competitive employment.

Description of the Intervention

SE was developed as a vocational rehabilitation service in response to a need for long-term services and supports for individuals with disabilities placed in competitive jobs. It is an evidence-based psychosocial intervention for people with schizophrenia and other serious mental illnesses wherein individuals are assisted by an employment specialist or job "coach" in obtaining and maintaining employment. SE can be provided in a variety of service contexts, including community mental health centers, community rehabilitation programs, and psychiatric rehabilitation centers, as well as in coordinated specialty care programs in combination with supported education for individuals in the early phase of schizophrenia (Humensky et al. 2017). The prevailing model of SE for schizophrenia is individual placement and support (IPS; Drake and Becker 1996); it has been disseminated across the United States and abroad.

Goals of Supported Employment and Treatment Principles

SE is based on principles of community integration. A distinguishing characteristic of SE is the focus on mainstream jobs in the competitive labor market. Eligibility for services is based on client interest in work without exclusion based on work readiness, substance use problems, poor motivation, or symptoms. The IPS model is characterized by a rapid job search with attention to client preferences and strengths, without extensive preemployment assessment or training. After placement, individuals are helped to learn skills and are provided with ongoing supports through an employment specialist. Client engagement, outreach, job development, benefits counseling, integration with other mental health services, and employment of a multidisciplinary team-based approach are key. The SE model views work as a means to promote recovery and wellness.

Research Support

RCTs have consistently demonstrated the effectiveness of SE with respect to helping clients achieve competitive employment, work more hours, and earn more wages than individuals receiving rehabilitative day treatment (e.g., Cook et al. 2005a; Drake et al. 1996) or other vocational services (Twamley et al. 2003). Data from a multisite longitudinal trial even suggest that SE confers greater advantage to people with schizophrenia spectrum disorders than to those with other psychiatric disabilities (Cook et al. 2016). Furthermore, evidence from over 20 RCTs indicates that the IPS model of SE is more effective than other vocational programs at reducing unemployment (Bond et al. 2012). Given that the effectiveness of individual components of SE has not been demonstrated, current practice guidelines recommend that the full SE model be implemented and that SE be offered to any individual with an interest in work (Dixon et al. 2010). Despite the overall effectiveness of SE for people with schizophrenia for achieving competitive employment and earned income, at least one-third of them do not achieve optimal work outcomes. The evidence that SE is superior to other vocational services is weak for long-term job retention and financial independence. A number of promising complementary approaches have been evaluated to target impairments in learning that may hinder the uptake and maintenance of new job skills.

One approach to facilitating skill acquisition during SE is the addition of *errorless learning*, a method of training through a series of discrete steps that are graduated in difficulty level and designed to minimize errors. Two independent studies compared IPS with errorless learning to IPS alone (Kern et al. 2018). Work behavior problems identified during the first weeks at work were targeted for intervention by breaking down target behaviors into hierarchically ordered constituent steps and implementing an individualized training plan. Instructional aids were used to facilitate skill mastery and then were gradually withdrawn to encourage functional independence. Across studies, both groups improved on targeted problems, with greater improvement in the errorless learning group. Although equivalent hours and earnings per week were reported, the addition of errorless learning yielded significant advantages with respect to job tenure and job retention at 12-month follow-up.

Another approach to enhance skill acquisition is to target the cognitive skills that underlie learning. A number of studies have sought to overcome deficits in cognition that are barriers to successful employment. The addition of computer-based cognitive training, work feedback, and a social information–processing group to a Veterans Affairs (VA) vocational intervention program significantly increased hours of work over 6 months (Bell et al. 2005) and increased the likelihood of sustained employment compared with those who received the vocational intervention alone (Bell et al. 2008). Integrating CR in the context of SE has supported successful job placement and retention for individuals with schizophrenia in a variety of community-based settings (McGurk et al. 2007). Cognitive assessment and job loss analysis is used to understand the specific cognitive problems that have impeded job performance, inform computer-based cognitive training sessions, and develop cognitive strategies to improve cognitive and work functioning. Collaboration between the client, cognitive training specialist, and SE specialist aims to provide continuous support to overcome employment barriers. Data indicating greater immediate cognitive gains and more jobs obtained, weeks worked, and wages earned (McGurk et al. 2015) underscore the importance of comprehensive programs using a multidisciplinary team approach.

Implications for Clinical Practice

The IPS learning community, created in 2001, facilitates the dissemination of SE and provides ongoing implementation supports to maintain a high quality of community-based SE services (Becker et al. 2014). There is clear evidence across SE approaches that higher-fidelity SE programs (Becker et al. 2001; Bond et al. 2016; McGurk et al. 2007) and programs with better integration of vocational and mental health services (Becker et al. 2006; Cook et al. 2005b) have better outcomes. Evidence indicating that having disability benefits and social, vocational, and functional limitations can impact individual-level employment outcomes (Harvey et al. 2012) suggests a need to integrate complementary skills-based approaches in routine practice settings in order to optimize and sustain SE outcomes.

Illness Management and Recovery

Intervention Rationale

The importance of the development and dissemination of a comprehensive, standardized program for individuals with serious mental illness has come to the forefront of mental health treatment. The concept of recovery has become a focus of the treatment of individuals with serious mental illness, and collaboration is necessary between treatment providers and individuals seeking treatment to help the individuals move toward their recovery goals. In 1997, members of the National Institute of Mental Health proposed that the various then-current psychosocial interventions for this population be consolidated into a standardized program. In response to this, Mueser and colleagues (2002) reviewed the literature on controlled trials of psychoeducational approaches to treatment and developed IMR.

Description of the Intervention

IMR is a program that consolidates various psychosocial interventions for helping people with mental illness manage their symptoms and prevent relapses within the context of pursuing personal goals. A number of empirically supported strategies are incorporated: psychoeducation about mental illness and its treatment, CBT techniques, motivational enhancement strategies, relapse prevention planning, SST to strengthen social support, and coping skills training for the management of persistent symptoms (Mueser et al. 2006). A structured curriculum is the basis of IMR sessions. IMR begins by personalizing the concept of recovery and setting personal recovery goals. Over the course of IMR, which can be between 3 and 10 months in duration, 10 curriculum topics are covered: recovery strategies, practical facts about mental illnesses, the stress-vulnerability model and treatment strategies, building social support, using medication effectively, drug and alcohol use, reducing relapses, coping with stress, coping with problems and persistent symptoms, and getting one's needs met by the mental health system. IMR is packaged as an "implementation resource kit" and is available for free online (https:// store.samhsa.gov/product/Illness-Management-and-Recovery-Evidence-Based-Practices-EBP-KIT/sma09-4463). It can be performed in an individual or small group setting in weekly sessions. Individuals are asked to complete homework and practice assignments throughout treatment, and family or other sources of support can be involved.

Goals of Illness Management and Recovery and Treatment Principles

The following are the primary goals of IMR:

- Teach individuals about mental illness and treatment strategies.
- Develop skills for self-management of symptoms (coping skills and stress management) to reduce relapse and hospitalization.
- Establish goals that are meaningful and personal to the individual's recovery.

The underlying theoretical models of IMR are the transtheoretical model and the stress-vulnerability model. These models guide the IMR curriculum as well as the techniques employed. The transtheoretical model posits that motivation to change occurs in a series of stages and interventions should be tailored to each stage. IMR addresses this by integrating motivational interviewing and goal setting throughout to help individuals develop a vision of their recovery, realize how new knowledge and developing skill sets apply to that vision, and take the necessary steps to move forward. The stress-vulnerability model suggests that the development of schizophrenia is a result of the relationship between biological vulnerability, stress, and coping difficulties. IMR is intended to interrupt the cycle of stress and vulnerability that often results in relapse. The curriculum includes skill building for medication adherence, reducing substance use, increasing social support, managing stress, and relapse prevention planning to lessen symptom severity and reduce instances of relapse and hospitalizations. Cognitive-behavioral and motivation enhancement techniques encourage individuals to use their knowledge and empower them to self-manage their illness and pursue recovery. In these ways, the core recovery values of hope, consumer empowerment, personal choice, respect, and collaboration are enacted.

Research Support

In an RCT, individuals with severe mental illness who participated in IMR, compared with individuals receiving treatment as usual, showed significant improvement in their knowledge of illness and their identification and attainment of personal goals, and they also received higher clinician ratings for IMR outcome. These findings indicate that IMR both helps individuals gain knowledge about their illness and facilitates their recovery (Hasson-Ohayon et al. 2007). A review of the literature echoed these findings. McGuire et al. (2014) showed that across three RCTs, three quasi-controlled trials, and three pre-post trials, individuals who received IMR reported improvement in key domains (i.e., progress toward goals, knowledge of mental illness, relapse prevention plan) and received improved ratings of psychiatric symptoms by clinicians and independent observers.

Implications for Clinical Practice

The IMR kit facilitates dissemination and implementation of this program, which is suitable for use in a variety of settings, including community mental health centers, supportive housing programs, state-operated psychiatric hospitals, and VA medical centers. Resources are available for training frontline staff and for program evaluation and implementation. Common factors that may limit success rates include agency support, the degree to which the agency culture embraces recovery-oriented programming, access to external consultation, and the availability of supervision specific to IMR. Evidence suggests that fidelity to the IMR model and provider competency are associated with improvement in consumer outcomes (Hasson-Ohayon et al. 2007; McGuire et al. 2016), thus underscoring the need for ongoing implementation support (i.e., training, consultation) to enhance recovery goal attainment for IMR consumers.

Psychoeducation

Intervention Rationale

Schizophrenia is a challenging condition to live with and impacts not only patients but also their families and the broader social system. Many patients and families lack information about the illness and the resources to manage it. Stigma, stress, isolation, and fear are commonly reported by patients and families. Psychoeducation is an evidence-based psychosocial intervention that uses education, skills training, and support to promote recovery and decrease family stress. Numerous efficacy and effectiveness trials support the role of psychoeducation as an adjunct and complement to pharmacological and other psychosocial treatments (Dixon et al. 2001).

Description of the Intervention

Psychoeducation may be defined as the process of educating about mental illness in a way that promotes learning, behavior change, and recovery. Because learning and behavior change are less likely to occur with approaches that simply impart didactic information, effective psychoeducation programs also provide guidance, skills training, and support. Psychoeducation can be provided individually, with the family, or with groups of patients and/or families. Psychoeducation curricula are widely available as manuals, online courses, and videos. Some curricula are intended for inpatient settings, whereas other approaches have been developed for outpatient, residential,

TABLE 9–3.	Common elements of psychoeducation programs

Engaging the patient and family as valued team members who participate in the planning and delivery of treatment

Providing relevant information about treatment options

Listening nonjudgmentally to concerns

Exploring expectations of the treatment

Assessing the strengths and limitations of the family's ability to provide support to the patient

Responding sensitively to emotional distress and feelings of loss

Assessing the social and clinical needs of the patient and family

Teaching effective strategies to communicate among family members

Providing an explicit crisis plan and professional response

Providing training in structured problem-solving techniques

Educating about and supporting involvement with social support networks, such as the National Alliance on Mental Illness

Facilitating access to relevant professional care

---

or community settings. The course of psychoeducation treatment can range from weeks to years, with a median duration of around 12 weekly sessions (Xia et al. 2011). Psychoeducation may be provided by mental health clinicians or community support organizations such as the National Alliance on Mental Illness.

Goals of Psychoeducation and Treatment Principles

Psychoeducation is intended to teach patients and their families about the illness so they can better manage symptoms and navigate treatment options. The ultimate goals of psychoeducation are to improve a person's community functioning, healthy behaviors, resilience, engagement in treatment as an active participant, and ability to seek help, as well as to reduce relapse and self-stigma. Table 9–3 lists the common elements of psychoeducation programs.

Psychoeducation is a learning activity; the basic principles of learning and teaching apply to psychoeducation. Individuals learn best when they feel supported, empowered, understood, and appropriately challenged and when they are provided with opportunities to practice new skills in an environment that provides constructive feedback.

Psychoeducation for Patients

Schizophrenia, like any serious illness, can be frightening and overwhelming to negotiate. Furthermore, the illness itself disrupts self-observation and insight so patients may not readily appreciate the need for treatment. Poor adherence to treatment recommendations, in particular medication, has been associated with relapses and more frequent hospitalizations (Haddad et al. 2014). Some psychoeducation programs are designed specifically for the person diagnosed with schizophrenia, with the goal of improving treatment outcomes and recovery. A trained mental health provider, who is familiar with the psychoeducational curriculum and recovery principles, provides the intervention. The basic principles of recovery guide the psychoeducational intervention—to value and promote hope, personal responsibility, and self-advocacy. Recovery is appreciated as a process with personal meaning and goals and is not simply defined as symptom relief. The goal of psychoeducation for patients is to engage them in a process of change through provision of education, support, and training.

Family Psychoeducation

Families often lack information and support as they negotiate multiple roles to care for someone with schizophrenia. They may not understand what schizophrenia is, how it manifests, how it is treated, and what is realistic to expect of their loved one. Often, they feel frightened, stigmatized, isolated, and overwhelmed. Family members need guidance as they negotiate competing demands to serve as advocate, counselor, crisis and medication manager, and income provider. Family psychoeducation programs use many therapeutic elements (e.g., cognitive, behavioral, supportive) to engage the family in a process of learning and change, with the goals of improving patient functional outcomes and ameliorating caregiver burden (McFarlane et al. 2003). Psychoeducation for families differs from family therapy in that the emphasis in the former is on providing education and support, whereas the emphasis in family therapy is on changing interpersonal dynamics. When families better understand the illness, signs of relapse, and treatment possibilities, it becomes easier for them to provide emotional support, clinical and crisis assistance, and advocacy, as well as to anticipate and provide the financial and housing assistance their loved one may need.

Research Support

The efficacy and effectiveness of family psychoeducation have been established in numerous RCTs (Armijo et al. 2013; Lucksted et al. 2012; Pharoah et al. 2010). A review of 32 RCTs including 2,981 participants found that family psychoeducation was more efficacious than standard treatment in decreasing relapse frequency, reducing hospital admission, promoting more consistent medication adherence, and reducing burden on family life for those in longer courses of family treatment (Pharoah et al. 2010). There are differences in response to family interventions; one of every eight patients treated with some form of family intervention is prevented from hospitalization (Pharoah et al. 2010). Providing family psychoeducation is associated with significant direct and indirect cost savings (Tarrier et al. 1988).

Xia and colleagues (2011) reviewed 44 RCTs of patient psychoeducation programs implemented with 5,142 participants over a median duration of 12 weeks. Compared with standard treatments, psychoeducation was better at improving patient compliance with treatment and at reducing rate of relapse and hospitalization in the short term (12 weeks). The efficacy and effectiveness of brief psychoeducation interventions for patients were supported in a review of 20 RCTs of 2,337 participants (Zhao et al. 2015). Brief psychoeducation interventions consisting of 10 sessions or fewer (ranging from 1 day to eight sessions over 1 year) were associated with greater medication compliance than routine care in the short term and with reduced relapse rates in the medium term (13–52 weeks).

Implications for Clinical Practice

Psychoeducation about mental health provides benefits to consumers and caregivers and can facilitate a productive partnership among the stakeholders involved in the care of someone with schizophrenia. That said, there can be barriers to acceptance of the service. Patients and families may feel hopeless that anything will help, or their concern about stigma and negative judgments may lead to reluctance to expose themselves. Patients may not understand why their families need help. A patient may worry about losing autonomy and confidentiality if the treatment team meets with his or her family. These barriers can be mitigated by sensitively engaging the patient and family in discussion about their feelings of hopelessness and their concerns about stigma, loss of autonomy, and privacy. Guidance and resources to help develop psychoeducation mental health programs can be found on the Substance Abuse and Mental Health Services Administration website (www.samhsa.gov).

Conclusion

Psychosocial interventions are intended to target the barriers to functional recovery and are therefore recognized as an important complement to pharmacological treatments. In this chapter, we describe six established psychosocial interventions: cognitive-behavioral therapy, cognitive remediation, SST, SE, IMR, and psychoeducation. All of these interventions use a combination of therapeutic approaches to engage the participants in a process of learning to better manage their illness. The efficacy research for each modality indicates that participants learn the most and apply their learning most successfully when the treatment is provided in a recovery context, in which the patient is empowered yet supported, and is given appropriate challenges and opportunities to practice the skills.

Provision of psychosocial interventions in a recovery context also appreciates the role of timing, so that treatment proceeds at a pace that suits each patient's learning style and fosters his or her intrinsic motivation to learn more and take positive, constructive control of his or her treatment. There needs to be congruence between the patient's goals, the patient's needs, and the specific intervention offered. If the goal is to return to school, yet the patient cannot pay attention, cognitive remediation may be a starting point. How the other interventions are woven into the treatment plan would then depend on a process of shared decision making, with the provider and patient considering what skills need to be strengthened next. As the research indicates, the specific psychosocial interventions combine well, and it is to be expected that patients may benefit from more than one of the approaches described.

References

Armijo J, Méndez E, Morales R, et al: Efficacy of community treatments for schizophrenia and other psychotic disorders: a literature review. Front Psychiatry 4:116, 2013 24130534

Becker DR, Smith J, Tanzman B, et al: Fidelity of supported employment programs and employment outcomes. Psychiatr Serv 52(6):834–836, 2001 11376236

Becker DR, Xie H, McHugo GJ, et al: What predicts supported employment program outcomes? Community Ment Health J 42(3):303–313, 2006 16532378

Becker DR, Drake RE, Bond GR: The IPS supported employment learning collaborative. Psychiatr Rehabil J 37(2):79–85, 2014 24512479

Bell MD, Bryson GJ, Greig TC, et al: Neurocognitive enhancement therapy with work therapy: productivity outcomes at 6- and 12-month follow-ups. J Rehabil Res Dev 42(6):829–838, 2005 16680620

Bell MD, Zito W, Greig T, et al: Neurocognitive enhancement therapy with vocational services: work outcomes at two-year follow-up. Schizophr Res 105(1–3):18–29, 2008 18715755

Bellack AS, Bennett ME, Gearon JS, et al: A randomized clinical trial of a new behavioral treatment for drug abuse in people with severe and persistent mental illness. Arch Gen Psychiatry 63(4):426–432, 2006 16585472

Best MW, Bowie CR: A review of cognitive remediation approaches for schizophrenia: from top-down to bottom-up, brain training to psychotherapy. Expert Rev Neurother 17(7):713–723, 2017 28511562

Bond GR, Becker DR, Drake RE, et al: Implementing supported employment as an evidence-based practice. Psychiatr Serv 52(3):313–322, 2001 11239097

Bond GR, Drake RE, Becker DR: Generalizability of the Individual Placement and Support (IPS) model of supported employment outside the U.S. World Psychiatry 11(1):32–39, 2012 22295007

Bond GR, Drake RE, Becker DR, Noel VA: The IPS learning community: a longitudinal study of sustainment, quality, and outcome. Psychiatr Serv 67(8):864–869, 2016 27032661

Bowie CR, Reichenberg A, Patterson TL, et al: Determinants of real-world functional performance in schizophrenia subjects: correlations with cognition, functional capacity, and symptoms. Am J Psychiatry 163(3):418–425, 2006 16513862

Bowie CR, McGurk SR, Mausbach B, et al: Combined cognitive remediation and functional skills training for schizophrenia: effects on cognition, functional competence, and real-world behavior. Am J Psychiatry 169(7):710–718, 2012 22581070

Brenner HD, Roder V, Hodel B, et al: Integrated Psychological Therapy for Schizophrenic Patients. Toronto, ON, Canada, Hogrefe & Huber, 1994

Burns AMN, Erickson DH, Brenner CA: Cognitive-behavioral therapy for medication-resistant psychosis: a meta-analytic review. Psychiatr Serv 65(7):874–880, 2014 24686725

Bustillo J, Lauriello J, Horan W, et al: The psychosocial treatment of schizophrenia: an update. Am J Psychiatry 158(2):163–175, 2001 11156795

Canadian Psychiatric Association Working Group: Clinical practice guidelines: treatment of schizophrenia. Can J Psychiatry 50 (suppl 1):1S–57S, 2005

Cella M, Wykes T: The nuts and bolts of cognitive remediation: exploring how different training components relate to cognitive and functional gains. Schizophr Res 203:12–16, 2019 28919130

Cognitive Remediation Expert Working Group: Minutes from the CREW meeting. Paper presented at the 3rd conference of the Schizophrenia International Research Society, Florence, Italy, April 2012

Cook JA, Leff HS, Blyler CR, et al: Results of a multisite randomized trial of supported employment interventions for individuals with severe mental illness. Arch Gen Psychiatry 62(5):505–512, 2005a 15867103

Cook JA, Lehman AF, Drake R, et al: Integration of psychiatric and vocational services: a multisite randomized, controlled trial of supported employment. Am J Psychiatry 162(10):1948–1956, 2005b 16199843

Cook JA, Burke-Miller JK, Roessel E: Long-term effects of evidence-based supported employment on earnings and on SSI and SSDI participation among individuals with psychiatric disabilities. Am J Psychiatry 173(10):1007–1014, 2016 27113123

Dixon L, McFarlane WR, Lefley H, et al: Evidence-based practices for services to families of people with psychiatric disabilities. Psychiatr Serv 52(7):903–910, 2001 11433107

Dixon LB, Dickerson F, Bellack AS, et al; Schizophrenia Patient Outcomes Research Team (PORT): The 2009 Schizophrenia PORT psychosocial treatment recommendations and summary statements. Schizophr Bull 36(1):48–70, 2010 19955389

Drake RE, Becker DR: The Individual Placement and Support model of supported employment. Psychiatr Serv 47(5):473–475, 1996 8740486

Drake RE, Becker DR, Biesanz JC, et al: Day treatment versus supported employment for persons with severe mental illness: a replication study. Psychiatr Serv 47(10):1125–1127, 1996 8890346

Ellis A, Harper RA: A New Guide to Rational Living. Oxford, UK, Prentice Hall, 1975

Glynn SM, Marder SR, Liberman RP, et al: Supplementing clinic-based skills training with manual-based community support sessions: effects on social adjustment of patients with schizophrenia. Am J Psychiatry 159(5):829–837, 2002 11986138

Haddad PM, Brain C, Scott J: Nonadherence with antipsychotic medication in schizophrenia: challenges and management strategies. Patient Relat Outcome Meas 5:43–62, 2014 25061342

Harvey PD, Heaton RK, Carpenter WT Jr, et al: Functional impairment in people with schizophrenia: focus on employability and eligibility for disability compensation. Schizophr Res 140(1–3):1–8, 2012 22503642

Hasson-Ohayon I, Roe D, Kravetz S: A randomized controlled trial of the effectiveness of the Illness Management and Recovery program. Psychiatr Serv 58(11):1461–1466, 2007 17978257

Hogarty GE, Flesher S: Practice principles of cognitive enhancement therapy for schizophrenia. Schizophr Bull 25(4):693–708, 1999 10667740

Humensky J, Scodes J, Wall M, et al: Disability enrollment in a community-based coordinated specialty care program. Am J Psychiatry 174(12):1224–1225, 2017 29191038

Jauhar S, McKenna PJ, Radua J, et al: Cognitive-behavioural therapy for the symptoms of schizophrenia: systematic review and meta-analysis with examination of potential bias. Br J Psychiatry 204(1):20–29, 2014 24385461

Kern RS, Zarate R, Glynn SM, et al: Improving work outcome in supported employment for serious mental illness: results from 2 independent studies of errorless learning. Schizophr Bull 44(1):38–45, 2018 28981901

Kopelowicz A, Zarate R, Gonzalez Smith V, et al: Disease management in Latinos with schizophrenia: a family assisted, skills training approach. Schizophr Bull 29(2):211–227, 2003 14552498

Kurtz MM, Mueser KT: A meta-analysis of controlled research on social skills training for schizophrenia. J Consult Clin Psychol 76(3):491–504, 2008 18540742

Kurtz MM, Richardson CL: Social cognitive training for schizophrenia: a meta-analytic investigation of controlled research. Schizophr Bull 38(5):1092–1104, 2012 21525166

Kurtz MM, Mueser KT, Thime WR, et al: Social skills training and computer-assisted cognitive remediation in schizophrenia. Schizophr Res 162(1–3):35–41, 2015 25640526

Liberman RP, Wallace CJ, Blackwell G, et al: Innovations in skills training for the seriously mentally ill: the UCLA Social and Independent Living Skills Modules. Innovations and Research 2:43–60, 1993

Liberman RP, Wallace CJ, Blackwell G, et al: Skills training versus psychosocial occupational therapy for persons with persistent schizophrenia. Am J Psychiatry 155(8):1087–1091, 1998 9699698

Liberman RP, Glynn S, Blair KE, et al: In vivo amplified skills training: promoting generalization of independent living skills for clients with schizophrenia. Psychiatry 65(2):137–155, 2002 12108138

Lucksted A, McFarlane W, Downing D, et al: Recent developments in family psychoeducation as an evidence-based practice. J Marital Fam Ther 38(1):101–121, 2012 22283383

Marwaha S, Johnson S: Schizophrenia and employment - a review. Soc Psychiatry Psychiatr Epidemiol 39(5):337–349, 2004 15133589

McFarlane WR, Dixon L, Lukens E, et al: Family psychoeducation and schizophrenia: a review of the literature. J Marital Fam Ther 29(2):223–245, 2003 12728780

McGuire AB, Kukla M, Green A, et al: Illness management and recovery: a review of the literature. Psychiatr Serv 65(2):171–179, 2014 24178191

McGuire AB, Bartholomew T, Anderson AI, et al: Illness management and recovery in community practice. Psychiatr Rehabil J 39(4):343–351, 2016 27505349

McGurk SR, Mueser KT, Feldman K, et al: Cognitive training for supported employment: 2–3 year outcomes of a randomized controlled trial. Am J Psychiatry 164(3):437–441, 2007 17329468

McGurk SR, Mueser KT, Xie H, et al: Cognitive enhancement treatment for people with mental illness who do not respond to supported employment: a randomized controlled trial. Am J Psychiatry 172(9):852–861, 2015 25998278

McGurk SR, Mueser KT, Xie H, et al: Cognitive remediation for vocational rehabilitation non-responders. Schizophr Res 175(1–3):48–56, 2016 27209526

Medalia A, Saperstein AM: Does cognitive remediation for schizophrenia improve functional outcomes? Curr Opin Psychiatry 26(2):151–157, 2013 23318663

Medalia A, Herlands T, Saperstein A, Revheim R: Cognitive Remediation for Psychological Disorders, 2nd Edition. New York, NY, Oxford University Press, 2017

Medalia A, Saperstein AM, Erlich M, et al: Cognitive remediation in large systems of psychiatric care. CNS Spectr 24(1):163–173, 2019 29716665

Mueser KT, Corrigan PW, Hilton DW, et al: Illness management and recovery: a review of the research. Psychiatr Serv 53(10):1272–1284, 2002 12364675

Mueser KT, Aalto S, Becker DR, et al: The effectiveness of skills training for improving outcomes in supported employment. Psychiatr Serv 56(10):1254–1260, 2005 16215191

Mueser KT, Meyer PS, Penn DL, et al: The Illness Management and Recovery program: rationale, development, and preliminary findings. Schizophr Bull 32 (suppl 1):S32–S43, 2006 16899534

Myhr G, Payne K: Cost-effectiveness of cognitive-behavioural therapy for mental disorders: implications for public health care funding policy in Canada. Can J Psychiatry 51(10):662–670, 2006 17052034

National Institute for Health and Care Excellence: Psychosis and Schizophrenia in Adults: Prevention and Management (Clinical Guideline 178). London, National Institute for Health and Care Excellence, 2014

O'Keeffe J, Conway R, McGuire B: A systematic review examining factors predicting favourable outcome in cognitive behavioural interventions for psychosis. Schizophr Res 183:22–30, 2017 27889383

Peña J, Ibarretxe-Bilbao N, Sánchez P, et al: Combining social cognitive treatment, cognitive remediation, and functional skills training in schizophrenia: a randomized controlled trial. NPJ Schizophr 2:16037, 2016 27868083

Pharoah F, Mari J, Rathbone J, et al: Family intervention for schizophrenia. Cochrane Database Syst Rev (12):CD000088, 2010 21154340

Roder V, Mueller DR, Mueser KT, et al: Integrated Psychological Therapy (IPT) for schizophrenia: is it effective? Schizophr Bull 32 (suppl 1):S81–S93, 2006 16916888

Sarin F, Wallin L, Widerlöv B: Cognitive behavior therapy for schizophrenia: a meta-analytical review of randomized controlled trials. Nord J Psychiatry 65(3):162–174, 2011 21563994

Silverstein SM, Spaulding WD, Menditto AA, et al: Attention shaping: a reward-based learning method to enhance skills training outcomes in schizophrenia. Schizophr Bull 35(1):222–232, 2009 18212327

Soumet-Leman C, Medalia A, Erlich MD: Acceptability and perceived effectiveness of cognitive remediation in clinical practice. Psychiatr Serv 69(4):493–494, 2018 29607773

Spaulding WD, Sullivan ME: Treatment of cognition in the schizophrenia spectrum: the context of psychiatric rehabilitation. Schizophr Bull 42 (suppl 1):S53–S61, 2016 27460619

Tarrier N, Barrowclough C, Vaughn C, et al: The community management of schizophrenia: a controlled trial of a behavioural intervention with families to reduce relapse. Br J Psychiatry 153:532–542, 1988 3074860

Twamley EW, Jeste DV, Lehman AF: Vocational rehabilitation in schizophrenia and other psychotic disorders: a literature review and meta-analysis of randomized controlled trials. J Nerv Ment Dis 191(8):515–523, 2003 12972854

van der Gaag M, Smit F, Bechdolf A, et al: Preventing a first episode of psychosis: meta-analysis of randomized controlled prevention trials of 12 month and longer-term follow-ups. Schizophr Res 149(1–3):56–62, 2013 23870806

Wallace CJ, Liberman RP, MacKain SJ, et al: Effectiveness and replicability of modules for teaching social and instrumental skills to the severely mentally ill. Am J Psychiatry 149(5):654–658, 1992 1575257

Wykes T, Steel C, Everitt B, Tarrier N: Cognitive behavior therapy for schizophrenia: effect sizes, clinical models, and methodological rigor. Schizophr Bull 34(3):523–537, 2008 17962231

Wykes T, Huddy V, Cellard C, et al: A meta-analysis of cognitive remediation for schizophrenia: methodology and effect sizes. Am J Psychiatry 168(5):472–485, 2011 21406461

Xia J, Merinder LB, Belgamwar MR: Psychoeducation for schizophrenia. Cochrane Database Syst Rev (6):CD002831, 2011 21678337

Zhao S, Sampson S, Xia J, et al: Psychoeducation (brief) for people with serious mental illness. Cochrane Database Syst Rev (4):CD010823, 2015 25854522

CHAPTER 10

Co-occurring Disorders and Conditions

Sarah Pratt, Ph.D.

Melanie Bennett, Ph.D.

Mary F. Brunette, M.D.

Over half of people with schizophrenia have at least one co-occurring behavioral health disorder (Bermanzohn et al. 2000; Bland et al. 1987; Cassano et al. 1998). Because co-occurring disorders have a negative impact on the course of schizophrenia (Bermanzohn et al. 2000; Bland et al. 1987; Cassano et al. 1998), detection and optimal treatment of co-occurring disorders will improve outcomes.

Some conditions that co-occur with schizophrenia may have overlapping biological foundations or genetic links to schizophrenia, and research aimed at establishing whether people with schizophrenia are at increased risk for other disorders could expand understanding of the causes of schizophrenia. A better understanding of co-occurring disorders may provide clues about the neurobiology of schizophrenia itself.

Although medications and psychosocial interventions are effective for treating the symptoms of schizophrenia, identifying and treating co-occurring conditions remain major clinical challenges. In this chapter, we review many co-occurring conditions experienced by people with schizophrenia: substance use disorders including tobacco use disorder, obesity, depression, suicide, panic disorder, social anxiety disorder, trauma/posttraumatic stress disorder (PTSD), and obsessive-compulsive disorder (OCD) (Table 10–1). We discuss their prevalence and impact, review causal theories, and provide current information on detection and on management with pharmacological and psychosocial treatments.

TABLE 10–1.   Co-occurring substance use and other psychiatric disorders in schizophrenia

Co-occurring disorder	Estimated lifetime prevalence	Recommended treatment approaches
Substance use disorders	47%–58.5%	Switch to second-generation antipsychotics, with more evidence for clozapine
		Addition of medications for substance use disorders
		Integrated treatments for mental illness and substance use disorder
Tobacco use disorder	50%–65%	Addition of FDA-approved cessation medications
		Addition of behavioral treatment for maintaining motivation and learning skills to cope with urges
Obesity	44.8%–53.3%	Switch to psychotropic medications with lower risk of weight gain
		Addition of combined exercise and diet interventions
		Addition of metformin and/or other antiobesity medications
Depressive disorders	Up to 81%	Switch to second-generation antipsychotics
		Addition of antidepressant medication
		Addition of psychosocial treatments for depression
Panic disorder	6%–30%	Addition of antipanic medications and cognitive-behavioral therapy, as suggested by case reports
Social phobia	15%–39.5%	Addition of antidepressants and cognitive-behavioral therapy, as suggested by case reports
Posttraumatic stress disorder	14%–43%	Addition of treatments effective in general population: antidepressant medications and cognitive-behavioral therapy
Obsessive-compulsive disorder	4%–23.5%	Addition of serotonin reuptake inhibitors and cognitive-behavioral therapy, as suggested by case reports

Co-occurring Substance Use Disorders

Population-based studies of the prevalence of alcohol or psychoactive drug use disorders (referred to in this chapter by the generic term "substance use disorders") have found lifetime comorbidity in 47%–58.5% of people with schizophrenia compared with 16% of the general population (Kendler et al. 1996; Regier et al. 1990). Alcohol is the psychoactive substance most commonly abused by people with schizophrenia, followed by cannabis and stimulants (Brunette et al. 2018a; Drake and Mueser 1996; Mueser et al. 1990; Selzer and Lieberman 1993). Although the prevalence of opioid use disorders has increased in the United States (Martins et al. 2017), it is unclear how commonly these are comorbid with schizophrenia (Chiappelli et al. 2018; Iyiewuare et al. 2017). Although tobacco use disorder has declined substantially in the general population, over half of people with schizophrenia remain dependent on nicotine in tobacco (Correll et al. 2014; Lasser et al. 2000).

Overview of Substance Use Disorders

Substance use disorders complicate the course and treatment of schizophrenia, even when the substance use pattern is modest (Drake and Wallach 1993; D'Souza et al. 2005). Substance use is associated with a range of negative clinical and health outcomes, including symptom exacerbation and greater risk for hospitalization, homelessness, victimization, and suicide (Hjorthøj et al. 2015; Hurlburt et al. 1996; Kerfoot et al. 2011; Kivimies et al. 2016; Lysaker et al. 1994; Neria et al. 2002; Painter et al. 2018; Rosenberg et al. 2001a; Sara et al. 2014; Swartz et al. 2006; Velligan et al. 2017). Heavy cannabis use and to a lesser extent stimulant and nicotine use, particularly early in adolescence, are associated with an earlier onset and greater risk for developing schizophrenia (Gurillo et al. 2015; Helle et al. 2016; Murray et al. 2017). Moreover, substance use disorders in first-episode patients may complicate assessment of psychosis and delay treatment (Addington 1999; Brunette et al. 2018a; Green et al. 2004).

Many theories have been proposed to explain the increased prevalence of substance use disorders in patients with schizophrenia. Studies examining comorbidity between psychiatric and substance use disorders have found that polygenic risk scores for schizophrenia were significantly associated with substance use disorder in general and most strongly associated with cannabis and cocaine use disorders (Carey et al. 2016; Hartz et al. 2017; Reginsson et al. 2018), suggesting shared genetic risk for psychosis and substance use disorders. However, family, twin, and genetic studies thus far indicate that the biological (presumed genetic) vulnerability for schizophrenia is mostly different from the vulnerability for substance use disorder.

The stress-vulnerability model proposes that a genetic vulnerability, modified by early environmental events, interacts with later environmental stressors to precipitate the onset of a psychiatric or substance use disorder. In this model, vulnerability to schizophrenia and to substance use disorders may be related: substance use may serve as the environmental stressor that precipitates onset of psychosis in vulnerable individuals (Degenhardt et al. 2003). This model is supported by data indicating that use of substances is associated with an earlier onset of schizophrenia (Helle et al. 2016), that people with schizophrenia are highly sensitive to the detrimental effects of low doses of substances (Drake and Wallach 1993; D'Souza et al. 2006; Lieberman et al. 1987), and that these patients experience negative clinical effects, such as relapse of psychosis, with substance use (Kerfoot et al. 2011).

Several authors have proposed a "self-medication" hypothesis that substances are used to lessen symptoms of the psychotic disorder or to reduce side effects of antipsychotic medications (Khantzian 1997; Siris 1990). However, most research does not support a causal relationship between substance use and level of psychiatric symptoms (Addington and Addington 1998; Brunette et al. 1997). Moreover, first-episode patients have high rates of substance use disorders prior to exposure to antipsychotic medications and their side effects (Brunette et al. 2018a). Instead, patients with schizophrenia may have natural reward-seeking, learning, and processing deficits (Cassidy et al. 2014a, 2014b; Gold et al. 2008) that may be ameliorated by substance use (Fischer et al. 2014), leading to ongoing substance use despite symptom exacerbations and other negative consequences.

The biological vulnerability to substance use disorders in individuals with schizophrenia may be an inherent part of the neurobiology of schizophrenia (Stone et al. 2001). Several authors (Chambers et al. 2001; Green et al. 1999) proposed a neurobiological formulation suggesting that the high rates of comorbid substance use disorders in patients with schizophrenia may relate to a deficiency in the dopamine-mediated mesocorticolimbic brain reward circuits and to the ability of substances of abuse to ameliorate this deficiency. This model suggests that alcohol and drug use may enhance the functioning of the brain reward circuit by improving the "signal detection" capability of dopamine-rich pathways (Chau et al. 2004; Fadda et al. 1989; Goeders and Smith 1986), resulting in a subjective improvement in how patients feel despite the negative impact they have on the illness.

Detection and Management of Substance Use Disorders

Substance use disorders in patients with schizophrenia are underdetected and undertreated in both mental health and addiction treatment settings (Gerra et al. 2006; Litz and Leslie 2017; Oiesvold et al. 2013; Sallaup et al. 2016), leading to inconsistent messages to patients about their disorders and fragmented care (Ridgely et al. 1990). To improve detection, clinicians should routinely assess and discuss substance use with all patients at regular intervals. Use of standardized measures such as the Web-based NIDA-Modified ASSIST (the National Institute on Drug Abuse Modified Alcohol, Smoking and Substance Involvement Screening Test) (Humeniuk et al. 2008; National Institute on Drug Abuse 2012) or instruments specifically developed for patients with mental illness (e.g., the Dartmouth Assessment of Lifestyle Instrument, the Alcohol Use Scale, and the Drug Use Scale [Mueser et al. 1995; Rosenberg et al. 1998]) can facilitate screening and assessment. Clinicians should supplement these self-report assessments with their observations of behaviors consistent with substance use (e.g., frequent missed appointments, difficulty managing components of daily life, financial or legal problems) and collateral information from family members and case managers. Checking prescription drug monitoring websites can assist with the detection of risky prescription drug use (Hackman et al. 2014).

An especially useful assessment is a functional analysis, which incorporates the individual's experience of both the positive and negative aspects of substance use and how these may help or complicate his or her life. This type of assessment actively involves the individual in the assessment process while simultaneously providing the foundation for cognitive-behavioral substance abuse counseling. The clinician's nonjudgmental attitude reinforces honest communication about substance use and improves detection and treatment (Miller and Rollnick 2002).

Integrated treatment for psychotic and substance use disorders allows for coordinated pharmacotherapy, rehabilitation, and substance abuse interventions in one comprehensive package that yields better patient outcomes (Barrowclough et al. 2001; De Witte et al. 2014; Drake et al. 2004, 2016) (Table 10–2). Important components of integrated treatment include 1) staged interventions—such as assertive outreach, motivational interviewing, and substance abuse counseling—that are tailored to an in-

TABLE 10–2. **Principles of integrated dual disorder treatment for patients with schizophrenia**

Integration of mental health and substance use disorder treatments

Stagewise treatment that is tailored to the patient's motivation for change

Comprehensive services that include medication, psychosocial rehabilitation, skills training, and residential and vocational services

Long-term perspective

dividual's motivation for substance use change; 2) comprehensive services (e.g., medication management, rehabilitation interventions); and 3) a long-term perspective (Drake et al. 2004). One such treatment program, integrated dual disorder treatment (Mueser et al. 2003a; Substance Abuse and Mental Health Services Administration 2009), recommends that multidisciplinary teams provide the components of integrated care through case management, individual counseling, treatment groups, and family interventions. Chapter 11, "Evidence-Based Models of Service Delivery," provides more information on integrated dual diagnosis treatment. Incentives such as vouchers for goods or drawings for prizes (Ledgerwood et al. 2008) can increase treatment attendance (Leontieva et al. 2008) and reduce substance use (Brunette et al. 2018c; McDonell et al. 2013, 2017). Ensuring access to residential services and vocational supports is also important. Although research has not yet established an effective strategy for treating substance use disorders in young people with first-episode psychosis, the same principles of care apply (McLoughlin et al. 2014; Wisdom et al. 2011).

Research on pharmacotherapy for schizophrenia and co-occurring substance use disorders has not yet established a standardized treatment approach (Akerman et al. 2014; Azorin et al. 2016). However, it is clear that pharmacotherapy should include medications to treat both the mental illness and the substance use disorder, and clinicians should take care to prescribe medications that are safe in the context of substance use. Although dangerous interactions between psychotropic medication and substances of abuse are of real concern, they seem to be rare (see Mueser et al. 2003a for a review of potential interactions). Antipsychotic agents decrease symptoms of schizophrenia, improve overall functioning, and enhance a patient's ability to participate in psychosocial treatments, and thus antipsychotics facilitate recovery from both substance use disorders and schizophrenia (Noordsy et al. 2002).

Research on the impact of second-generation antipsychotics on substance use disorders that co-occur with schizophrenia is still developing but appears to suggest that some of these medications may be particularly helpful. Second-generation antipsychotics are generally safer and have fewer side effects than older medications and may be more useful than first-generation agents in individuals with these comorbid disorders. For example, clozapine use has been associated with reduced alcohol and cannabis use in naturalistic studies (Brunette et al. 2006; Green et al. 2003), and a randomized trial showed that switching to clozapine led to a lower level of cannabis use compared with continuing a patient's current antipsychotic (Brunette et al. 2011a). In population-based studies, clozapine was associated with better overall outcomes than other oral antipsychotics (Taipale et al. 2018; Tiihonen et al. 2017). Green and colleagues (1999) have suggested that clozapine may be uniquely effective for individuals with schizophrenia and co-occurring substance use disorders because of its unusual pharmacological profile. Clozapine potently blocks α_2-noradrenergic receptors, increases norepinephrine levels, and weakly blocks dopamine D_2 receptors, all of which may allow clozapine to normalize the signal detection capability of dysfunctional mesocorticolimbic brain reward circuits (Green et al. 1999).

Studies on the effects of other antipsychotics, such as risperidone and olanzapine, on substance use disorders that co-occur with schizophrenia had mixed results (Albanese 2000; Green et al. 2003; Littrell et al. 2001; Noordsy et al. 2001; Smelson et al. 2002; van Nimwegen et al. 2008). In a naturalistic study of patients with psychotic disorder and opioid use disorder taking methadone or buprenorphine, patients treated with olanzapine compared with those treated with haloperidol had significantly fewer positive urine samples and better symptom control (Gerra et al. 2007). A large randomized trial of olanzapine plus placebo compared with olanzapine plus an opioid antagonist demonstrated a significant reduction in alcohol use in both groups (Brunette et al. 2017a). Two open trials of quetiapine showed decreased stimulant craving or alcohol use (Brown et al. 2002; Brunette et al. 2009). Two small, uncontrolled studies of aripiprazole, a partial dopamine agonist, demonstrated reduced symptoms, reduced cocaine and alcohol craving, and fewer cocaine-positive urine samples in patients with schizophrenia and cocaine use disorder (Beresford et al. 2005) and patients with schizoaffective and substance use disorders (Brown et al. 2005). To our knowledge, no reports have been published on the impact of ziprasidone, lurasidone, iloperidone, or cariprazine on substance use disorders in patients with schizophrenia, although testing in animal models suggests that cariprazine and iloperidone warrant further investigation (Khokhar and Green 2016; Román et al. 2013).

Long-acting injectable (LAI) formulations of antipsychotics simplify medication taking and enable clinicians to be aware of when patients discontinue antipsychotic medications. Because use of LAI formulations leads to steady drug levels, lower doses of medications may be possible. Three studies indicate that patients assigned to LAI risperidone had better alcohol-related outcomes than did patients assigned to oral medications (A.I. Green et al. 2015; Rosenheck et al. 2011; Rubio et al. 2006). Three prospective studies of LAI paliperidone reported better adherence, delayed treatment failure, or reduced substance use disorder treatment utilization among patients with co-occurring disorders (Joshi et al. 2018; Lefebvre et al. 2017; Lynn Starr et al. 2018). Given the additional evidence indicating overall better outcomes with LAI antipsychotics (Taipale et al. 2018; Tiihonen et al. 2017), their use should be considered for people with schizophrenia and co-occurring substance use disorder.

Several medications shown to be effective for the treatment of substance use disorders in the general population also show promise in treating schizophrenia and should be used in addition to antipsychotic treatment (Batki 2015). The tricyclic antidepressants desipramine and imipramine have been related to positive outcomes in the treatment of cocaine use disorder (Siris et al. 1993; Ziedonis et al. 1992). Disulfiram has been used safely and with some success in patients with schizophrenia (Petrakis et al. 2006), although it must be used with caution because of its potential to increase psychosis (Kingsbury and Salzman 1990). A retrospective uncontrolled study of disulfiram in 33 patients with alcohol use disorder and serious mental illness (23 with schizophrenia) showed a 64% rate of sustained remission (Mueser et al. 2003b). Five preliminary studies reported that naltrexone, which has U.S. Food and Drug Administration (FDA) approval for alcohol use disorder (O'Malley et al. 1992), may also be effective for schizophrenia (Batki et al. 2008; Dougherty 1997; Maxwell and Shinderman 1997, 2000; Petrakis et al. 2004). A controlled trial of acamprosate in patients with schizophrenia and alcohol use disorder showed reduced thoughts of alcohol drinking but no impact on alcohol drinking behavior (Ralevski et al. 2011). Varenicline, which has FDA approval for treating tobacco use disorder and is considered safe in schizophrenia (Anthenelli et al. 2016), reduces drinking in people with alcohol use disorder (Litten et al. 2013; O'Malley et al. 2018). One small trial of varenicline was promising in people with schizophrenia and alcohol use disorder but low tolerability was demonstrated (Meszaros et al. 2013). Opioid agonists and antagonists are effective for the treatment of opioid use disorder but have not been systematically studied in patients with comorbid schizophrenia and opioid use disorder. Although prescription benzodiazepines are effective for alcohol withdrawal, outpatient use of benzodiazepines does not appear to improve outcomes, is associated with increased risk of mortality (Tiihonen et al. 2016), and is also associated with the development of benzodiazepine use disorders (Brunette et al. 2003). Therefore, they should be avoided in patients with schizophrenia.

With the trend toward legalization of medical and/or recreational cannabis in the United States, there is interest in whether cannabinoids may be useful in the treatment of co-occurring substance use disorder and schizophrenia (Boggs et al. 2018a; Iseger and Bossong 2015). In early research, a small case series of a medicinal, low-tetrahydrocannabinol (THC)/high-cannabidiol form of cannabis among inpatients with co-occurring disorders showed that this type of cannabis was not effective in treating symptoms of schizophrenia or cannabis use disorder (Schipper et al. 2018).

A shared decision-making approach to prescribing medications supports recovery from both disorders (Noordsy et al. 2000). Clinicians should encourage patients to take antipsychotics and other appropriate psychotropic medication despite ongoing substance use in order to stabilize symptoms of schizophrenia, which then facilitates participation in treatment for substance use disorders. A multidisciplinary team approach to comprehensive, integrated psychosocial and psychopharmacological treatments for both disorders can increase treatment engagement and improve outcomes (Brunette and Mueser 2006; De Witte et al. 2014; Drake 2007; Mueser et al. 2003a).

Overview of Tobacco Use Disorder

Currently, 50%–65% of people with schizophrenia smoke tobacco (Correll et al. 2014; Dickerson et al. 2018b), a rate that is substantially higher than the national rate of 15.5% for people without serious mental illness (Jamal et al. 2018). Nicotine withdrawal can worsen agitation (Schechter and Rand 1974) and complicate management of psychosis in the emergency room (Allen et al. 2011). Because hydrocarbons in smoke inhibit cytochrome P450 1A1, 1A2, and 2E1, change between states of smoking and abstinence shifts some antipsychotic serum levels (e.g., clozapine, olanzapine, haloperidol), complicating transitions between inpatient and outpatient treatment (Lowe and Ackman 2010). Furthermore, because toxins in smoke cause cancers, cardiovascular disease, lung diseases, and diabetes, smoking is a significant cause of early mortality in people with schizophrenia who smoke tobacco (Auquier et al. 2006; Bushe et al. 2010; Dickerson et al. 2014; Kelly et al. 2011). Consequently, addressing tobacco use disorder among smokers is an important component of treatment (Williams et al. 2013).

Biological, psychological, social, and environmental factors contribute to the high rates of smoking initiation and low rates of quitting in individuals with schizophrenia. Studies suggest that there may be a shared genetic liability to tobacco use disorder and schizophrenia (Chen et al. 2016; de Leon and Diaz 2012; Wing et al. 2012). For example, some types of nicotinic acetylcholine receptors may be dysfunctional or abnormally expressed in people with schizophrenia (Kunii et al. 2015; Parikh et al. 2016). Many studies (Ahnallen et al. 2012; Avila et al. 2003; Dépatie et al. 2002; Featherstone and Siegel 2015; Gehricke et al. 2007; Myers et al. 2004; Olincy et al. 2003), but not all (Boggs et al. 2018b), have shown that nicotine can improve aspects of impaired cognition and reward function in this group, potentially leading to greater positive reinforcement for smoking and negative reinforcement for smoking during withdrawal in patients with schizophrenia compared with smokers without schizophrenia (Berg et al. 2014). Beliefs about the perceived benefits of smoking as well as concerns about quitting held by many patients, families, and clinicians may inhibit quitting in people with schizophrenia and tobacco use disorder (Aschbrenner et al. 2017a, 2017b; Brown et al. 2015; Himelhoch and Daumit 2003). Yet, most people with schizophrenia have periods of wanting to quit and have made quit attempts; furthermore, many have successfully quit (Aschbrenner et al. 2015; Bennett et al. 2013; Dickerson et al. 2011; Ferron et al. 2011). Notably, psychosis, mood, and anxiety symptoms do not worsen when patients quit smoking; in fact, symptoms often improve after quitting (e.g., Cather et al. 2017a; Sankaranarayanan et al. 2016).

Detection and Management of Tobacco Use Disorder

Patients with schizophrenia should be screened and assessed for tobacco use at every treatment visit (Agency for Healthcare Research and Quality 2012; Fiore et al. 2008). Clinicians can then provide clear advice to quit and active intervention or referral to resources for smoking cessation, as standardized in the "5 A's":

- Ask about smoking.
- Advise to quit.
- Assess for readiness to try.
- Assist with cessation treatment.
- Arrange follow-up.

Use of the 5 A's in mental health settings is associated with decreased smoking (Dixon et al. 2009).

Clinical practice guidelines and evidence reviews recommend using both psychosocial (skills-based, problem-solving, and motivational enhancement approaches) and pharmacological (bupropion, varenicline, or nicotine replacement therapies) interventions for all smokers, including those with schizophrenia (Cather et al. 2017b; Fiore et al. 2008; Tidey and Miller 2015). Health care settings are increasingly implementing tobacco screening and referral to state-sponsored telephone quit lines that provide counseling (usually 3–5 sessions) and pharmacotherapy (usually a brief supply of nicotine replacement therapy [NRT]) when on-site resources are not available. Although studies have reported that between 20% and 30% of those with mental health conditions using telephone quit lines self-report quitting smoking at follow-up (Kerkvliet et al. 2015; Lukowski et al. 2015; Mathew et al. 2015; Vickerman et al. 2015), rates of verified quitting among people with schizophrenia using quit lines are much lower (Brunette et al. 2018b;

Morris et al. 2011) than rates reported with more intensive and longer behavioral interventions with pharmacotherapy (for review, see Cather et al. 2017b).

The best evidence for psychosocial interventions for smoking cessation among patients with schizophrenia supports the use of behavioral and motivational approaches, together with pharmacological interventions (discussed in the next paragraph), to help patients who are psychiatrically stable to identify personal reasons for quitting, learn alternative coping strategies, and utilize pharmacotherapy to address cravings (Bennett et al. 2013). Similar to addressing other substance use disorders, a stage-based approach is warranted (Bennett et al. 2013). Motivational approaches that include personalized feedback about smoking and quitting can improve engagement in smoking cessation treatment and increase quit attempts (Steinberg et al. 2004, 2016). Assessment and motivational education about smoking and its financial, social, and health impacts lead to abstinence in 10%–20% of young people with schizophrenia without further intervention (Brunette et al. 2018a; Coletti et al. 2015; Prochaska et al. 2015), possibly because young people tend to have lower levels of nicotine dependence (Brunette et al. 2017b). Adaptations to skills-based behavioral interventions for smokers with schizophrenia include breaking down skills into concrete steps, implementing skills via action planning and role-playing, and reviewing content repeatedly for those who experience impairments in learning and memory (Bennett et al. 2015). Such tailored behavioral interventions can be delivered via mobile technology (smartphones, tablets, or computers) (Brunette et al. 2011b, 2013; Vilardaga et al. 2018), an approach that may be especially appealing to young adults (Brunette et al. 2018a). Incentives for abstinence, when offered with cessation treatment, also may increase rates of abstinence among smokers with schizophrenia (Brunette et al. 2018c). People with schizophrenia and tobacco use disorder are open to working with supportive family members, friends, and peer specialists around smoking cessation (Aschbrenner et al. 2017b, 2018; Dickerson et al. 2016), which can increase utilization of effective cessation treatments (Aschbrenner et al. 2017b). Strategies to engage these smokers in cessation services are critically important because use of and retention in services predict cessation (Ferron et al. 2016).

All FDA-approved medications for treating tobacco use disorder have been shown to be effective in people with comorbid schizophrenia. One placebo-controlled trial has evaluated the use of NRT in individuals with comorbid tobacco use disorder and schizophrenia, demonstrating an odds ratio of 3.40 for the efficacy of NRT patch over placebo patch (Evins et al. 2019). Additionally, 11 published studies have included at least one study arm of treatment with NRT. For example, when NRT was used with frequent medical management visits, 26.2% of the smokers were able to achieve verified abstinence (Williams et al. 2010). NRT is also useful for reducing symptoms of withdrawal, including agitation, in acute treatment settings (Allen et al. 2011). Bupropion, an antidepressant with FDA approval for smoking cessation, was tested in at least four studies in people with schizophrenia and was found to be most effective when combined with NRT among patients participating in group therapy with motivational and cognitive-behavioral components (Evins et al. 2007; George et al. 2008). Varenicline is the most effective cessation medication in people with schizophrenia (Evins et al. 2014; Williams et al. 2012). In a controlled trial designed to assess safety (Anthenelli et al. 2016), there were no differences in suicidality and agitation between placebo and varenicline among over 1,000 smokers with mental illness who took this medication. The FDA approved removal of a black box warning in 2016, thereby supporting use of varenicline in people with schizophrenia. Anthenelli et al. (2016) reported the following rates of moderate and severe neuropsychiatric side effects in over 4,000 smokers with psychiatric disorders: 6.5% in the varenicline group, 6.7% in the bupropion group, 5.2% in the nicotine patch group, and 4.9% in the placebo group. Because relapse is high after discontinuing medications (Evins et al. 2007, 2014), clinicians should consider maintaining these medications with relapse prevention counseling for a year or more after cessation.

There is rationale for and interest in using repetitive transcranial magnetic stimulation (rTMS) for the treatment of people with severe addiction (Salling and Martinez 2016; Spagnolo and Goldman 2017). Small rTMS studies have provided mixed results for reducing cigarette smoking in patients with schizophrenia (Kozak et al. 2018; Prikryl et al. 2014).

Finally, environmental approaches such as banning smoking in hospitals are safe and may reduce initiation of smoking (El-Guebaly et al. 2002; Lawn and Pols 2005), but hospital bans do not lead to quitting unless they are paired with cessation interventions during the hospital stay and following discharge (Metse et al. 2017; Prochaska et al. 2014). In the future, population-based approaches such as reducing nicotine levels in cigarettes may reduce smoking (Tidey et al. 2016) and possibly promote switching to lower-harm tobacco products. One pilot study suggested that some chronic smokers with schizophrenia can use electronic cigarettes to reduce or quit smoking (Pratt et al. 2016).

In summary, settings that provide care to smokers with schizophrenia can take a holistic, long-term approach that incorporates evidence-based screening, assessment, cessation interventions, and attention to environmental and social factors that can reduce smoking and enhance quitting. Nicotine withdrawal should be treated in acute treatment settings, and antipsychotic doses may need to be changed during hospital stays. Use of both behavioral and pharmacological interventions results in optimal cessation outcomes, and long-term treatments reduce relapse.

Obesity

Overview of Obesity

The mean prevalence of obesity in people with schizophrenia is 49.4% (Mitchell et al. 2013), a rate that is twice that in the general U.S. population (Allison et al. 2009; Daumit et al. 2003; Dickerson et al. 2006). Although young patients with first-episode psychosis are already more likely to show signs of impaired glucose homeostasis than are young people without schizophrenia (Pillinger et al. 2017), differences in obesity are often not yet apparent (Correll et al. 2014). The degree to which risk for obesity is intrinsic to schizophrenia or due to altered lifestyle and psychotropic medications is still under investigation (Freyberg et al. 2017); however, it is clear that multiple factors contribute to risk for obesity in this group, including physical inactivity (Brown et al. 1999), poor dietary practices (Jakobsen et al. 2018; Manu et al. 2015; McCreadie et al. 1998; Nenke et al. 2015), and the impact of antipsychotics, especially clozapine, olanzapine, and iloperidone (Leucht et al. 2013). Several neurobiological mechanisms have been proposed to explain the propensity for and individual variation in weight gain with antipsychotics, including changes in the expression of immunity genes and resulting changes in inflammatory cytokines (Chase et al. 2015; Fonseka et al. 2016). Genetic polymorphisms among multiple other genes have also been associated with antipsychotic-induced weight gain, including common variants in the melanocortin 4 receptor, α_{2A} adrenoceptor, dopamine D_2 receptor, serotonin 5-HT$_{2C}$ receptor, and brain-derived neurotrophic factor (Zhang et al. 2016).

Obesity in patients with schizophrenia is associated with poor psychological health, high levels of distress, low levels of functioning, and poor quality of life (Malhotra et al. 2016). Most concerning, obesity is a component of metabolic syndrome (Mitchell et al. 2013) and contributes to the development of a variety of diseases (Leucht et al. 2007), including diabetes, cancer, and cardiovascular diseases, which lead to early mortality (Olfson et al. 2015). Attention to comorbid obesity and cardiovascular disease is critical as the gap between life expectancy in the general population and those with schizophrenia has widened in recent years (Saha et al. 2007).

Detection and Management of Obesity

Current guidelines recommend that clinicians regularly assess body weight and girth in people with schizophrenia, especially those taking second-generation antipsychotics (American Diabetes Association et al. 2004). Given the evidence demonstrating a strong association between self-monitoring and weight loss (Burke et al. 2011; Vanwormer et al. 2008), as well as weight maintenance (Laitner et al. 2016), all patients with schizophrenia who are overweight or obese should be encouraged to track their weight at home (at least weekly) and taught to track food intake. Individuals who are severely obese (defined as a body mass index [BMI] >40 or weight >400 lb) will require a specialized scale.

Patients with schizophrenia benefit from education about the risks of obesity; the advantages of healthy weight, exercise, and a healthy diet; the impact of medications on body metabolism and satiety; and medication strategies to mitigate obesity. It is particularly important for individuals to understand that medications can prevent a feeling of fullness, leading to greater food intake and weight gain. Many patients need training in how to shop for, prepare, or buy premade foods that are high in fiber and low in calories. The Mediterranean-style diet, for example, may benefit individuals by increasing short-chain fatty acids; it might also target immune and metabolic dysfunction in schizophrenia (Joseph et al. 2017).

Strategies to prevent and address obesity in patients with schizophrenia include interventions that assist with adopting a healthy lifestyle (diet and exercise); switching to antipsychotics with low cardiometabolic risk; and taking medications that may lower weight, as well as avoid or rectify abnormal glucose and lipid parameters. Several literature reviews have reported on the multitude of studies investigating these three strategies to prevent antipsychotic-associated weight gain and/or obesity (Aschbrenner et al. 2017b; Correll et al. 2013; Das et al. 2012; Manu et al. 2015; McGinty et al. 2016; Siskind et al. 2016; Teasdale et al. 2017; Zimbron et al. 2016). Each of these strategies similarly lowers weight approximately 6.6–13.2 lb over 3–6 months.

An emerging evidence base supports the effectiveness of combined exercise and diet interventions developed specifically for overweight and obese people with schizophrenia (Bartels et al. 2013, 2015; Daumit et al. 2013; C.A. Green et al. 2015). The most effective interventions utilize behavioral approaches to encourage calorie reduction, dietary restructuring, and increase of physical activity with at least moderate-intensity exercise (Manu et al. 2015). The most widely implemented intervention is a program of weekly fitness coaching integrated into community mental health treatment (Bartels et al. 2013, 2015). Patients with high levels of negative symptoms may not respond as well to behavioral interventions (Storch Jakobsen et al. 2018) and should also receive pharmacological strategies.

Most patients with schizophrenia and obesity are able to lose weight by switching to antipsychotics (and other medications) with lower weight gain liability, such as aripiprazole, ziprasidone, or perphenazine (Chen et al. 2012; Meyer et al. 2008; Mukundan et al. 2010; Newcomer et al. 2008; Stroup et al. 2011). There is no clear evidence that one switching strategy is better than another (Mukundan et al. 2010).

Adding medications can also be beneficial. Metformin is used for the treatment of type 2 diabetes and has been used in concert with antipsychotics to prevent weight gain. Its effects are attributed to suppression of hepatic gluconeogenesis and increased peripheral insulin sensitivity (Kirpichnikov et al. 2002). It also increases production of glucagon-like peptide, which stimulates insulin secretion while inhibiting glucagon secretion (Kappe et al. 2013). Multiple studies have demonstrated that metformin can reduce or prevent weight gain in patients with schizophrenia taking antipsychotic medications with high weight gain propensity (Siskind et al. 2016). For example, four randomized controlled trials (RCTs) indicated that patients who used metformin with olanzapine weighed 11 lb less than did those who were assigned to placebo with olanzapine (Praharaj et al. 2011).

Additionally, six drugs have received FDA approval to treat people with obesity (BMI >30), and these can be considered for patients with a BMI over 27 and obesity-related comorbidities (Saunders et al. 2018). Overall, in general population studies, these medications result in at least 5% weight loss among 44%–75% of patients taking them (Khera et al. 2016). Here we review medications with evidence for efficacy in patients with schizophrenia. Liraglutide, the glucagon-like peptide-1 receptor agonist administered as a subcutaneous injection, has been shown to be effective in people with obesity and schizophrenia (Larsen et al. 2017). The combination drug naltrexone sustained release (SR)/bupropion SR is suggested for patients with craving or addictive eating patterns who do not need and are not abusing opioid medications or street drugs. Although this combination has not been studied in patients with schizophrenia, initial studies have begun to evaluate naltrexone and other opioid receptor blockers alone for antipsychotic-associated weight gain (Silverman et al. 2018). Meta-analyses of 22 studies (2–24 weeks in duration) demonstrated efficacy for topiramate (mean weight loss of about 6–8 lbs, usually over 12 weeks) in patients treated with antipsychotics who have schizophrenia (Goh et al. 2019; Zheng et al. 2016). Topiramate is more effective when used preemptively (e.g., when antipsychotics are initiated) (Zheng et al. 2016) and has the advantage of also improving positive, negative, and general symptoms of psychosis. Orlistat (available over the counter) is a lipase inhibitor that is suggested for patients with hypercholesterolemia who can limit their intake of fatty foods. One 16-week trial of orlistat without behavioral intervention for obesity in patients with schizophrenia taking clozapine or olanzapine showed significant weight loss only among male participants (5.2 lb) (Joffe et al. 2008; Tchoukhine et al. 2011). Use of orlistat can be limited by side effects, including diarrhea and incontinence, but it was reasonably tolerated among participants in this study.

Combination treatments are commonly used to address obesity in patients with schizophrenia. For example, metformin is typically studied in combination with behavioral lifestyle interventions (Zheng et al. 2019). However, the level of additive benefit of combinations of interventions for obesity is not known. Given the negative consequences of obesity, clinicians can use shared decision making to select and implement a tailored combination of behavioral and pharmacotherapeutic strategies for patients who are at risk for or currently experiencing obesity.

Depressive Symptoms and Disorders

Overview of Depression

Although schizophrenia is viewed primarily as a psychotic disorder, rates of co-occurring depressive disorders are high (Bosanac and Castle 2013). Most people with schizophrenia experience a clinically significant depressive episode at least once in their lives, with lifetime risk up to 80% (Bland et al. 1987; Häfner et al. 1999; Kendler et al. 1996; Koreen et al. 1993; Martin et al. 1985) and point prevalence of major depression ranging from 20% (in patients with chronic schizophrenia) to 50% (in first-episode samples) (Baynes et al. 2000; Delahanty et al. 2001; Häfner et al. 1999; Herbener and Harrow 2002; Jin et al. 2001; Krynicki et al. 2018; Messias et al. 2001; Upthegrove et al. 2017). Depression rates tend to be underestimated, especially among African Americans, in part due to the overlap between negative symptoms of schizophrenia and depression symptoms (Delahanty et al. 2001; Elk et al. 1986).

Symptoms of depression are common during exacerbations of psychosis (Baynes et al. 2000; Häfner et al. 1999; Jin et al. 2001; Oosthuizen et al. 2002) and often improve as the psychosis remits (Birchwood et al. 2000; Häfner et al. 1999; Koreen et al. 1993; Tollefson et al. 1999). Depression can be especially problematic during the prodromal and early phases of the illness. Although the presence of mood symptoms during a psychotic episode of schizophrenia has been considered a positive prognostic indicator, depression during remission of psychosis is associated with worse outcomes (Upthegrove et al. 2017). Depression is associated with completed suicides (Hor and Taylor 2010), risk of relapse of psychosis (Mandel et al. 1982), hospital readmission (Shepherd et al. 1989), worse functioning (Jin et al. 2001), lower quality of life (Dixon et al. 2001), violence (Krakowski and Czobor 2014), and medication nonadherence (Upthegrove et al. 2017). Consequently, symptoms of depression should be carefully monitored and treated (Conley et al. 2007; Upthegrove et al. 2017).

Depression in schizophrenia may be an intrinsic part of the disorder. Regions critical to emotional processing, such as the hippocampus, insula, and prefrontal cortex, are implicated in both disorders (Upthegrove et al. 2017). Depression also may occur as a psychological reaction to developing and living with schizophrenia (Bosanac and Castle 2013; Upthegrove et al. 2017). Demoralization, which occurs as people struggle with their illness and its effect on their functioning (Siris 2000a), seems to be associated with better insight into the illness (Bartels and Drake 1988). Some people develop a sense of hopelessness and helplessness (Hoffmann et al. 2000) that predicts poor outcome in rehabilitation.

Detection and Management of Depression

Determining the temporal appearance, duration, quality, and severity of depressive symptoms is necessary for diagnosis and formulation of an appropriate treatment plan. Symptoms of depression can be mistaken for negative symptoms, including affective flattening, alogia, avolition, apathy, anhedonia, and asociality (Birchwood et al. 2000; Sax et al. 1996; Siris 2000a), or for medication side effects, such as sedation, akinesia, and other extrapyramidal system symptoms, particularly parkinsonism (Norman et al. 1998; Siris 1987). Key features of major depression that distinguish it from negative symptoms include the presence of depressed mood, nondelusional guilt, and neurovegetative symptoms. A recent literature review found that symptoms related to expressive deficits (e.g., alogia, blunted affect) were specific to negative symptoms, whereas symptoms such as avolition, anergia, and amotivation occurred in both the depressive and negative domains, and hopelessness and consummatory anhedonia represented specific symptoms of depression (Krynicki et al. 2018).

Use of standardized scales can enhance the assessment of depression in patients with schizophrenia. The Calgary Depression Scale for Schizophrenia (Addington et al. 1990), a nine-item, clinician-rated measure, performs better in assessing patients with established schizophrenia (Lako et al. 2012) and those at high risk for psychosis (Addington et al. 2014) than scales used for general population samples. Clinicians should also assess risk factors for depression such as family history of depressive disorders (Subotnik et al. 1997) and should rule out medications or medical conditions that can cause depression, such as thyroid dysfunction, sleep apnea, stimulant withdrawal, or side effects from antihypertensive medications (Bosanac and Castle 2013).

Optimal treatment of psychosis is an important step in treating depression in patients with schizophrenia. Both first- and second-generation antipsychotic medications reduce symptoms of depression in patients with schizophrenia (Kjelby et al. 2011; Lieberman et al. 2005), but second-generation medications generally have a lower risk for side effects that may mimic depression (Furtado and Srihari 2008; Galling et al. 2017; Rybakowski et al. 2012). Adding a second antipsychotic to the first does not improve depressive symptoms (Galling et al. 2017). People with schizophrenia and major depression responded better to quetiapine than to risperidone (Addington et al. 2011; Kasper et al. 2015), but in people with treatment-refractory schizophrenia, clozapine outperformed quetiapine for improving depressive symptoms (Nakajima et al. 2015).

Adding antidepressant medication or electroconvulsive therapy (ECT) treats major depression directly in patients with schizophrenia. A large study demonstrated the efficacy of citalopram over placebo for depression symptoms and suicidal ideation in patients with schizophrenia, as well as its safety in older adults (Kasckow et al. 2010; Zisook et al. 2009, 2010). A naturalistic population-level study found that antidepressant treatment was associated with reduced mortality among people with schizophrenia who had made prior suicide attempts (Haukka et al. 2008). Combined findings from smaller studies of antidepressant medications indicate a modest reduction in depression symptoms and good tolerability (Galling et al. 2018; Gregory et al. 2017). ECT may be used safely for treatment-resistant depression in patients with schizophrenia (Nothdurfter et al. 2006).

Although psychosocial interventions that are effective for the treatment of depression in the general population have not been carefully studied in patients with schizophrenia, effective interventions that can be used include cognitive-behavioral therapy (CBT), problem-solving training, coping skills training, acceptance and commitment therapy, mindfulness therapy, relaxation training, exercise, family therapy, and support (Gumley et al. 2017; Moritz et al. 2015; Siris 1990, 2000b). Two studies indicate that providing CBT for psychosis may be effective for reducing symptoms of depression in the long term among people with schizophrenia (Jones et al. 2012; Lincoln et al. 2012). For people who are demoralized and hopeless, interventions geared toward developing meaningful daytime activities can be helpful (Provencher et al. 2002).

In summary, further research is needed to establish the most effective combination of interventions for depressive symptoms in patients with schizophrenia. Nevertheless, treatment may include pharmacological and/or psychosocial interventions (van Rooijen et al. 2019). The choice of a strategy to manage depressive symptoms depends to some extent on when such symptoms appear during the course of the disorder as well as on their severity and their persistence. For brief depressive reactions to stressful life events, supportive counseling and monitoring may be effective. If symptoms persist or are severe, further interventions should be considered. Symptoms should be carefully differentiated from neurological side effects, and a trial of dose reduction or a switch from a first-generation to a second-generation agent should be considered to reduce the side effects that can mimic depression (Hogarty et al. 1995). Because depressive symptoms may herald psychotic relapse, people should be monitored carefully for the emergence or exacerbation of psychosis. If the depression is part of a psychotic exacerbation, antipsychotic medication should be increased or replaced with another agent. If depressive symptoms persist or worsen in the absence of a psychotic exacerbation, use of an antidepressant medication and/or behavioral interventions can be considered.

Overview of Suicide

The most recently published rate of suicide among people with schizophrenia is 52 per 100,000 person-years, four times that of the general population (Olfson et al. 2015), with a significantly higher rate for males (63.7) than females (38.5). Suicide was the leading cause of death for people with schizophrenia ages 15–24 years (Lin et al. 2018) and for individuals ages 16–30 years with a new psychotic illness diagnosis (Simon et al. 2018). Depressive symptoms, active hallucinations and delusions, prior suicide attempts, substance misuse, and greater illness insight are associated with death from suicide by individuals with schizophrenia (Bornheimer 2019; Hor and Taylor 2010). Research is beginning to evaluate potential biological risk factors for suicide in schizophrenia, including low cholesterol, cytomegalovirus, and neurotropic human herpesvirus, but there is not sufficient evidence to support routine screening for these factors (Ayesa-Arriola et al. 2018; Dickerson et al. 2018a; Shrivastava et al. 2017). Additionally, researchers are applying computer "machine learning" to better predict suicide using multiple clinical features in people with schizophrenia (Hettige et al. 2017); these approaches may be useful in the future.

Detection and Management of Suicidality

The detection of suicidal ideation and prevention of suicide in people with schizophrenia can be difficult, in part because many suicide attempts are impulsive (Allebeck et al. 1987; Gut-Fayand et al. 2001), and also because lethal methods may be used (Breier and Astrachan 1984; Heilä et al. 1997), with no advance disclosure (Earle et al. 1994). Optimal treatment includes careful assessment of suicide risk factors (Hor and Taylor 2010), active outreach to engage individuals meaningfully in treatment, psychosocial rehabilitation and skills training to improve coping skills, and effective pharmacotherapy for psychosis and depression symptoms.

Listening to and responding to the reports of distress, especially overt suicidal ideation, is especially crucial (Cohen et al. 1990). Hospitalization can maintain safety with monitoring, structure, and support, as well as provide an opportunity for intensive review and adjustment of psychopharmacological treatments to address symptoms of psychosis and depression. However, because discharge from the hospital can lead to social isolation and increased stress, follow-up treatment and supports must be in place prior to discharge. Intensive monitoring with in-person interventions such as with intensive case management (Dieterich et al. 2017) or via telehealth tools (Kasckow et al. 2016; Pratt et al. 2015) may provide even more opportunities to prevent suicide.

Adequate psychopharmacological treatment of psychosis and depression is also essential (Hasan et al. 2015). In a study of 88 individuals with schizophrenia who died from suicide, more than half either were prescribed inadequate doses of antipsychotic medication or were not compliant with treatment; an additional 23% were considered to be not responsive to medication (Heilä et al. 1999). Psychoeducation and close monitoring may increase compliance with pharmacological treatment. Studies suggest that clozapine may decrease suicidal ideation, suicide attempts, and suicide completion in people with schizophrenia more effectively than first-generation antipsychotic medications (Meltzer and Okayli 1995; Reid et al. 1998; Walker et al. 1997) and olanzapine (Meltzer et al. 2003), and analysis of death rates reported in multiple studies indicated that long-term treatment with clozapine was associated with a lower overall crude mortality ratio (0.56) (Vermeulen et al. 2019).

Anxiety Symptoms and Disorders

Overview of Anxiety Symptoms and Disorders

Anxiety symptoms and disorders are common in people with schizophrenia, with lifetime prevalence rates higher than in the general population (Achim et al. 2011). Although published prevalence rates vary due to differences in assessment methods and diagnostic methodology, anxiety symptoms have been found to occur in up to 65% of people with schizophrenia (Temmingh and Stein 2015), and anxiety diagnoses have been reported in up to 38% (Achim et al. 2011). To be diagnosed as a co-occurring anxiety disorder, symptoms occurring during psychotic episodes must be differentiated from paranoia, reactions to delusions, and agitation related to psychosis. Additionally, anxiety should be differentiated from antipsychotic medication–induced side effects, such as akathisia, as well as other comorbid syndromes, such as substance-induced symptoms (e.g., cocaine intoxication, alcohol withdrawal), and depressive disorders (Zisook et al. 1999). Female gender, younger age, higher level of education, and marriage have been associated with anxiety symptoms in people with schizophrenia (Dixon et al. 2001). Comorbid anxiety disorders tend to be underdiagnosed, and therefore undertreated, especially in ethnic or racial minorities (Dixon et al. 2001). The negative impact of anxiety on course and prognosis of schizophrenia necessitates recognition and appropriate treatment (Temmingh and Stein 2015). In this section, we review the literature on the most common comorbid anxiety disorders, including panic and social anxiety disorder. In subsequent sections, we review the literature on PTSD and OCD, which are no longer classified as anxiety disorders in DSM-5 (American Psychiatric Association 2013).

Panic Attacks and Panic Disorder

A meta-analysis of the published literature on anxiety disorders in people with schizophrenia reported a mean prevalence rate of 9.8% for comorbid panic disorder (Achim et al. 2011). An earlier review of the literature estimated that panic attacks occurred in 25% and panic disorder in 15% of people with schizophrenia (Buckley et al. 2009). Buckley et al. (2009) also noted that comorbid panic symptoms were associated with more severe psychopathology, increased risk of suicidal ideation and behavior, and increased vulnerability to substance abuse. Panic symptoms and panic disorder can develop before, during, or after the onset of the psychotic disorder (Baylé et al. 2001; Craig et al. 2002). The association between panic attacks and increased risk of developing schizophrenia had led some to suggest that panic could be a part of the prodrome of schizophrenia (Goodwin et al. 2004). Panic attacks are associated with female gender, Caucasian race, and lower level of education (Goodwin et al. 2002).

Detection and Management of Panic

People with comorbid schizophrenia and panic experience the full spectrum of classic panic symptoms (Goodwin et al. 2002), with prominent trembling, feelings of unreality, and fear of dying, which can be experienced with psychotic symptoms, such as auditory hallucinations (Gabínio et al. 2017). Panic is dramatically underrecognized in individuals with schizophrenia (Craig et al. 2002); therefore, systematic screening and assessment can improve care for people with this comorbidity. The Panic Disorder Severity Scale (PDSS) is a widely used measure to assess symptoms of panic disorder (Shear et al. 1997).

CBT is effective for the treatment of panic disorder in the general population (Barlow et al. 2000). Two very small, uncontrolled pilot studies of CBT for panic in patients with schizophrenia demonstrated that 75% of those who completed the treatment experienced symptom improvement (Arlow et al. 1997; Hofmann et al. 2000). Exercise may reduce anxiety symptoms among general population patients with panic disorder (Jayakody et al. 2014; Lattari et al. 2018); however, this approach has not been tested among people with comorbid schizophrenia and panic.

Although antipsychotic medications generally reduce anxiety—as measured by subscales of symptom rating measures, such as the Positive and Negative Syndrome Scale (PANSS) (Marder et al. 1997)—no controlled studies have assessed the impact of antipsychotic medications on panic. One case report indicated that three patients with schizophrenia experienced improvement in their panic attacks when switched from first-generation antipsychotics to quetiapine (Takahashi et al. 2004). Moreover, although antidepressants and benzodiazepines are effective medications for people with primary panic disorder in the general population, no controlled studies have assessed their effectiveness for panic disorder in patients with schizophrenia. A report of two people showed that panic symptoms responded to imipramine augmentation of fluphenazine (Siris et al. 1989). In addition, two small studies showed that benzodiazepines reduced panic attacks in 10 people with schizophrenia (Argyle 1990; Kahn et al. 1988). Further research is needed to assess the impact of panic disorder on people with schizophrenia, as well to assess the effectiveness of treatments.

Social Anxiety Disorder

A meta-analysis reported a pooled prevalence rate of 25% of outpatients and 9% of inpatients for social phobia (now social anxiety disorder in DSM-5) in individuals with schizophrenia (McEnery et al. 2019b), although much higher rates have been reported among small samples (e.g., Lowengrub et al. 2015). Comorbid social anxiety in schizophrenia is associated with worse prognosis, including greater likelihood of early relapse and, not surprisingly, greater levels of social disability (McEnery et al. 2019b). Symptoms of social anxiety can negatively impact not only engagement in basic day-to-day tasks such as grocery shopping but also pursuit of school and work (McEnery et al. 2019b).

Detection and Management of Social Anxiety Disorder

People with schizophrenia and social anxiety exhibit levels of social fear (Penn et al. 1994) and social phobia (Pallanti et al. 2004) similar to those of people with primary social anxiety disorder. However, social anxiety and fear of social situations may be confused with the avoidance and withdrawal associated with psychotic symptoms (Pallanti et al. 2004; Penn et al. 1994) and must be carefully delineated from paranoia, withdrawal, and apathy. The key identifying features of social anxiety disorder are the *fear of* or *anxiety about social situations* where the individual might be scrutinized by others and the *avoidance* of those situations or *endurance* of them with intense anxiety. Evidence of embarrassment regarding scrutiny, rather than fear of persecution, will help identify people with schizophrenia and social anxiety.

The most widely used standardized measures of social anxiety include the self-reported Social Phobia Scale (Mattick and Clarke 1998), which assesses fears of being scrutinized during routine activities (eating, drinking, writing); the self-reported Social Interaction Anxiety Scale (Mattick and Clarke 1998), which assesses fears of social situations; and the observer-rated Brief Social Phobia Scale (Davidson et al. 1997), which assesses fear, avoidance, and physiological arousal.

CBT, which includes education, cognitive restructuring, social skills training, and gradual exposure to feared social situations, is effective for people with social anxiety disorder in the general population (Taylor 1996). Two studies of group-based CBT for people with schizophrenia and social anxiety disorder demonstrated improvements in the treatment group compared with the wait-list groups (Michail et al. 2017). Cognitive bias modification, a computerized attention task designed to train individuals to reduce attention to threatening stimuli, has also shown early promise as a method to treat social anxiety disorder in people with schizophrenia (Macleod and Holmes 2012). Social skills training improves social dysfunction in individuals with schizophrenia (Kurtz and Mueser 2008), but this approach has not been tested to address comorbid social anxiety disorder per se. An online group approach for young people with schizophrenia and co-occurring social anxiety disorder has been developed but not yet tested (McEnery et al. 2019a).

Regarding pharmacological interventions, antipsychotics alone may not always be helpful. Pallanti and colleagues described 12 people treated with clozapine whose social anxiety symptoms became clinically detectable when their psychosis remitted during clozapine treatment (Pallanti et al. 1999). The same group has suggested that serotonin reuptake inhibitors (SRIs), which are effective for the treatment of social anxiety disorder in the general population (Blanco et al. 2003), may be helpful for people with schizophrenia and social phobia (Pallanti et al. 1999), but no controlled trials have been completed. Further studies are needed to assess the impact and interactions of social anxiety disorder on people with schizophrenia, as well as to systematically test behavioral and pharmacological treatments.

Posttraumatic Stress Disorder

Overview of Posttraumatic Stress Disorder

Individuals with serious mental illnesses including schizophrenia report high rates of childhood abuse, with estimates ranging from 10% to 61% for physical abuse and 13% to 61% for sexual abuse (Bendall et al. 2008; Grubaugh et al. 2011). A meta-analysis of 36 studies found that the experience of childhood trauma greatly elevates the risk for development of psychosis (Varese et al. 2012). Many patients experience multiple traumatic events over their lifetime (Gearon et al. 2003; Goodman et al. 2001; Lu et al. 2013), experiences that may be associated with the identification of and hospitalization for psychosis (Mueser et al. 2010).

Given these rates of trauma, it is not surprising that lifetime prevalence rates of PTSD in schizophrenia range from 14% to 53% (Calhoun et al. 2007; Goodman et al. 2001; Grubaugh et al. 2011; Mueser et al. 2002; Resnick et al. 2003; Sautter et al. 1999), compared with 7%–12% in the general population (Kessler et al. 2005). People with schizophrenia and PTSD experience greater impairment in social and community functioning, higher risk for substance use disorders, more severe psychotic illness, and increased risk for suicide relative to people with schizophrenia alone (Calhoun et al. 2006; Fan et al. 2008; Ford and Fournier 2007; Misiak and Frydecka 2016; Mueser et al. 1998, 2002, 2004; Sautter et al. 1999; Seow et al. 2016; Strauss et al. 2006). Models of PTSD in schizophrenia suggest that PTSD symptoms have a direct effect on functioning but also impact mental illness symptoms and correlates including depression and substance abuse (Mueser et al. 2002; Subica et al. 2012).

Detection and Management of Posttraumatic Stress Disorder

Although clinicians are often wary of discussing trauma with schizophrenia patients (Becker et al. 2004; Salyers et al. 2004), assessment and treatment of PTSD are generally well tolerated by patients when clinicians use person-centered explanation prior to assessment (van den Berg et al. 2016). Gold standard measures such as the PTSD Checklist (PCL) (Blevins et al. 2015; Weathers et al. 1993), the Traumatic Life Events Questionnaire (TLEQ) (Kubany et al. 2000), and the Clinician-Administered PTSD Scale (CAPS) (Weathers et al. 2001, 2018) show good psychometric properties in schizophrenia samples (Gearon et al. 2004; Grubaugh et al. 2007; Mueser et al. 2001), as do other measures of sexual and physical abuse (Fisher et al. 2011; Ford et al. 2017; Goodman et al. 1999; Grubaugh et al. 2007). Assessment should begin with the TLEQ to confirm the experience of a traumatic life event, followed by the PCL to determine symptom severity. For those individuals who screen positive, the CAPS can be used to establish a PTSD diagnosis. For clinicians who have not completed CAPS training,

PCL scores can be used as a starting point for reviewing DSM-5 criteria. The PCL should be administered regularly to monitor symptoms of PTSD.

PTSD treatment can be successfully integrated with comprehensive services for psychosis, depression, and substance use disorder (Rosenberg et al. 2001b). Evidence-based psychotherapies for PTSD, including prolonged exposure and cognitive processing therapy (Resick et al. 2002, 2008), have been tested with promising results in several open trials and smaller feasibility studies in patients with schizophrenia and other serious mental illnesses (de Bont et al. 2013; Frueh et al. 2009; Mueser et al. 2007; van den Berg and van der Gaag 2012). Using cognitive restructuring as the main treatment component (Mueser et al. 2015; Rosenberg et al. 2001b), two RCTs tested a 12- to 16-session individual CBT program that includes cognitive restructuring targeting trauma-related thoughts and beliefs, breathing retraining, and psychoeducation about PTSD. These studies showed that participants in the CBT condition improved in both PTSD and depressive symptoms, and changes were maintained 3 and 6 months later (Mueser et al. 2008, 2015). Mueser and colleagues (Mueser et al. 2015; Nishith et al. 2015) also developed a brief, manualized intervention consisting of psychoeducation about trauma and PTSD and instruction in breathing retraining, but initial testing did not show symptom improvement over routine care (Steel et al. 2017). Others have found that PTSD treatment for patients with comorbid psychiatric conditions and its integration within mental health services is feasible and can be effective (van den Berg et al. 2015, 2016; van Minnen et al. 2015). The most recent update of the Veterans Affairs/Department of Defense Clinical Practice Guideline for PTSD (U.S. Department of Veterans Affairs 2017) provides guidance on using CBT with individuals with serious mental illness.

Antidepressants reduce PTSD symptoms and are the current standard of pharmacological care (Bernardy and Friedman 2015). Even though they are prescribed to people with schizophrenia and co-occurring PTSD (Himelhoch et al. 2012), antidepressants have not been studied in individuals with schizophrenia and co-occurring PTSD.

Although additional research on treatment for PTSD in patients with schizophrenia is needed (Sin et al. 2017), current research supports assessment and treatment using CBT principles. The mental health clinician should assess for trauma and PTSD and then discuss the patient's desire to address these issues. If a patient is not ready for or interested in focusing on trauma, the clinician can work with the patient on general strategies for managing anxiety and provide pharmacotherapy for PTSD.

Obsessive-Compulsive Symptoms and Disorder

Overview of Obsessive-Compulsive Symptoms and Disorder

Approximately 30% of people with schizophrenia have comorbid obsessive-compulsive symptoms (OCS) and 12% have OCD (Achim et al. 2011; Grover et al. 2017; Swets et al. 2014), rates that are substantially higher than those in the general population (1.6%). Clinical factors most consistently correlated with OCS and OCD are earlier age at schizophrenia onset, comorbid depression, suicidal ideation, and suicide attempts (Buckley et al. 2009; Grover et al. 2017; Swets et al. 2014). OCS may precede the onset of psychosis, begin at or after the onset of schizophrenia, or occur transiently over time (Craig et al. 2002; de Haan et al. 2013; Hwang et al. 2000). OCS are important to identify because they may have prognostic significance and may respond to specialized treatments, as discussed below.

Although obsessions and compulsions of people with schizophrenia are similar to those of people without psychosis (e.g., contamination/washing, checking/repeating) (Eisen et al. 1997; Fenton and McGlashan 1986; Ohta et al. 2003; Poyurovsky et al. 2001), distinguishing between delusions and obsessions can be difficult (Schirmbeck et al. 2018). Classically, *delusions* are described as fixed, false beliefs that are ego-syntonic and actively embraced, whereas *obsessions* are perceived at some point as intrusive and unwanted and cause anxiety or distress (Hwang et al. 2000). However, this distinction does not always hold true in clinical interviews of patients with primary OCD or in patients with psychosis. Approximately 15% of patients with primary OCD have poor insight (Attiullah et al. 2000; Marazziti et al. 2002); moreover, there appears to be a continuum of insight in patients with schizophrenia, and for some patients, obsessions and delusions may be overlapping (Bermanzohn et al. 1997).

Results from some studies, but not all (de Haan et al. 2013; Devi et al. 2015; Frías et al. 2014a, 2014b), indicate that OCS in people with schizophrenia may be associated with poor outcomes. Those with comorbid OCS tend to be more socially isolated and less treatment responsive than those without this symptom complex (Berman et al. 1995; Fenton and McGlashan 1986; Hwang and Opler 2000). Moreover, research suggests that the presence of OCS in people with schizophrenia is associated with more neurocognitive dysfunction and greater disability (Berman et al. 1998; Buckley et al. 2009; Hwang et al. 2000; Lysaker et al. 2000; Schirmbeck et al. 2013, 2018; Schmidtke et al. 1998; Swets et al. 2014). OCS may be preceded by depressive symptoms, wax and wane with psychosis symptoms, and, if persistent, are associated with greater symptoms and lower function over time (Schirmbeck et al. 2018).

Comorbid OCD and OCS in patients with schizophrenia may have heterogeneous causes (Zink 2014). Supersensitivity of serotonin 5-HT receptors may occur during antipsychotic treatment, inducing OCS. OCS occurred in 10%–28% of patients prospectively treated with second-generation antipsychotic medications, with the highest prevalence among those treated with clozapine (Fonseka et al. 2014). However, OCS also occurred in a substantial proportion (19.6%) of patients with schizophrenia who were not taking antipsychotics (Scheltema Beduin et al. 2012), and OCS predated psychotic symptoms in over half of individuals with co-occurring OCD and schizophrenia (Craig et al. 2002; Hwang et al. 2000; Ohta et al. 2003), leading to the proposal of a schizo-obsessive subtype of schizophrenia (Schulz 1986; Scotti-Muzzi and Saide 2017). Common neurobiological mechanisms have been proposed to underlie both OCD and schizophrenia, and some evidence suggests a shared genetic vulnerability (Scotti-Muzzi and Saide 2017; Zink 2014). Further research is needed to understand the cause of OCS in people with schizophrenia, as well as the impact of OCS on these individuals.

Detection and Management of Obsessive-Compulsive Symptoms

Although the types of obsessions and compulsions in people with schizophrenia are similar to those found in individuals with classic OCD—contamination obsessions, hand-washing rituals, and counting and checking compulsions (Tibbo et al. 2000)—OCS are typically underdiagnosed and undertreated (Craig et al. 2002; Swets et al. 2014). Standardized scales, such as the Yale-Brown Obsessive Compulsive Scale (Goodman et al. 1989; Storch et al. 2010), enhance assessment and have been reliably used for patients with schizophrenia.

First-generation antipsychotic medications used alone appear to be ineffective in the treatment of OCD in schizophrenia (Poyurovsky et al. 2000), although SRIs added adjunctively to first-generation antipsychotics may be effective (Berman et al. 1995). In several small (and mostly open-label) trials using adjunctive clomipramine, imipramine, or fluoxetine, 67.2% of people showed improvement in OCS with no worsening of psychosis, whereas 19% showed worsening of psychosis (Chang and Berman 1999). Similar results were found in case series of fluvoxamine augmentation (Poyurovsky et al. 1999; Reznik and Sirota 2000a). In small, prospective controlled trials, clomipramine augmentation (Berman et al. 1995) and fluvoxamine augmentation (Reznik and Sirota 2000b) were superior to placebo or no augmentation for reducing obsessions and compulsions.

Research on the use of second-generation antipsychotic medications alone in individuals with schizophrenia and OCS varies among medications. Although reports suggest that risperidone (McDougle et al. 2000; Veznedaroglu et al. 2003) and aripiprazole (Glick et al. 2008) may enhance treatment response for psychotic and obsessive-compulsive symptoms, other prospective reports suggest that clozapine and olanzapine may worsen OCS in a minority of patients in a manner similar to that seen with first-generation agents (Fonseka et al. 2014; Schirmbeck et al. 2013). SRIs used in combination with second-generation antipsychotics have been reported to reduce OCS in case reports and prospective, small uncontrolled trials of people with schizophrenia (Patel et al. 1997; Poyurovsky et al. 2003; Strous et al. 1999; Stryjer et al. 2013). Because some SRIs can increase serum levels of some antipsychotics in the blood due to a decreased rate of antipsychotic metabolism, this combination should be used carefully. Finally, several case reports and a small, uncontrolled prospective trial ($N=11$) of lamotrigine added to patients' current schizophrenia pharmacotherapy demonstrated reduced OCS (Poyurovsky et al. 2010; Rodriguez et al. 2010; Zink et al. 2007).

Multiple RCTs have demonstrated modest improvement of OCS with use of rTMS in people with OCD, with largest effects when used over the supplementary motor area (Rehn et al. 2018). In three patients with schizophrenia and treatment-refractory OCD, rTMS (1 Hz over supplementary motor area) transiently improved treatment-refractory OCD symptoms (Mendes-Filho et al. 2013), but a subsequent small RCT did not show benefit of this approach over sham treatment (Mendes-Filho et al. 2016). rTMS over other locations has not been tested in comorbid schizophrenia and OCD.

CBT, including systematic exposure to obsessions and response (compulsion) prevention, is effective for the treatment of OCD in people in the general population (van Balkom et al. 1998) but has not been systematically studied in people with schizophrenia and co-occurring OCS or OCD. In a small open trial, 22 individuals with schizophrenia and OCD experienced significant reductions in obsessions and compulsions after 30 hours of CBT (Tundo et al. 2007). Larger controlled trials are needed to establish the efficacy of treatments for co-occurring OCD in those with schizophrenia.

Conclusion

Co-occurring conditions are very common in people with schizophrenia. Periodic, comprehensive screening and assessments can identify people with comorbid symptoms and disorders. Coordinated and integrated treatment of these co-occurring disorders with additional behavioral and pharmacological approaches can improve symptoms, illness course, and quality of life for patients with schizophrenia.

References

Achim AM, Maziade M, Raymond E, et al: How prevalent are anxiety disorders in schizophrenia? A meta-analysis and critical review on a significant association. Schizophr Bull 37(4):811–821, 2011 19959704

Addington D, Addington J, Schissel B: A depression rating scale for schizophrenics. Schizophr Res 3(4):247–251, 1990 2278986

Addington DE, Mohamed S, Rosenheck RA, et al: Impact of second-generation antipsychotics and perphenazine on depressive symptoms in a randomized trial of treatment for chronic schizophrenia. J Clin Psychiatry 72(1):75–80, 2011 20868641

Addington J: Early intervention strategies for co-morbid cannabis use and psychosis. Presented at the Inaugural International Cannabis and Psychosis Conference, Melbourne, Australia, February 16–17, 1999

Addington J, Addington D: Effect of substance misuse in early psychosis. Br J Psychiatry Suppl 172(33):134–136, 1998 9764140

Addington J, Shah H, Liu L, et al: Reliability and validity of the Calgary Depression Scale for Schizophrenia (CDSS) in youth at clinical high risk for psychosis. Schizophr Res 153(1–3):64–67, 2014 24439270

Agency for Healthcare Research and Quality: Five major steps to intervention (the "5 A's"). December 2012. Available at: https://www.ahrq.gov/professionals/clinicians-providers/guidelines-recommendations/tobacco/5steps.html. Accessed May 30, 2019.

Ahnallen CG, Liverant GI, Gregor KL, et al: The relationship between reward-based learning and nicotine dependence in smokers with schizophrenia. Psychiatry Res 196(1):9–14, 2012 22342123

Akerman SC, Brunette MF, Noordsy DL, Green AI: Pharmacotherapy of co-occurring schizophrenia and substance use disorders. Curr Addict Rep 1(4):251–260, 2014 27226947

Albanese MJ: Risperidone in substance abusers with bipolar disorder. Presented at the 39th annual meeting of the American College of Neuropsychopharmacology, San Juan, Puerto Rico, December 10–14, 2000

Allebeck P, Varla A, Kristjansson E, et al: Risk factors for suicide among patients with schizophrenia. Acta Psychiatr Scand 76(4):414–419, 1987 3425368

Allen MH, Debanné M, Lazignac C, et al: Effect of nicotine replacement therapy on agitation in smokers with schizophrenia: a double-blind, randomized, placebo-controlled study. Am J Psychiatry 168(4):395–399, 2011 21245085

Allison DB, Newcomer JW, Dunn AL, et al: Obesity among those with mental disorders: a National Institute of Mental Health meeting report. Am J Prev Med 36(4):341–350, 2009 19285199

American Diabetes Association; American Psychiatric Association; American Association of Clinical Endocrinologists; et al: Consensus development conference on antipsychotic drugs and obesity and diabetes. J Clin Psychiatry 65(2):267–272, 2004 15003083

American Psychiatric Association: Diagnostic and Statistical Manual of Mental Disorders, 5th Edition. Arlington, VA, American Psychiatric Association, 2013

Anthenelli RM, Benowitz NL, West R, et al: Neuropsychiatric safety and efficacy of varenicline, bupropion, and nicotine patch in smokers with and without psychiatric disorders (EAGLES): a double-blind, randomised, placebo-controlled clinical trial. Lancet 387(10037):2507–2520, 2016 27116918

Argyle N: Panic attacks in chronic schizophrenia. Br J Psychiatry 157:430–433, 1990 2245278

Arlow PB, Moran ME, Bermanzohn PC, et al: Cognitive-behavioral treatment of panic attacks in chronic schizophrenia. J Psychother Pract Res 6(2):145–150, 1997 9071665

Aschbrenner KA, Brunette MF, McElvery R, et al: Cigarette smoking and interest in quitting among overweight and obese adults with serious mental illness enrolled in a fitness intervention. J Nerv Ment Dis 203(6):473–476, 2015 26034872

Aschbrenner KA, Dixon LB, Naslund JA, et al: An online survey of family members' beliefs and attitudes about smoking and mental illness. J Dual Diagn 13(3):179–183, 2017a 28481179

Aschbrenner KA, Naslund JA, Gill L, et al: Preferences for smoking cessation support from family and friends among adults with serious mental illness. Psychiatr Q 88(4):701–710, 2017b 28091796

Aschbrenner KA, Patten CA, Brunette MF: Feasibility of a support person intervention to promote smoking cessation treatment use among smokers with mental illness. Transl Behav Med 8(5):785–792, 2018 29385555

Attiullah N, Eisen JL, Rasmussen SA: Clinical features of obsessive-compulsive disorder. Psychiatr Clin North Am 23(3):469–491, 2000 10986722

Auquier P, Lançon C, Rouillon F, et al: Mortality in schizophrenia. Pharmacoepidemiol Drug Saf 15(12):873–879, 2006 17058327

Avila MT, Sherr JD, Hong E, et al: Effects of nicotine on leading saccades during smooth pursuit eye movements in smokers and nonsmokers with schizophrenia. Neuropsychopharmacology 28(12):2184–2191, 2003 12968127

Ayesa-Arriola R, Canal Rivero M, Delgado-Alvarado M, et al: Low-density lipoprotein cholesterol and suicidal behaviour in a large sample of first-episode psychosis patients. World J Biol Psychiatry 19 (suppl 3):S158–S161, 2018 29235890

Azorin JM, Simon N, Adida M, et al: Pharmacological treatment of schizophrenia with comorbid substance use disorder. Expert Opin Pharmacother 17(2):231–253, 2016 26635059

Barlow DH, Gorman JM, Shear MK, et al: Cognitive-behavioral therapy, imipramine, or their combination for panic disorder: a randomized controlled trial. JAMA 283(19):2529–2536, 2000 10815116

Barrowclough C, Haddock G, Tarrier N, et al: Randomized controlled trial of motivational interviewing, cognitive behavior therapy, and family intervention for patients with comorbid schizophrenia and substance use disorders. Am J Psychiatry 158(10):1706–1713, 2001 11579006

Bartels SJ, Drake RE: Depressive symptoms in schizophrenia: comprehensive differential diagnosis. Compr Psychiatry 29(5):467–483, 1988 3053027

Bartels SJ, Pratt SI, Aschbrenner KA, et al: Clinically significant improved fitness and weight loss among overweight persons with serious mental illness. Psychiatr Serv 64(8):729–736, 2013 23677386

Bartels SJ, Pratt SI, Aschbrenner KA, et al: Pragmatic replication trial of health promotion coaching for obesity in serious mental illness and maintenance of outcomes. Am J Psychiatry 172(4):344–352, 2015 25827032

Batki SL: What is the right pharmacotherapy for alcohol use disorder in patients with schizophrenia? J Clin Psychiatry 76(10):e1336–e1337, 2015 26528663

Batki SL, Leontieva L, Dimmock JA, et al: Negative symptoms are associated with less alcohol use, craving, and "high" in alcohol dependent patients with schizophrenia. Schizophr Res 105(1–3):201–207, 2008 18701256

Baylé FJ, Krebs MO, Epelbaum C, et al: Clinical features of panic attacks in schizophrenia. Eur Psychiatry 16(6):349–353, 2001 11585715

Baynes D, Mulholland C, Cooper SJ, et al: Depressive symptoms in stable chronic schizophrenia: prevalence and relationship to psychopathology and treatment. Schizophr Res 45(1–2):47–56, 2000 10978872

Becker CB, Zayfert C, Anderson E: A survey of psychologists' attitudes towards and utilization of exposure therapy for PTSD. Behav Res Ther 42(3):277–292, 2004 14975770

Bendall S, Jackson HJ, Hulbert CA, et al: Childhood trauma and psychotic disorders: a systematic, critical review of the evidence. Schizophr Bull 34(3):568–579, 2008 18003630

Bennett ME, Wilson AL, Genderson M, et al: Smoking cessation in people with schizophrenia. Curr Drug Abuse Rev 6(3):180–190, 2013 23721094

Bennett ME, Brown CH, Li L, et al: Smoking cessation in individuals with serious mental illness: a randomized controlled trial of two psychosocial interventions. J Dual Diagn 11(3–4):161–173, 2015 26457385

Beresford TP, Clapp L, Martin B, et al: Aripiprazole in schizophrenia with cocaine dependence: a pilot study. J Clin Psychopharmacol 25(4):363–366, 2005 16012280

Berg SA, Sentir AM, Cooley BS, et al: Nicotine is more addictive, not more cognitively therapeutic in a neurodevelopmental model of schizophrenia produced by neonatal ventral hippocampal lesions. Addict Biol 19(6):1020–1031, 2014 23919443

Berman I, Sapers BL, Chang HH, et al: Treatment of obsessive-compulsive symptoms in schizophrenic patients with clomipramine. J Clin Psychopharmacol 15(3):206–210, 1995 7635998

Berman I, Merson A, Viegner B, et al: Obsessions and compulsions as a distinct cluster of symptoms in schizophrenia: a neuropsychological study. J Nerv Ment Dis 186(3):150–156, 1998 9521350

Bermanzohn PC, Porto L, Arlow PB, et al: Obsessions and delusions: separate and distinct, or overlapping? CNS Spectr 2(3):58–61, 1997

Bermanzohn PC, Porto L, Arlow PB, et al: Hierarchical diagnosis in chronic schizophrenia: a clinical study of co-occurring syndromes. Schizophr Bull 26(3):517–525, 2000 10993392

Bernardy NC, Friedman MJ: Psychopharmacological strategies in the management of posttraumatic stress disorder (PTSD): what have we learned? Curr Psychiatry Rep 17(4):564, 2015 25749751

Birchwood M, Iqbal Z, Chadwick P, et al: Cognitive approach to depression and suicidal thinking in psychosis, 1: ontogeny of post-psychotic depression. Br J Psychiatry 177:516–521, 2000 11102326

Blanco C, Schneier FR, Schmidt A, et al: Pharmacological treatment of social anxiety disorder: a meta-analysis. Depress Anxiety 18(1):29–40, 2003 12900950

Bland RC, Newman SC, Orn H: Schizophrenia: lifetime co-morbidity in a community sample. Acta Psychiatr Scand 75(4):383–391, 1987 3495958

Blevins CA, Weathers FW, Davis MT, et al: The Posttraumatic Stress Disorder Checklist for DSM-5 (PCL-5): development and initial psychometric evaluation. J Trauma Stress 28(6):489–498, 2015 26606250

Boggs DL, Nguyen JD, Morgenson D, et al: Clinical and preclinical evidence for functional interactions of cannabidiol and Δ^9-tetrahydrocannabinol. Neuropsychopharmacology 43(1):142–154, 2018a 28875990

Boggs DL, Surti TS, Esterlis I, et al: Minimal effects of prolonged smoking abstinence or resumption on cognitive performance challenge the "self-medication" hypothesis in schizophrenia. Schizophr Res 194:62–69, 2018b 28392208

Bornheimer LA: Suicidal ideation in first-episode psychosis (FEP): examination of symptoms of depression and psychosis among individuals in an early phase of treatment. Suicide Life Threat Behav 49(2):423–431, 2019 29444349

Bosanac P, Castle DJ: Schizophrenia and depression. Med J Aust 199(6)(suppl):S36–S39, 2013 25370284

Breier A, Astrachan BM: Characterization of schizophrenic patients who commit suicide. Am J Psychiatry 141(2):206–209, 1984 6691481

Brown CH, Medoff D, Dickerson FB, et al: Factors influencing implementation of smoking cessation treatment within community mental health centers. J Dual Diagn 11(2):145–150, 2015 25985201

Brown ES, Nejtek VA, Perantie DC: Neuroleptics and quetiapine in psychiatric illness with comorbid stimulant abuse. Presented at the 57th annual convention of the Society of Biological Psychiatry, Philadelphia, PA, May 16–18, 2002

Brown ES, Jeffress J, Liggin JD, et al: Switching outpatients with bipolar or schizoaffective disorders and substance abuse from their current antipsychotic to aripiprazole. J Clin Psychiatry 66(6):756–760, 2005 15960570

Brown S, Birtwistle J, Roe L, et al: The unhealthy lifestyle of people with schizophrenia. Psychol Med 29(3):697–701, 1999 10405091

Brunette MF, Mueser KT: Psychosocial interventions for the long-term management of patients with severe mental illness and co-occurring substance use disorder. J Clin Psychiatry 67 (suppl 7):10–17, 2006 16961419

Brunette MF, Mueser KT, Xie H, et al: Relationships between symptoms of schizophrenia and substance abuse. J Nerv Ment Dis 185(1):13–20, 1997 9040528

Brunette MF, Noordsy DL, Xie H, et al: Benzodiazepine use and abuse among patients with severe mental illness and co-occurring substance use disorders. Psychiatr Serv 54(10):1395–1401, 2003 14557527

Brunette MF, Drake RE, Xie H, et al: Clozapine use and relapses of substance use disorder among patients with co-occurring schizophrenia and substance use disorders. Schizophr Bull 32(4):637–643, 2006 16782758

Brunette MF, O'Keefe C, Dawson R, et al: An open label study of quetiapine in patients with schizophrenia and alcohol disorders. J Ment Health Subst Use 2(3):203–211, 2009

Brunette MF, Dawson R, O'Keefe CD, et al: A randomized trial of clozapine vs. other antipsychotics for cannabis use disorder in patients with schizophrenia. J Dual Diagn 7(1–2):50–63, 2011a 25914610

Brunette MF, Ferron JC, McHugo GJ, et al: An electronic decision support system to motivate people with severe mental illnesses to quit smoking. Psychiatr Serv 62(4):360–366, 2011b 21459986

Brunette MF, Ferron JC, Drake RE, et al: Carbon monoxide feedback in a motivational decision support system for nicotine dependence among smokers with severe mental illnesses. J Subst Abuse Treat 45(4):319–324, 2013 23706623

Brunette MF, Correll CU, Silverman BL, et al: A phase II, randomized, double-blind study of ALKS 3831 in schizophrenia and co-occurring alcohol use disorder. Presented at the 56th annual meeting of theAmerican College of Neuropsychopharmacology, Palm Springs, CA, December 3–7, 2017a

Brunette MF, Feiron JC, Aschbrenner K, et al: Characteristics and predictors of intention to use cessation treatment among smokers with schizophrenia: young adults compared to older adults. J Subst Abus Alcohol 5(1):1055, 2017b 29881770

Brunette MF, Ferron JC, Robinson D, et al: Brief Web-based interventions for young adult smokers with severe mental illnesses: a randomized, controlled pilot study. Nicotine Tob Res 20(10):1206–1214, 2018a 29059417

Brunette MF, Mueser KT, Babbin S, et al: Demographic and clinical correlates of substance use disorders in first episode psychosis. Schizophr Res 194:4–12, 2018b 28697856

Brunette MF, Pratt SI, Bartels SJ, et al: Randomized trial of interventions for smoking cessation among Medicaid beneficiaries with mental illness. Psychiatr Serv 69(3):274–280, 2018c 29137560

Buckley PF, Miller BJ, Lehrer DS, Castle DJ: Psychiatric comorbidities and schizophrenia. Schizophr Bull 35(2):383–402, 2009 19011234

Burke RM, Morin RJ, Perlyn CA, et al: Special considerations in vascular anomalies: operative management of craniofacial osseous lesions. Clin Plast Surg 38(1):133–142, 2011 21095478

Bushe CJTM, Taylor M, Haukka J: Mortality in schizophrenia: a measurable clinical endpoint. J Psychopharmacol 24(4)(suppl):17–25, 2010 20923917

Calhoun PS, Bosworth HB, Stechuchak KA, et al: The impact of posttraumatic stress disorder on quality of life and health service utilization among veterans who have schizophrenia. J Trauma Stress 19(3):393–397, 2006 16789002

Calhoun PSSK, Stechuchak KM, Strauss J, et al: Interpersonal trauma, war zone exposure, and posttraumatic stress disorder among veterans with schizophrenia. Schizophr Res 91(1–3):210–216, 2007 17276658

Carey CE, Agrawal A, Bucholz KK, et al: Associations between polygenic risk for psychiatric disorders and substance involvement. Front Genet 7:149, 2016 27574527

Cassano GB, Pini S, Saettoni M, et al: Occurrence and clinical correlates of psychiatric comorbidity in patients with psychotic disorders. J Clin Psychiatry 59(2):60–68, 1998 9501887

Cassidy CM, Brodeur MB, Lepage M, et al: Do reward-processing deficits in schizophrenia-spectrum disorders promote cannabis use? An investigation of physiological response to natural rewards and drug cues. J Psychiatry Neurosci 39(5):339–347, 2014a 24913137

Cassidy CM, Lepage M, Malla A: Do motivation deficits in schizophrenia-spectrum disorders promote cannabis use? An investigation of behavioural response to natural rewards and drug cues. Psychiatry Res 215(3):522–527, 2014b 24398065

Cather C, Hoeppner S, Pachas G, et al: Improved depressive symptoms in adults with schizophrenia during a smoking cessation attempt with varenicline and behavioral therapy. J Dual Diagn 13(3):168–178, 2017a 28414583

Cather C, Pachas GN, Cieslak KM, et al: Achieving smoking cessation in individuals with schizophrenia: special considerations. CNS Drugs 31(6):471–481, 2017b 28550660

Chambers RA, Krystal JH, Self DW: A neurobiological basis for substance abuse comorbidity in schizophrenia. Biol Psychiatry 50(2):71–83, 2001 11526998

Chang HH, Berman I: Treatment issues for patients with schizophrenia who have obsessive-compulsive symptoms. Psychiatr Ann 29(9):529–532, 1999

Chase KA, Rosen C, Gin H, et al: Metabolic and inflammatory genes in schizophrenia. Psychiatry Res 225(1–2):208–211, 2015 25433960

Chau DT, Roth RM, Green AI: The neural circuitry of reward and its relevance to psychiatric disorders. Curr Psychiatry Rep 6(5):391–399, 2004 15355762

Chen J, Bacanu SA, Yu H, et al; cotinine meta-analysis group; FTND meta-analysis group: Genetic relationship between schizophrenia and nicotine dependence. Sci Rep 6:25671, 2016 27164557

Chen Y, Bobo WV, Watts K, et al: Comparative effectiveness of switching antipsychotic drug treatment to aripiprazole or ziprasidone for improving metabolic profile and atherogenic dyslipidemia: a 12-month, prospective, open-label study. J Psychopharmacol 26(9):1201–1210, 2012 22234928

Chiappelli J, Chen S, Hackman A, et al: Evidence for differential opioid use disorder in schizophrenia in an addiction treatment population. Schizophr Res 194:26–31, 2018 28487076

Cohen LJ, Test MA, Brown RL: Suicide and schizophrenia: data from a prospective community treatment study. Am J Psychiatry 147(5):602–607, 1990 2327487

Coletti DJ, Brunette M, John M, et al: Responses to tobacco smoking-related health messages in young people with recent-onset schizophrenia. Schizophr Bull 41(6):1256–1265, 2015 26316595

Conley RR, Ascher-Svanum H, Zhu B, et al: The burden of depressive symptoms in the long-term treatment of patients with schizophrenia. Schizophr Res 90(1–3):186–197, 2007 17110087

Correll CU, Sikich L, Reeves G, et al: Metformin for antipsychotic-related weight gain and metabolic abnormalities: when, for whom, and for how long? Am J Psychiatry 170(9):947–952, 2013 24030606

Correll CU, Robinson DG, Schooler NR, et al: Cardiometabolic risk in patients with first-episode schizophrenia spectrum disorders: baseline results from the RAISE-ETP study. JAMA Psychiatry 71(12):1350–1363, 2014 25321337

Craig T, Hwang MY, Bromet EJ: Obsessive-compulsive and panic symptoms in patients with first-admission psychosis. Am J Psychiatry 159(4):592–598, 2002 11925297

Das C, Mendez G, Jagasia S, et al: Second-generation antipsychotic use in schizophrenia and associated weight gain: a critical review and meta-analysis of behavioral and pharmacologic treatments. Ann Clin Psychiatry 24(3):225–239, 2012 22860242

Daumit GL, Clark JM, Steinwachs DM, et al: Prevalence and correlates of obesity in a community sample of individuals with severe and persistent mental illness. J Nerv Ment Dis 191(12):799–805, 2003 14671456

Daumit GL, Dickerson FB, Wang NY, et al: A behavioral weight-loss intervention in persons with serious mental illness. N Engl J Med 368(17):1594–1602, 2013 23517118

Davidson JR, Miner CM, De Veaugh-Geiss J, et al: The Brief Social Phobia Scale: a psychometric evaluation. Psychol Med 27(1):161–166, 1997 9122296

de Bont PA, van Minnen A, de Jongh A: Treating PTSD in patients with psychosis: a within-group controlled feasibility study examining the efficacy and safety of evidence-based PE and EMDR protocols. Behav Ther 44(4):717–730, 2013 24094795

Degenhardt L, Hall W, Lynskey M: Testing hypotheses about the relationship between cannabis use and psychosis. Drug Alcohol Depend 71(1):37–48, 2003 12821204

de Haan L, Sterk B, Wouters L, et al: The 5-year course of obsessive-compulsive symptoms and obsessive-compulsive disorder in first-episode schizophrenia and related disorders. Schizophr Bull 39(1):151–160, 2013 21799212

Delahanty J, Ram R, Postrado L, et al: Differences in rates of depression in schizophrenia by race. Schizophr Bull 27(1):29–38, 2001 11215547

de Leon J, Diaz FJ: Genetics of schizophrenia and smoking: an approach to studying their comorbidity based on epidemiological findings. Hum Genet 131(6):877–901, 2012 22190153

Dépatie L, O'Driscoll GA, Holahan AL, et al: Nicotine and behavioral markers of risk for schizophrenia: a double-blind, placebo-controlled, cross-over study. Neuropsychopharmacology 27(6):1056–1070, 2002 12464463

Devi S, Rao NP, Badamath S, et al: Prevalence and clinical correlates of obsessive-compulsive disorder in schizophrenia. Compr Psychiatry 56:141–148, 2015 25308405

De Witte NA, Crunelle CL, Sabbe B, et al: Treatment for outpatients with comorbid schizophrenia and substance use disorders: a review. Eur Addict Res 20(3):105–114, 2014 24192558

Dickerson FB, Brown CH, Kreyenbuhl JA, et al: Obesity among individuals with serious mental illness. Acta Psychiatr Scand 113(4):306–313, 2006 16638075

Dickerson F, Bennett M, Dixon L, et al: Smoking cessation in persons with serious mental illnesses: the experience of successful quitters. Psychiatr Rehabil J 34(4):311–316, 2011 21459747

Dickerson F, Stallings C, Origoni A, et al: Mortality in schizophrenia: clinical and serological predictors. Schizophr Bull 40(4):796–803, 2014 23943410

Dickerson FB, Savage CL, Schweinfurth LA, et al: The use of peer mentors to enhance a smoking cessation intervention for persons with serious mental illnesses. Psychiatr Rehabil J 39(1):5–13, 2016 26461436

Dickerson F, Origoni A, Schweinfurth LAB, et al: Clinical and serological predictors of suicide in schizophrenia and major mood disorders. J Nerv Ment Dis 206(3):173–178, 2018a 29474231

Dickerson F, Schroeder J, Katsafanas E, et al: Cigarette smoking by patients with serious mental illness, 1999–2016: an increasing disparity. Psychiatr Serv 69(2):147–153, 2018b 28945183

Dieterich M, Irving CB, Bergman H, et al: Intensive case management for severe mental illness. Cochrane Database Syst Rev 1:CD007906, 2017 28067944

Dixon L, Green-Paden L, Delahanty J, et al: Variables associated with disparities in treatment of patients with schizophrenia and comorbid mood and anxiety disorders. Psychiatr Serv 52(9):1216–1222, 2001 11533396

Dixon LB, Medoff D, Goldberg R, et al: Is implementation of the 5 A's of smoking cessation at community mental health centers effective for reduction of smoking by patients with serious mental illness? Am J Addict 18(5):386–392, 2009 19874158

Dougherty RJ: Naltrexone in the treatment of alcohol dependent dual diagnosed patients (abstract). J Addict Dis 16:107, 1997

Drake RE: Management of substance use disorder in schizophrenia patients: current guidelines. CNS Spectr 12(10) (suppl 17):27–32, 2007 17934387

Drake RE, Mueser KT: Alcohol-use disorder and severe mental illness. Alcohol Health Res World 20(2):87–93, 1996

Drake RE, Wallach MA: Moderate drinking among people with severe mental illness. Hosp Community Psychiatry 44(8):780–782, 1993 8375841

Drake RE, Mueser KT, Brunette MF, et al: A review of treatments for people with severe mental illnesses and co-occurring substance use disorders. Psychiatr Rehabil J 27(4):360–374, 2004 15222148

Drake RE, Luciano AE, Mueser KT, et al: Longitudinal course of clients with co-occurring schizo-phrenia-spectrum and substance use disorders in urban mental health centers: a 7-year pro-spective study. Schizophr Bull 42(1):202–211, 2016 26294706

D'Souza DC, Abi-Saab WM, Madonick S, et al: Delta-9-tetrahydrocannabinol effects in schizo-phrenia: implications for cognition, psychosis, and addiction. Biol Psychiatry 57(6):594–608, 2005 15780846

D'Souza DC, Gil RB, Madonick S, et al: Enhanced sensitivity to the euphoric effects of alcohol in schizophrenia. Neuropsychopharmacology 31(12):2767–2775, 2006 16985503

Earle KA, Forquer SL, Volo AM, et al: Characteristics of outpatient suicides. Hosp Community Psychiatry 45(2):123–126, 1994 8168789

Eisen JL, Beer DA, Pato MT, et al: Obsessive-compulsive disorder in patients with schizophre-nia or schizoaffective disorder. Am J Psychiatry 154(2):271–273, 1997 9016282

El-Guebaly N, Cathcart J, Currie S, et al: Public health and therapeutic aspects of smoking bans in mental health and addiction settings. Psychiatr Serv 53(12):1617–1622, 2002 12461225

Elk R, Dickman BJ, Teggin AF: Depression in schizophrenia: a study of prevalence and treat-ment. Br J Psychiatry 149:228–229, 1986 3779279

Evins AE, Cather C, Culhane MA, et al: A 12-week double-blind, placebo-controlled study of bupropion SR added to high-dose dual nicotine replacement therapy for smoking cessa-tion or reduction in schizophrenia. J Clin Psychopharmacol 27(4):380–386, 2007 17632223

Evins AE, Cather C, Pratt SA, et al: Maintenance treatment with varenicline for smoking cessa-tion in patients with schizophrenia and bipolar disorder: a randomized clinical trial. JAMA 311(2):145–154, 2014 24399553

Evins AE, Benowitz NL, West R, et al: Neuropsychiatric safety and efficacy of varenicline, bu-propion, and nicotine patch in smokers with psychotic, anxiety, and mood disorders in the EAGLES trial. J Clin Psychopharmacol 39(2):108–116, 2019 30811371

Fadda F, Mosca E, Colombo G, et al: Effect of spontaneous ingestion of ethanol on brain dopa-mine metabolism. Life Sci 44(4):281–287, 1989 2915601

Fan X, Henderson DC, Nguyen DD, et al: Posttraumatic stress disorder, cognitive function and quality of life in patients with schizophrenia. Psychiatry Res 159(1–2):140–146, 2008 18423611

Featherstone RE, Siegel SJ: The role of nicotine in schizophrenia. Int Rev Neurobiol 124:23–78, 2015 26472525

Fenton WS, McGlashan TH: The prognostic significance of obsessive-compulsive symptoms in schizophrenia. Am J Psychiatry 143(4):437–441, 1986 3953886

Ferron JC, Brunette MF, He X, et al: Course of smoking and quit attempts among clients with co-occurring severe mental illness and substance use disorders. Psychiatr Serv 62(4):353–359, 2011 21459985

Ferron JC, Devitt T, McHugo GJ, et al: Abstinence and use of community-based cessation treat-ment after a motivational intervention among smokers with severe mental illness. Com-munity Ment Health J 52(4):446–456, 2016 26932324

Fiore MC, Jaén CR, Baker TB, et al; 2008 PHS Guideline Update Panel, Liaisons, and Staff: Treat-ing tobacco use and dependence: 2008 update U.S. Public Health Service Clinical Practice Guideline executive summary. Respir Care 53(9):1217–1222, 2008 18807274

Fischer AS, Whitfield-Gabrieli S, Roth RM, et al: Impaired functional connectivity of brain re-ward circuitry in patients with schizophrenia and cannabis use disorder: effects of canna-bis and THC. Schizophr Res 158(1–3):176–182, 2014 25037524

Fisher HL, Craig TK, Fearon P, et al: Reliability and comparability of psychosis patients' retro-spective reports of childhood abuse. Schizophr Bull 37(3):546–553, 2011 19776204

Fonseka TM, Richter MA, Müller DJ: Second generation antipsychotic-induced obsessive-compulsive symptoms in schizophrenia: a review of the experimental literature. Curr Psy-chiatry Rep 16(11):510, 2014 25256097

Fonseka TM, Müller DJ, Kennedy SH: Inflammatory cytokines and antipsychotic-induced weight gain: review and clinical implications. Mol Neuropsychiatry 2(1):1–14, 2016 27606316

Ford JD, Fournier D: Psychological trauma and posttraumatic stress disorder among women in community mental health aftercare following psychiatric intensive care. Journal of Psychi-atric Intensive Care 3(1):27–34, 2007

Ford JD, Schneeberger AR, Komarovskaya I, et al: The Symptoms of Trauma Scale (SOTS): psychometric evaluation and gender differences with adults diagnosed with serious mental illness. J Trauma Dissociation 18(4):559–574, 2017 27732452

Freyberg Z, Aslanoglou D, Shah R, et al: Intrinsic and antipsychotic drug-induced metabolic dysfunction in schizophrenia. Front Neurosci 11:432, 2017 28804444

Frías Á, Palma C, Farriols N, et al: Neuropsychological profile and treatment-related features among patients with comorbidity between schizophrenia spectrum disorder and obsessive-compulsive disorder: is there evidence for a "schizo-obsessive" subtype? Psychiatry Res 220(3):846–854, 2014a 25453638

Frías A, Palma C, Farriols N, et al: Psychopathology and quality of life among patients with comorbidity between schizophrenia spectrum disorder and obsessive-compulsive disorder: no evidence for a "schizo-obsessive" subtype. Compr Psychiatry 55(5):1165–1173, 2014b 24794642

Frueh BC, Grubaugh AL, Cusack KJ, et al: Exposure-based cognitive-behavioral treatment of PTSD in adults with schizophrenia or schizoaffective disorder: a pilot study. J Anxiety Disord 23(5):665–675, 2009 19342194

Furtado VA, Srihari V: Atypical antipsychotics for people with both schizophrenia and depression. Cochrane Database Syst Rev (1):CD005377, 2008 18254078

Gabínio T, Ricci TG, Kahn JP, et al: Panic psychosis: paroxysmal panic anxiety concomitant with auditory hallucinations in schizophrenia. Br J Psychiatry 39(1):85–86, 2017 28273271

Galling B, Roldán A, Hagi K, et al: Antipsychotic augmentation vs. monotherapy in schizophrenia: systematic review, meta-analysis and meta-regression analysis. World Psychiatry 16(1):77–89, 2017 28127934

Galling B, Vernon JA, Pagsberg AK, et al: Efficacy and safety of antidepressant augmentation of continued antipsychotic treatment in patients with schizophrenia. Acta Psychiatr Scand 137(3):187–205, 2018 29431197

Gearon JS, Kaltman SI, Brown C, et al: Traumatic life events and PTSD among women with substance use disorders and schizophrenia. Psychiatr Serv 54(4):523–528, 2003 12663840

Gearon JS, Bellack AS, Tenhula WN: Preliminary reliability and validity of the Clinician-Administered PTSD Scale for schizophrenia. J Consult Clin Psychol 72(1):121–125, 2004 14756621

Gehricke JG, Loughlin SE, Whalen CK, et al: Smoking to self-medicate attentional and emotional dysfunctions. Nicotine Tob Res 9 (suppl 4):S523–S536, 2007 18067030

George TP, Vessicchio JC, Sacco KA, et al: A placebo-controlled trial of bupropion combined with nicotine patch for smoking cessation in schizophrenia. Biol Psychiatry 63(11):1092–1096, 2008 18096137

Gerra G, Leonardi C, D'Amore A, et al: Buprenorphine treatment outcome in dually diagnosed heroin dependent patients: a retrospective study. Prog Neuropsychopharmacol Biol Psychiatry 30(2):265–272, 2006 16309810

Gerra G, Di Petta G, D'Amore A, et al: Combination of olanzapine with opioid-agonists in the treatment of heroin-addicted patients affected by comorbid schizophrenia spectrum disorders. Clin Neuropharmacol 30(3):127–135, 2007 17545747

Glick ID, Poyurovsky M, Ivanova O, et al: Aripiprazole in schizophrenia patients with comorbid obsessive-compulsive symptoms: an open-label study of 15 patients. J Clin Psychiatry 69(12):1856–1859, 2008 19026264

Goeders NE, Smith JE: Reinforcing properties of cocaine in the medial prefrontal cortex: primary action on presynaptic dopaminergic terminals. Pharmacol Biochem Behav 25(1):191–199, 1986 3018792

Goh KK, Chen CH, Lu ML: Topiramate mitigates weight gain in antipsychotic-treated patients with schizophrenia: meta-analysis of randomised controlled trials. Int J Psychiatry Clin Pract 23(1):14–32, 2019 29557263

Gold JM, Waltz JA, Prentice KJ, et al: Reward processing in schizophrenia: a deficit in the representation of value. Schizophr Bull 34(5):835–847, 2008 18591195

Goodman LA, Thompson KM, Weinfurt K, et al: Reliability of reports of violent victimization and posttraumatic stress disorder among men and women with serious mental illness. J Trauma Stress 12(4):587–599, 1999 10646178

Goodman LA, Salyers MP, Mueser KT, et al; 5 Site Health and Risk Study Research Committee: Recent victimization in women and men with severe mental illness: prevalence and correlates. J Trauma Stress 14(4):615–632, 2001 11776413

Goodman WK, Price LH, Rasmussen SA, et al: The Yale-Brown Obsessive Compulsive Scale, I: development, use, and reliability. Arch Gen Psychiatry 46(11):1006–1011, 1989 2684084

Goodwin R, Lyons JS, McNally RJ: Panic attacks in schizophrenia. Schizophr Res 58(2–3):213–220, 2002 12409161

Goodwin RD, Fergusson DM, Horwood LJ: Panic attacks and psychoticism. Am J Psychiatry 161(1):88–92, 2004 14702255

Green AI, Zimmet SV, Strous RD, et al: Clozapine for comorbid substance use disorder and schizophrenia: do patients with schizophrenia have a reward-deficiency syndrome that can be ameliorated by clozapine? Harv Rev Psychiatry 6(6):287–296, 1999 10370435

Green AI, Burgess ES, Dawson R, et al: Alcohol and cannabis use in schizophrenia: effects of clozapine vs. risperidone. Schizophr Res 60(1):81–85, 2003 12505141

Green AI, Tohen MF, Hamer RM, et al; HGDH Research Group: First episode schizophrenia-related psychosis and substance use disorders: acute response to olanzapine and haloperidol. Schizophr Res 66(2–3):125–135, 2004 15061244

Green AI, Brunette MF, Dawson R, et al: Long-acting injectable vs oral risperidone for schizophrenia and co-occurring alcohol use disorder: a randomized trial. J Clin Psychiatry 76(10):1359–1365, 2015 26302441

Green CA, Yarborough BJ, Leo MC, et al: Weight maintenance following the STRIDE lifestyle intervention for individuals taking antipsychotic medications. Obesity (Silver Spring) 23(10):1995–2001, 2015 26334929

Gregory A, Mallikarjun P, Upthegrove R: Treatment of depression in schizophrenia: systematic review and meta-analysis. Br J Psychiatry 211(4):198–204, 2017 28882827

Grover S, Dua D, Chakrabarti S, et al: Obsessive compulsive symptoms/disorder in patients with schizophrenia: prevalence, relationship with other symptom dimensions and impact on functioning. Psychiatry Res 250:277–284, 2017 28189922

Grubaugh AL, Elhai JD, Cusack KJ, et al: Screening for PTSD in public-sector mental health settings: the diagnostic utility of the PTSD Checklist. Depress Anxiety 24(2):124–129, 2007 16892418

Grubaugh AL, Zinzow HM, Paul L, et al: Trauma exposure and posttraumatic stress disorder in adults with severe mental illness: a critical review. Clin Psychol Rev 31(6):883–899, 2011 21596012

Gumley A, White R, Briggs A, et al: A parallel group randomised open blinded evaluation of Acceptance and Commitment Therapy for depression after psychosis: pilot trial outcomes (ADAPT). Schizophr Res 183:143–150, 2017 27894822

Gurillo P, Jauhar S, Murray RM, et al: Does tobacco use cause psychosis? Systematic review and meta-analysis. Lancet Psychiatry 2(8):718–725, 2015 26249303

Gut-Fayand A, Dervaux A, Olié JP, et al: Substance abuse and suicidality in schizophrenia: a common risk factor linked to impulsivity. Psychiatry Res 102(1):65–72, 2001 11368841

Hackman DT, Greene MS, Fernandes TJ, et al: Prescription drug monitoring program inquiry in psychiatric assessment: detection of high rates of opioid prescribing to a dual diagnosis population. J Clin Psychiatry 75(7):750–756, 2014 25093472

Häfner H, Löffler W, Maurer K, et al: Depression, negative symptoms, social stagnation and social decline in the early course of schizophrenia. Acta Psychiatr Scand 100(2):105–118, 1999 10480196

Hartz SM, Horton AC, Oehlert M, et al: Association between substance use disorder and polygenic liability to schizophrenia. Biol Psychiatry 82(10):709–715, 2017 28739213

Hasan A, Falkai P, Wobrock T, et al; WFSBP Task Force on Treatment Guidelines for Schizophrenia: World Federation of Societies of Biological Psychiatry (WFSBP) Guidelines for Biological Treatment of Schizophrenia, Part 3: Update 2015 Management of special circumstances: depression, suicidality, substance use disorders and pregnancy and lactation. World J Biol Psychiatry 16(3):142–170, 2015 25822804

Haukka J, Tiihonen J, Härkänen T, et al: Association between medication and risk of suicide, attempted suicide and death in nationwide cohort of suicidal patients with schizophrenia. Pharmacoepidemiol Drug Saf 17(7):686–696, 2008 18327869

Heilä H, Isometsä ET, Henriksson MM, et al: Suicide and schizophrenia: a nationwide psychological autopsy study on age- and sex-specific clinical characteristics of 92 suicide victims with schizophrenia. Am J Psychiatry 154(9):1235–1242, 1997 9286182

Heilä H, Isometsä ET, Henriksson MM, et al: Suicide victims with schizophrenia in different treatment phases and adequacy of antipsychotic medication. J Clin Psychiatry 60(3):200–208, 1999 10192600

Helle S, Ringen PA, Melle I, et al: Cannabis use is associated with 3 years earlier onset of schizophrenia spectrum disorder in a naturalistic, multi-site sample (N=1119). Schizophr Res 170(1):217–221, 2016 26682958

Herbener ES, Harrow M: The course of anhedonia during 10 years of schizophrenic illness. J Abnorm Psychol 111(2):237–248, 2002 12003446

Hettige NC, Nguyen TB, Yuan C, et al: Classification of suicide attempters in schizophrenia using sociocultural and clinical features: a machine learning approach. Gen Hosp Psychiatry 47:20–28, 2017 28807134

Himelhoch S, Daumit G: To whom do psychiatrists offer smoking-cessation counseling? Am J Psychiatry 160(12):2228–2230, 2003 14638595

Himelhoch S, Slade E, Kreyenbuhl J, et al: Antidepressant prescribing patterns among VA patients with schizophrenia. Schizophr Res 136(1–3):32–35, 2012 22325077

Hjorthøj C, Østergaard ML, Benros ME, et al: Association between alcohol and substance use disorders and all-cause and cause-specific mortality in schizophrenia, bipolar disorder, and unipolar depression: a nationwide, prospective, register-based study. Lancet Psychiatry 2(9):801–808, 2015 26277044

Hoffmann H, Kupper Z, Kunz B: Hopelessness and its impact on rehabilitation outcome in schizophrenia—an exploratory study. Schizophr Res 43(2–3):147–158, 2000 10858633

Hofmann SG, Bufka LF, Brady KM, et al: Cognitive-behavioral treatment of panic in patients with schizophrenia: preliminary findings. J Cogn Psychother 14:27–37, 2000

Hogarty GE, McEvoy JP, Ulrich RF, et al: Pharmacotherapy of impaired affect in recovering schizophrenic patients. Arch Gen Psychiatry 52(1):29–41, 1995 7811160

Hor K, Taylor M: Suicide and schizophrenia: a systematic review of rates and risk factors. J Psychopharmacol 24(4) (suppl):81–90, 2010 20923923

Humeniuk R, Ali R, Babor TF, et al: Validation of the Alcohol, Smoking and Substance Involvement Screening Test (ASSIST). Addiction 103(6):1039–1047, 2008 18373724

Hurlburt MS, Hough RL, Wood PA: Effects of substance abuse on housing stability of homeless mentally ill persons in supported housing. Psychiatr Serv 47(7):731–736, 1996 8807687

Hwang M, Opler L: Management of schizophrenia with obsessive-compulsive disorder. Psychiatr Clin North Am 32(4):835–851, 2000 19944887

Hwang MY, Morgan JE, Losconzcy MF: Clinical and neuropsychological profiles of obsessive-compulsive schizophrenia: a pilot study. J Neuropsychiatry Clin Neurosci 12(1):91–94, 2000 10678519

Iseger TA, Bossong MG: A systematic review of the antipsychotic properties of cannabidiol in humans. Schizophr Res 162(1–3):153–161, 2015 25667194

Iyiewuare PO, McCullough C, Ober A, et al: Demographic and mental health characteristics of individuals who present to community health clinics with substance misuse. Health Serv Res Manag Epidemiol 4:2333392817734523, 2017 29124080

Jakobsen AS, Speyer H, Nørgaard HCB, et al: Dietary patterns and physical activity in people with schizophrenia and increased waist circumference. Schizophr Res 199:109–115, 2018 29555213

Jamal A, Phillips E, Gentzke AS, et al: Current cigarette smoking among adults—United States, 2016. MMWR Morb Mortal Wkly Rep 67(2):53–59, 2018 29346338

Jayakody K, Gunadasa S, Hosker C: Exercise for anxiety disorders: systematic review. Br J Sports Med 48(3):187–196, 2014 23299048

Jin H, Zisook S, Palmer BW, et al: Association of depressive symptoms with worse functioning in schizophrenia: a study in older outpatients. J Clin Psychiatry 62(10):797–803, 2001 11816869

Joffe G, Takala P, Tchoukhine E, et al: Orlistat in clozapine- or olanzapine-treated patients with overweight or obesity: a 16-week randomized, double-blind, placebo-controlled trial. J Clin Psychiatry 69(5):706–711, 2008 18426261

Jones C, Hacker D, Cormac I, et al: Cognitive behaviour therapy versus other psychosocial treatments for schizophrenia. Cochrane Database Syst Rev (4):CD008712, 2012 22513966

Joseph J, Depp C, Shih PB, et al: Modified Mediterranean diet for enrichment of short chain fatty acids: potential adjunctive therapeutic to target immune and metabolic dysfunction in schizophrenia? Front Neurosci 11:155, 2017 28396623

Joshi K, Lafeuille MH, Kamstra R, et al: Real-world adherence and economic outcomes associated with paliperidone palmitate versus oral atypical antipsychotics in schizophrenia patients with substance-related disorders using Medicaid benefits. J Comp Eff Res 7(2):121–133, 2018 28809128

Kahn JP, Puertollano MA, Schane MD, et al: Adjunctive alprazolam for schizophrenia with panic anxiety: clinical observation and pathogenetic implications. Am J Psychiatry 145(6):742–744, 1988 2897166

Kappe C, Patrone C, Holst JJ, et al: Metformin protects against lipoapoptosis and enhances GLP-1 secretion from GLP-1-producing cells. J Gastroenterol 48(3):322–332, 2013 22850868

Kasckow J, Lanouette N, Patterson T, et al: Treatment of subsyndromal depressive symptoms in middle-aged and older adults with schizophrenia: effect on functioning. Int J Geriatr Psychiatry 25(2):183–190, 2010 19711335

Kasckow J, Zickmund S, Gurklis J, et al: Using telehealth to augment an intensive case monitoring program in veterans with schizophrenia and suicidal ideation: a pilot trial. Psychiatry Res 239:111–116, 2016 27137970

Kasper S, Montagnani G, Trespi G, et al: Treatment of depressive symptoms in patients with schizophrenia: a randomized, open-label, parallel-group, flexible-dose subgroup analysis of patients treated with extended-release quetiapine fumarate or risperidone. Int Clin Psychopharmacol 30(1):14–22, 2015 25356632

Keane TM, Pratt EM, Miller MW: Assessment of PTSD and its comorbidities in adults, in Handbook of PTSD: Science and Practice. Edited by Friedman MJ, Keane TM, Resick PA. New York, Guilford, 2007, pp 279–305

Kelly DL, McMahon RP, Wehring HJ, et al: Cigarette smoking and mortality risk in people with schizophrenia. Schizophr Bull 37(4):832–838, 2011 20019128

Kendler KS, Gallagher TJ, Abelson JM, et al: Lifetime prevalence, demographic risk factors, and diagnostic validity of nonaffective psychosis as assessed in a U.S. community sample. The National Comorbidity Survey. Arch Gen Psychiatry 53(11):1022–1031, 1996 8911225

Kerfoot KE, Rosenheck RA, Petrakis IL, et al; CATIE Investigators: Substance use and schizophrenia: adverse correlates in the CATIE study sample. Schizophr Res 132(2–3):177–182, 2011 21872443

Kerkvliet JL, Wey H, Fahrenwald NL: Cessation among state quitline participants with a mental health condition. Nicotine Tob Res 17(6):735–741, 2015 25385874

Kessler RC, Berglund P, Demler O, et al: Lifetime prevalence and age-of-onset distributions of DSM-IV disorders in the National Comorbidity Survey Replication. Arch Gen Psychiatry 62(6):593–602, 2005 15939837

Khantzian EJ: The self-medication hypothesis of substance use disorders: a reconsideration and recent applications. Harv Rev Psychiatry 4(5):231–244, 1997 9385000

Khera R, Murad MH, Chandar AK, et al: Association of pharmacological treatments for obesity with weight loss and adverse events: a systematic review and meta-analysis. JAMA 315(22):2424–2434, 2016 27299618

Khokhar JY, Green AI: Effects of iloperidone, combined with desipramine, on alcohol drinking in the Syrian golden hamster. Neuropharmacology 105:25–34, 2016 26796639

Kingsbury SJ, Salzman C: Disulfiram in the treatment of alcoholic patients with schizophrenia. Hosp Community Psychiatry 41(2):133–134, 1990 2303214

Kirpichnikov D, McFarlane SI, Sowers JR: Metformin: an update. Ann Intern Med 137(1):25–33, 2002 12093242

Kivimies K, Repo-Tiihonen E, Kautiainen H, et al: Opioid abuse and hospitalization rates in patients with schizophrenia. Nord J Psychiatry 70(2):128–132, 2016 26313367

Kjelby E, Jørgensen HA, Kroken RA, et al: Anti-depressive effectiveness of olanzapine, quetiapine, risperidone and ziprasidone: a pragmatic, randomized trial. BMC Psychiatry 11:145, 2011 21884578

Koreen AR, Siris SG, Chakos M, et al: Depression in first-episode schizophrenia. Am J Psychiatry 150(11):1643–1648, 1993 8105706

Kozak K, Sharif-Razi M, Morozova M, et al: Effects of short-term, high-frequency repetitive transcranial magnetic stimulation to bilateral dorsolateral prefrontal cortex on smoking behavior and cognition in patients with schizophrenia and non-psychiatric controls. Schizophr Res Feb 24, 2018 [Epub ahead of print] 29486960

Krakowski MI, Czobor P: Depression and impulsivity as pathways to violence: implications for antiaggressive treatment. Schizophr Bull 40(4):886–894, 2014 23943412

Krynicki CR, Upthegrove R, Deakin JF, et al: The relationship between negative symptoms and depression in schizophrenia: a systematic review. Acta Psychiatr Scand 137(5):380–390, 2018 29532909

Kubany ES, Haynes SN, Leisen MB, et al: Development and preliminary validation of a brief broad-spectrum measure of trauma exposure: the Traumatic Life Events Questionnaire. Psychol Assess 12(2):210–224, 2000 10887767

Kunii Y, Zhang W, Xu Q, et al: CHRNA7 and CHRFAM7A mRNAs: co-localized and their expression levels altered in the postmortem dorsolateral prefrontal cortex in major psychiatric disorders. Am J Psychiatry 172(11):1122–1130, 2015 26206074

Kurtz MM, Mueser KT: A meta-analysis of controlled research on social skills training for schizophrenia. J Consult Clin Psychol 76(3):491–504, 2008 18540742

Laitner MH, Minski SA, Perri MG: The role of self-monitoring in the maintenance of weight loss success. Eat Behav 21:193–197, 2016 26974582

Lako IM, Bruggeman R, Knegtering H, et al: A systematic review of instruments to measure depressive symptoms in patients with schizophrenia. J Affect Disord 140(1):38–47, 2012 22099566

Larsen JR, Vedtofte L, Jakobsen MS, et al: Effect of liraglutide treatment on prediabetes and overweight or obesity in clozapine- or olanzapine-treated patients with schizophrenia spectrum disorder: a randomized clinical trial. JAMA Psychiatry 74(7):719–728, 2017 28601891

Lasser K, Boyd JW, Woolhandler S, et al: Smoking and mental illness: a population-based prevalence study. JAMA 284(20):2606–2610, 2000 11086367

Lattari E, Budde H, Paes F, et al: Effects of aerobic exercise on anxiety symptoms and cortical activity in patients with panic disorder: a pilot study. Clin Pract Epidemiol Ment Health 14:11–25, 2018 29515644

Lawn S, Pols R: Smoking bans in psychiatric inpatient settings? A review of the research. Aust NZ J Psychiatry 39(10):866–885, 2005 16168014

Ledgerwood DM, Alessi SM, Hanson T, et al: Contingency management for attendance to group substance abuse treatment administered by clinicians in community clinics. J Appl Behav Anal 41(4):517–526, 2008 19192856

Lefebvre P, Muser E, Joshi K, et al: Impact of paliperidone palmitate versus oral atypical antipsychotics on health care resource use and costs in veterans with schizophrenia and comorbid substance abuse. Clin Ther 39(7):1380.e4–1395.e4, 2017 28641996

Leontieva L, Dimmock JA, Gately PW, et al: Voucher-based incentives for naltrexone treatment attendance in schizophrenia and alcohol use disorders. Psychiatr Serv 59(3):310–314, 2008 18308913

Leucht S, Burkard T, Henderson J, et al: Physical illness and schizophrenia: a review of the literature. Acta Psychiatr Scand 116(5):317–333, 2007 17919153

Leucht S, Cipriani A, Spineli L, et al: Comparative efficacy and tolerability of 15 antipsychotic drugs in schizophrenia: a multiple-treatments meta-analysis. Lancet 382(9896):951–962, 2013 23810019

Lieberman JA, Kane JM, Alvir J: Provocative tests with psychostimulant drugs in schizophrenia. Psychopharmacology (Berl) 91(4):415–433, 1987 2884687

Lieberman JA, Stroup TS, McEvoy JP, et al; Clinical Antipsychotic Trials of Intervention Effectiveness (CATIE) Investigators: Effectiveness of antipsychotic drugs in patients with chronic schizophrenia. N Engl J Med 353(12):1209–1223, 2005 16172203

Lin JJ, Liang FW, Li CY, et al: Leading causes of death among decedents with mention of schizophrenia on the death certificates in the United States. Schizophr Res Jan 30, 2018 [Epub ahead of print] 29395608

Lincoln TM, Ziegler M, Mehl S, et al: Moving from efficacy to effectiveness in cognitive behavioral therapy for psychosis: a randomized clinical practice trial. J Consult Clin Psychol 80(4):674–686, 2012 22663901

Litten RZ, Ryan ML, Fertig JB, et al; NCIG (National Institute on Alcohol Abuse and Alcoholism Clinical Investigations Group) Study Group: A double-blind, placebo-controlled trial assessing the efficacy of varenicline tartrate for alcohol dependence. J Addict Med 7(4):277–286, 2013 23728065

Littrell KH, Petty RG, Hilligoss NM, et al: Olanzapine treatment for patients with schizophrenia and substance abuse. J Subst Abuse Treat 21(4):217–221, 2001 11777671

Litz M, Leslie D: The impact of mental health comorbidities on adherence to buprenorphine: a claims based analysis. Am J Addict 26(8):859–863, 2017 29143483

Lowe EJ, Ackman ML: Impact of tobacco smoking cessation on stable clozapine or olanzapine treatment. Ann Pharmacother 44(4):727–732, 2010 20233914

Lowengrub KM, Stryjer R, Birger M, et al: Social anxiety disorder comorbid with schizophrenia: the importance of screening for this under recognized and under treated condition. Isr J Psychiatry Relat Sci 52(1):40–45, 2015 25841109

Lu W, Yanos PT, Silverstein SM, et al: Public mental health clients with severe mental illness and probable posttraumatic stress disorder: trauma exposure and correlates of symptom severity. J Trauma Stress 26(2):266–273, 2013 23508645

Lukowski AV, Morris CD, Young SE, et al: Quitline outcomes for smokers in 6 states: rates of successful quitting vary by mental health status. Nicotine Tob Res 17(8):924–930, 2015 26180216

Lynn Starr H, Bermak J, Mao L, et al: Comparison of long-acting and oral antipsychotic treatment effects in patients with schizophrenia, comorbid substance abuse, and a history of recent incarceration: an exploratory analysis of the PRIDE study. Schizophr Res 194:39–46, 2018 28601497

Lysaker P, Bell M, Beam-Goulet J, et al: Relationship of positive and negative symptoms to cocaine abuse in schizophrenia. J Nerv Ment Dis 182(2):109–112, 1994 8308528

Lysaker PH, Marks KA, Picone JB, et al: Obsessive and compulsive symptoms in schizophrenia: clinical and neurocognitive correlates. J Nerv Ment Dis 188(2):78–83, 2000 10695835

Macleod C, Holmes EA: Cognitive bias modification: an intervention approach worth attending to. Am J Psychiatry 169(2):118–120, 2012 22318791

Malhotra N, Kulhara P, Chakrabarti S, et al: Lifestyle related factors and impact of metabolic syndrome on quality of life, level of functioning and self-esteem in patients with bipolar disorder and schizophrenia. Indian J Med Res 143(4):434–442, 2016 27377499

Mandel MR, Severe JB, Schooler NR, et al: Development and prediction of postpsychotic depression in neuroleptic-treated schizophrenics. Arch Gen Psychiatry 39(2):197–203, 1982 6121543

Manu P, Dima L, Shulman M, et al: Weight gain and obesity in schizophrenia: epidemiology, pathobiology, and management. Acta Psychiatr Scand 132(2):97–108, 2015 26016380

Marazziti D, Dell'Osso L, Di Nasso E, et al: Insight in obsessive-compulsive disorder: a study of an Italian sample. Eur Psychiatry 17(7):407–410, 2002 12547307

Marder SR, Davis JM, Chouinard G: The effects of risperidone on the five dimensions of schizophrenia derived by factor analysis: combined results of the North American trials. J Clin Psychiatry 58(12):538–546, 1997 9448657

Martin RL, Cloninger CR, Guze SB, et al: Frequency and differential diagnosis of depressive syndromes in schizophrenia. J Clin Psychiatry 46(11 Pt 2):9–13, 1985 2865255

Martins SS, Sarvet A, Santaella-Tenorio J, et al: Changes in U.S. lifetime heroin use and heroin use disorder: prevalence from the 2001–2002 to 2012–2013 National Epidemiologic Survey on Alcohol and Related Conditions. JAMA Psychiatry 74(5):445–455, 2017 28355458

Mathew AR, Burris JL, Alberg AJ, et al: Impact of a brief telephone referral on quitline use, quit attempts and abstinence. Health Educ Res 30(1):134–139, 2015 25092882

Mattick RP, Clarke JC: Development and validation of measures of social phobia scrutiny fear and social interaction anxiety. Behav Res Ther 36(4):455–470, 1998 9670605

Maxwell S, Shinderman MS: Naltrexone in the treatment of dually diagnosed patients. J Addict Dis 16:125, 1997

Maxwell S, Shinderman MS: Use of naltrexone in the treatment of alcohol use disorders in patients with concomitant major mental illness. J Addict Dis 19(3):61–69, 2000 11076120

McCreadie R, Macdonald E, Blacklock C, et al: Dietary intake of schizophrenic patients in Nithsdale, Scotland: case-control study. BMJ 317(7161):784–785, 1998 9740565

McDonell MG, Srebnik D, Angelo F, et al: Randomized controlled trial of contingency management for stimulant use in community mental health patients with serious mental illness. Am J Psychiatry 170(1):94–101, 2013 23138961

McDonell MG, Leickly E, McPherson S, et al: A randomized controlled trial of ethyl glucuronide-based contingency management for outpatients with co-occurring alcohol use disorders and serious mental illness. Am J Psychiatry 174(4):370–377, 2017 28135843

McDougle CJ, Epperson CN, Pelton GH, et al: A double-blind, placebo-controlled study of risperidone addition in serotonin reuptake inhibitor-refractory obsessive-compulsive disorder. Arch Gen Psychiatry 57(8):794–801, 2000 10920469

McEnery C, Lim MH, Knowles A, et al: Development of a moderated online intervention to treat social anxiety in first-episode psychosis. Front Psychiatry 10:581, 2019a 31474889

McEnery C, Lim MH, Tremain H, et al: Prevalence rate of social anxiety disorder in individuals with a psychotic disorder: A systematic review and meta-analysis. Schizophr Res 208:25–33, 2019b 30722947

McGinty EE, Baller J, Azrin ST, et al: Interventions to address medical conditions and health-risk behaviors among persons with serious mental illness: a comprehensive review. Schizophr Bull 42(1):96–124, 2016 26221050

McLoughlin BC, Pushpa-Rajah JA, Gillies D, et al: Cannabis and schizophrenia. Cochrane Database Syst Rev (10):CD004837, 2014 25314586

Meltzer HY, Okayli G: Reduction of suicidality during clozapine treatment of neuroleptic-resistant schizophrenia: impact on risk-benefit assessment. Am J Psychiatry 152(2):183–190, 1995 7840350

Meltzer HY, Alphs L, Green AI, et al; International Suicide Prevention Trial Study Group: Clozapine treatment for suicidality in schizophrenia: International Suicide Prevention Trial (InterSePT). Arch Gen Psychiatry 60(1):82–91, 2003 12511175

Mendes-Filho VA, Belmonte-de-Abreu P, Pedrini M, et al: rTMS as an add-on treatment for resistant obsessive-compulsive symptoms in patients with schizophrenia: report of three cases. Br J Psychiatry 35(2):210–211, 2013 23904031

Mendes-Filho VA, de Jesus DR, Belmonte-de-Abreu P, et al: Effects of repetitive transcranial magnetic stimulation over supplementary motor area in patients with schizophrenia with obsessive-compulsive-symptoms: a pilot study. Psychiatry Res 242:34–38, 2016 27254652

Messias E, Kirkpatrick B, Ram R, Tien AY: Suspiciousness as a specific risk factor for major depressive episodes in schizophrenia. Schizophr Res 47(2–3):159–165, 2001 11278133

Meszaros ZS, Abdul-Malak Y, Dimmock JA, et al: Varenicline treatment of concurrent alcohol and nicotine dependence in schizophrenia: a randomized, placebo-controlled pilot trial. J Clin Psychopharmacol 33(2):243–247, 2013 23422399

Metse AP, Wiggers J, Wye P, et al: Efficacy of a universal smoking cessation intervention initiated in inpatient psychiatry and continued post-discharge: a randomised controlled trial. Aust NZ J Psychiatry 51(4):366–381, 2017 28195010

Meyer JM, Davis VG, Goff DC, et al: Change in metabolic syndrome parameters with antipsychotic treatment in the CATIE Schizophrenia Trial: prospective data from Phase 1. Schizophr Res 101(1–3):273–286, 2008 18258416

Michail M, Birchwood M, Tait L: Systematic review of cognitive-behavioural therapy for social anxiety disorder in psychosis. Brain Sci 7(5) pii: E45, 2017 28441335

Miller WR, Rollnick S: Motivational Interviewing: Preparing People for Change. New York, Guilford, 2002

Misiak B, Frydecka D: A history of childhood trauma and response to treatment with antipsychotics in first-episode schizophrenia patients: preliminary results. J Nerv Ment Dis 204(10):787–792, 2016 27441460

Mitchell AJ, Vancampfort D, Sweers K, et al: Prevalence of metabolic syndrome and metabolic abnormalities in schizophrenia and related disorders—a systematic review and meta-analysis. Schizophr Bull 39(2):306–318, 2013 22207632

Moritz S, Cludius B, Hottenrott B, et al: Mindfulness and relaxation treatment reduce depressive symptoms in individuals with psychosis. Eur Psychiatry 30(6):709–714, 2015 26163302

Morris CD, Waxmonsky JA, May MG, et al: Smoking reduction for persons with mental illnesses: 6-month results from community-based interventions. Community Ment Health J 47(6):694–702, 2011 21556784

Mueser KT, Yarnold PR, Levinson DF, et al: Prevalence of substance abuse in schizophrenia: demographic and clinical correlates. Schizophr Bull 16(1):31–56, 1990 2333480

Mueser KT, Drake RE, Clark RE, et al: Toolkit for Evaluating Substance Abuse in Persons With Severe Mental Illness. Cambridge, MA, Evaluation Center at HSRI, 1995

Mueser KT, Goodman LB, Trumbetta SL, et al: Trauma and posttraumatic stress disorder in severe mental illness. J Consult Clin Psychol 66(3):493–499, 1998 9642887

Mueser KT, Salyers MP, Rosenberg SD, et al: Psychometric evaluation of trauma and posttraumatic stress disorder assessments in persons with severe mental illness. Psychol Assess 13(1):110–117, 2001 11281032

Mueser KT, Rosenberg SD, Goodman LA, et al: Trauma, PTSD, and the course of severe mental illness: an interactive model. Schizophr Res 53(1–2):123–143, 2002 11728845

Mueser KT, Noordsy DL, Drake RE, et al: Integrated Treatment for Dual Disorders: A Guide to Effective Practice. New York, Guilford, 2003a

Mueser KT, Noordsy DL, Fox L, et al: Disulfiram treatment for alcoholism in severe mental illness. Am J Addict 12(3):242–252, 2003b 12851020

Mueser KT, Essock SM, Haines M, et al: Posttraumatic stress disorder, supported employment, and outcomes in people with severe mental illness. CNS Spectr 9(12):913–925, 2004 15616477

Mueser KT, Bolton E, Carty PC, et al: The Trauma Recovery Group: a cognitive-behavioral program for post-traumatic stress disorder in persons with severe mental illness. Community Ment Health J 43(3):281–304, 2007 17235698

Mueser KT, Rosenberg SD, Xie H, et al: A randomized controlled trial of cognitive-behavioral treatment for posttraumatic stress disorder in severe mental illness. J Consult Clin Psychol 76(2):259–271, 2008 18377122

Mueser KT, Lu W, Rosenberg SD, et al: The trauma of psychosis: posttraumatic stress disorder and recent onset psychosis. Schizophr Res 116(2–3):217–227, 2010 19939633

Mueser KT, Gottlieb JD, Xie H, et al: Evaluation of cognitive restructuring for post-traumatic stress disorder in people with severe mental illness. Br J Psychiatry 206(6):501–508, 2015 25858178

Mukundan A, Faulkner G, Cohn T, et al: Antipsychotic switching for people with schizophrenia who have neuroleptic-induced weight or metabolic problems. Cochrane Database Syst Rev (12):CD006629, 2010 21154372

Murray RM, Englund A, Abi-Dargham A, et al: Cannabis-associated psychosis: neural substrate and clinical impact. Neuropharmacology 124:89–104, 2017 28634109

Myers CS, Robles O, Kakoyannis AN, et al: Nicotine improves delayed recognition in schizo-phrenic patients. Psychopharmacology (Berl) 174(3):334–340, 2004 14997272

Nakajima S, Takeuchi H, Fervaha G, et al: Comparative efficacy between clozapine and other atypical antipsychotics on depressive symptoms in patients with schizophrenia: analysis of the CATIE phase 2E data. Schizophr Res 161(2–3):429–433, 2015 25556080

National Institute on Drug Abuse: The NIDA Quick Screen: the NIDA-Modified ASSIST. March 2012. Available at: https://www.drugabuse.gov/sites/default/files/pdf/nmassist.pdf. Accessed May 31, 2019.

Nenke MA, Hahn LA, Thompson CH, et al: Psychosis and cardiovascular disease: is diet the missing link? Schizophr Res 161(2–3):465–470, 2015 25560938

Neria Y, Bromet EJ, Sievers S, et al: Trauma exposure and posttraumatic stress disorder in psychosis: findings from a first-admission cohort. J Consult Clin Psychol 70(1):246–251, 2002 11860051

Newcomer JW, Campos JA, Marcus RN, et al: A multicenter, randomized, double-blind study of the effects of aripiprazole in overweight subjects with schizophrenia or schizoaffective disorder switched from olanzapine. J Clin Psychiatry 69(7):1046–1056, 2008 18605811

Nishith P, Mueser KT, Morse GA: A brief intervention for posttraumatic stress disorder in persons with a serious mental illness. Psychiatr Rehabil J 38(4):314–319, 2015 26414747

Noordsy DL, Torrey WC, Mead S, et al: Recovery-oriented psychopharmacology: redefining the goals of antipsychotic treatment. J Clin Psychiatry 61 (suppl 3):22–29, 2000 10724130

Noordsy DL, O'Keefe C, Mueser KT, et al: Six-month outcomes for patients who switched to olanzapine treatment. Psychiatr Serv 52(4):501–507, 2001 11274497

Noordsy DL, Torrey WC, Mueser KT, et al: Recovery from severe mental illness: an interpersonal and functional outcome definition. Int Rev Psychiatry 14:318–326, 2002

Norman RM, Malla AK, Cortese L, Diaz F: Aspects of dysphoria and symptoms of schizophrenia. Psychol Med 28(6):1433–1441, 1998 9854284

Nothdurfter C, Eser D, Schüle C, et al: The influence of concomitant neuroleptic medication on safety, tolerability and clinical effectiveness of electroconvulsive therapy. World J Biol Psychiatry 7(3):162–170, 2006 16861142

Ohta M, Kokai M, Morita Y: Features of obsessive-compulsive disorder in patients primarily diagnosed with schizophrenia. Psychiatry Clin Neurosci 57(1):67–74, 2003 12519457

Oiesvold T, Nivison M, Hansen V, et al: Diagnosing comorbidity in psychiatric hospital: challenging the validity of administrative registers. BMC Psychiatry 13:13, 2013 23297686

Olfson M, Gerhard T, Huang C, et al: Premature mortality among adults with schizophrenia in the United States. JAMA Psychiatry 72(12):1172–1181, 2015 26509694

Olincy A, Johnson LL, Ross RG: Differential effects of cigarette smoking on performance of a smooth pursuit and a saccadic eye movement task in schizophrenia. Psychiatry Res 117(3):223–236, 2003 12686365

O'Malley SS, Jaffe AJ, Chang G, et al: Naltrexone and coping skills therapy for alcohol dependence: a controlled study. Arch Gen Psychiatry 49(11):881–887, 1992 1444726

O'Malley SS, Zweben A, Fucito LM, et al: Effect of varenicline combined with medical management on alcohol use disorder with comorbid cigarette smoking: a randomized clinical trial. JAMA Psychiatry 75(2):129–138, 2018 29261824

Oosthuizen P, Emsley RA, Roberts MC, et al: Depressive symptoms at baseline predict fewer negative symptoms at follow-up in patients with first-episode schizophrenia. Schizophr Res 58(2–3):247–252, 2002 12409165

Painter JM, Malte CA, Rubinsky AD, et al: High inpatient utilization among Veterans Health Administration patients with substance-use disorders and co-occurring mental health conditions. Am J Drug Alcohol Abuse 44(3):386–394, 2018 29095057

Pallanti S, Quercioli L, Pazzagli A: Effects of clozapine on awareness of illness and cognition in schizophrenia. Psychiatry Res 86(3):239–249, 1999 10482343

Pallanti S, Quercioli L, Hollander E: Social anxiety in outpatients with schizophrenia: a relevant cause of disability. Am J Psychiatry 161(1):53–58, 2004 14702250

Parikh V, Kutlu MG, Gould TJ: nAChR dysfunction as a common substrate for schizophrenia and comorbid nicotine addiction: current trends and perspectives. Schizophr Res 171(1–3):1–15, 2016 26803692

Patel JK, Salzman C, Green AI, et al: Chronic schizophrenia: response to clozapine, risperidone, and paroxetine. Am J Psychiatry 154(4):543–546, 1997 9090343

Penn DL, Hope DA, Spaulding W, et al: Social anxiety in schizophrenia. Schizophr Res 11(3):277–284, 1994 8193064

Petrakis IL, O'Malley S, Rounsaville B, et al; VA Naltrexone Study Collaboration Group: Naltrexone augmentation of neuroleptic treatment in alcohol abusing patients with schizophrenia. Psychopharmacology (Berl) 172(3):291–297, 2004 14634716

Petrakis IL, Nich C, Ralevski E: Psychotic spectrum disorders and alcohol abuse: a review of pharmacotherapeutic strategies and a report on the effectiveness of naltrexone and disulfiram. Schizophr Bull 32(4):644–654, 2006 16887890

Pillinger T, Beck K, Gobjila C, et al: Impaired glucose homeostasis in first-episode schizophrenia: a systematic review and meta-analysis. JAMA Psychiatry 74(3):261–269, 2017 28097367

Poyurovsky M, Isakov V, Hromnikov S, et al: Fluvoxamine treatment of obsessive-compulsive symptoms in schizophrenic patients: an add-on open study. Int Clin Psychopharmacol 14(2):95–100, 1999 10220124

Poyurovsky M, Dorfman-Etrog P, Hermesh H, et al: Beneficial effect of olanzapine in schizophrenic patients with obsessive-compulsive symptoms. Int Clin Psychopharmacol 15(3):169–173, 2000 10870875

Poyurovsky M, Hramenkov S, Isakov V, et al: Obsessive-compulsive disorder in hospitalized patients with chronic schizophrenia. Psychiatry Res 102(1):49–57, 2001 11368839

Poyurovsky M, Kurs R, Weizman A: Olanzapine-sertraline combination in schizophrenia with obsessive-compulsive disorder (letter). J Clin Psychiatry 64(5):611, 2003 12755669

Poyurovsky M, Glick I, Koran LM: Lamotrigine augmentation in schizophrenia and schizoaffective patients with obsessive-compulsive symptoms. J Psychopharmacol 24(6):861–866, 2010 19074541

Praharaj SK, Jana AK, Goyal N, et al: Metformin for olanzapine-induced weight gain: a systematic review and meta-analysis. Br J Clin Pharmacol 71(3):377–382, 2011 21284696

Pratt SI, Naslund JA, Wolfe RS, et al: Automated telehealth for managing psychiatric instability in people with serious mental illness. J Ment Health 24(5):261–265, 2015 24988132

Pratt SI, Sargent J, Daniels L, et al: Appeal of electronic cigarettes in smokers with serious mental illness. Addict Behav 59:30–34, 2016 27043170

Prikryl R, Ustohal L, Kucerova HP, et al: Repetitive transcranial magnetic stimulation reduces cigarette consumption in schizophrenia patients. Prog Neuropsychopharmacol Biol Psychiatry 49:30–35, 2014 24211840

Prochaska JJ, Hall SE, Delucchi K, et al: Efficacy of initiating tobacco dependence treatment in inpatient psychiatry: a randomized controlled trial. Am J Public Health 104(8):1557–1565, 2014 23948001

Prochaska JJ, Fromont SC, Ramo DE, et al: Gender differences in a randomized controlled trial treating tobacco use among adolescents and young adults with mental health concerns. Nicotine Tob Res 17(4):479–485, 2015 25762759

Provencher HL, Gregg R, Mead S, et al: The role of work in the recovery of persons with psychiatric disabilities. Psychiatr Rehabil J 26(2):132–144, 2002 12433216

Ralevski E, O'Brien E, Jane JS, et al: Treatment with acamprosate in patients with schizophrenia spectrum disorders and comorbid alcohol dependence. J Dual Diagn 7(1–2):64–73, 2011 26954912

Regier DA, Farmer ME, Rae DS, et al: Comorbidity of mental disorders with alcohol and other drug abuse: results from the Epidemiologic Catchment Area (ECA) Study. JAMA 264(19):2511–2518, 1990 2232018

Reginsson GW, Ingason A, Euesden J, et al: Polygenic risk scores for schizophrenia and bipolar disorder associate with addiction. Addict Biol 23(1):485–492, 2018 28231610

Rehn S, Eslick GD, Brakoulias V: A meta-analysis of the effectiveness of different cortical targets used in repetitive transcranial magnetic stimulation (rTMS) for the treatment of obsessive-compulsive disorder (OCD). Psychiatr Q 89(3):645–665, 2018 29423665

Reid WH, Mason M, Hogan T: Suicide prevention effects associated with clozapine therapy in schizophrenia and schizoaffective disorder. Psychiatr Serv 49(8):1029–1033, 1998 9712207

Resick PA, Nishith P, Weaver TL, et al: A comparison of cognitive-processing therapy with prolonged exposure and a waiting condition for the treatment of chronic posttraumatic stress disorder in female rape victims. J Consult Clin Psychol 70(4):867–879, 2002 12182270

Resick PA, Galovski TE, Uhlmansiek MO, et al: A randomized clinical trial to dismantle components of cognitive processing therapy for posttraumatic stress disorder in female victims of interpersonal violence. J Consult Clin Psychol 76(2):243–258, 2008 18377121

Resnick SG, Bond GR, Mueser KT: Trauma and posttraumatic stress disorder in people with schizophrenia. J Abnorm Psychol 112(3):415–423, 2003 12943020

Reznik I, Sirota P: Obsessive and compulsive symptoms in schizophrenia: a randomized controlled trial with fluvoxamine and neuroleptics. J Clin Psychopharmacol 20(4):410–416, 2000a 10917401

Reznik I, Sirota P: An open study of fluvoxamine augmentation of neuroleptics in schizophrenia with obsessive and compulsive symptoms. Clin Neuropharmacol 23(3):157–160, 2000b 10895399

Ridgely MS, Goldman HH, Willenbring M: Barriers to the care of persons with dual diagnoses: organizational and financing issues. Schizophr Bull 16(1):123–132, 1990 2185535

Rodriguez CI, Corcoran C, Simpson HB: Diagnosis and treatment of a patient with both psychotic and obsessive-compulsive symptoms. Am J Psychiatry 167(7):754–761, 2010 20595428

Román V, Gyertyán I, Sághy K, et al: Cariprazine (RGH-188), a D3-preferring dopamine D3/D2 receptor partial agonist antipsychotic candidate demonstrates anti-abuse potential in rats. Psychopharmacology (Berl) 226(2):285–293, 2013 23138433

Rosenberg SD, Drake RE, Wolford GL, et al: Dartmouth Assessment of Lifestyle Instrument (DALI): a substance use disorder screen for people with severe mental illness. Am J Psychiatry 155(2):232–238, 1998 9464203

Rosenberg SD, Goodman LA, Osher FC, et al: Prevalence of HIV, hepatitis B, and hepatitis C in people with severe mental illness. Am J Public Health 91(1):31–37, 2001a 11189820

Rosenberg SD, Mueser KT, Friedman MJ, et al: Developing effective treatments for posttraumatic disorders among people with severe mental illness. Psychiatr Serv 52(11):1453–1461, 2001b 11684740

Rosenheck RA, Krystal JH, Lew R, et al; CSP555 Research Group: Long-acting risperidone and oral antipsychotics in unstable schizophrenia. N Engl J Med 364(9):842–851, 2011 21366475

Rubio G, Martínez I, Ponce G, et al: Long-acting injectable risperidone compared with zuclopenthixol in the treatment of schizophrenia with substance abuse comorbidity. Can J Psychiatry 51(8):531–539, 2006 16933590

Rybakowski JK, Vansteelandt K, Szafranski T, et al; EUFEST Study Group: Treatment of depression in first episode of schizophrenia: results from EUFEST. Eur Neuropsychopharmacol 22(12):875–882, 2012 22627166

Saha S, Chant D, McGrath J: A systematic review of mortality in schizophrenia: is the differential mortality gap worsening over time? Arch Gen Psychiatry 64(10):1123–1131, 2007 17909124

Sallaup TV, Vaaler AE, Iversen VC, et al: Challenges in detecting and diagnosing substance use in women in the acute psychiatric department: a naturalistic cohort study. BMC Psychiatry 16(1):406, 2016 27855664

Salling MC, Martinez D: Brain stimulation in addiction. Neuropsychopharmacology 41(12):2798–2809, 2016 27240657

Salyers MP, Evans LJ, Bond GR, et al: Barriers to assessment and treatment of posttraumatic stress disorder and other trauma-related problems in people with severe mental illness: clinician perspectives. Community Ment Health J 40(1):17–31, 2004 15077726

Sankaranarayanan A, Clark V, Baker A, et al: Reducing smoking reduces suicidality among individuals with psychosis: complementary outcomes from a Healthy Lifestyles intervention study. Psychiatry Res 243:407–412, 2016 27450743

Sara GE, Burgess PM, Malhi GS, et al: Stimulant and other substance use disorders in schizophrenia: prevalence, correlates and impacts in a population sample. Aust NZ J Psychiatry 48(11):1036–1047, 2014 24819935

Saunders KH, Umashanker D, Igel LI, et al: Obesity pharmacotherapy. Med Clin North Am 102(1):135–148, 2018 29156182

Sautter FJ, Brailey K, Uddo MM, et al: PTSD and comorbid psychotic disorder: comparison with veterans diagnosed with PTSD or psychotic disorder. J Trauma Stress 12(1):73–88, 1999 10027143

Sax KW, Strakowski SM, Keck PE Jr, et al: Relationships among negative, positive, and depressive symptoms in schizophrenia and psychotic depression. Br J Psychiatry 168(1):68–71, 1996 8770431

Schechter MD, Rand MJ: Effect of acute deprivation of smoking on aggression and hostility. Psychopharmacology (Berl) 35(1):19–28, 1974

Scheltema Beduin AA, Swets M, Machielsen M, et al: Obsessive-compulsive symptoms in patients with schizophrenia: a naturalistic cross-sectional study comparing treatment with clozapine, olanzapine, risperidone, and no antipsychotics in 543 patients. J Clin Psychiatry 73(11):1395–1402, 2012 23218156

Schipper R, Dekker M, de Haan L, et al: Medicinal cannabis (Bedrolite) substitution therapy in inpatients with a psychotic disorder and a comorbid cannabis use disorder: a case series. J Psychopharmacol 32(3):353–356, 2018 29039260

Schirmbeck F, Rausch F, Englisch S, et al: Stable cognitive deficits in schizophrenia patients with comorbid obsessive-compulsive symptoms: a 12-month longitudinal study. Schizophr Bull 39(6):1261–1271, 2013 23104864

Schirmbeck F, Swets M, Meijer CJ, et al; GROUP investigators: Obsessive-compulsive symptoms and overall psychopathology in psychotic disorders: longitudinal assessment of patients and siblings. Eur Arch Psychiatry Clin Neurosci 268(3):279–289, 2018 27988852

Schmidtke K, Schorb A, Winkelmann G, Hohagen F: Cognitive frontal lobe dysfunction in obsessive-compulsive disorder. Biol Psychiatry 43(9):666–673, 1998 9583000

Schulz SC: The use of low-dose neuroleptics in the treatment of "schizo-obsessive" patients. Am J Psychiatry 143(10):1318–1319, 1986 2876650

Scotti-Muzzi E, Saide OL: Schizo-obsessive spectrum disorders: an update. CNS Spectr 22(3):258–272, 2017 27669819

Selzer JA, Lieberman JA: Schizophrenia and substance abuse. Psychiatr Clin North Am 16(2):401–412, 1993 8332568

Seow LSE, Ong C, Mahesh MV, et al: A systematic review on comorbid post-traumatic stress disorder in schizophrenia. Schizophr Res 176(2–3):441–451, 2016 27230289

Shear MK, Brown TA, Barlow DH, et al: Multicenter collaborative panic disorder severity scale. Am J Psychiatry 154(11):1571–1575, 1997 9356566

Shepherd M, Watt D, Falloon I, et al: The natural history of schizophrenia: a five-year follow-up study of outcome and prediction in a representative sample of schizophrenics. Psychol Med Monogr Suppl 15:1–46, 1989 2798648

Shrivastava A, Johnston M, Campbell R, et al: Serum cholesterol and suicide in first episode psychosis: a preliminary study. Indian J Psychiatry 59(4):478–482, 2017 29497191

Silverman BL, Martin W, Memisoglu A, et al: A randomized, double-blind, placebo-controlled proof of concept study to evaluate samidorphan in the prevention of olanzapine-induced weight gain in healthy volunteers. Schizophr Res 195:245–251, 2018 29158012

Simon GE, Stewart C, Yarborough BJ, et al: Mortality rates after the first diagnosis of psychotic disorder in adolescents and young adults. JAMA Psychiatry 75(3):254–260, 2018 29387876

Sin J, Spain D, Furuta M, et al: Psychological interventions for post-traumatic stress disorder (PTSD) in people with severe mental illness. Cochrane Database Syst Rev 1:CD011464, 2017 28116752

Siris SG: Akinesia and postpsychotic depression: a difficult differential diagnosis. J Clin Psychiatry 48(6):240–243, 1987 2884213

Siris SG: Pharmacological treatment of substance-abusing schizophrenic patients. Schizophr Bull 16(1):111–122, 1990 1970669

Siris SG: Depression in schizophrenia: perspective in the era of "atypical" antipsychotic agents. Am J Psychiatry 157(9):1379–1389, 2000a 10964850

Siris SG: Management of depression in schizophrenia. Psychiatr Ann 30:13–19, 2000b

Siris SG, Aronson A, Sellew AP: Imipramine-responsive panic-like symptomatology in schizophrenia/schizoaffective disorder. Biol Psychiatry 25(4):485–488, 1989 2649158

Siris SG, Mason SE, Bermanzohn PC, et al: Adjunctive imipramine in substance-abusing dysphoric schizophrenic patients. Psychopharmacol Bull 29(1):127–133, 1993 8378506

Siskind DJ, Leung J, Russell AW, et al: Metformin for clozapine associated obesity: a systematic review and meta-analysis. PLoS One 11(6):e0156208, 2016 27304831

Smelson DA, Losonczy MF, Davis CW, et al: Risperidone decreases craving and relapses in individuals with schizophrenia and cocaine dependence. Can J Psychiatry 47(7):671–675, 2002 12355680

Spagnolo PA, Goldman D: Neuromodulation interventions for addictive disorders: challenges, promise, and roadmap for future research. Brain 140(5):1183–1203, 2017 28082299

Steel C, Hardy A, Smith B, et al: Cognitive-behaviour therapy for post-traumatic stress in schizophrenia: a randomized controlled trial. Psychol Med 47(1):43–51, 2017 27650432

Steinberg ML, Ziedonis DM, Krejci JA, et al: Motivational interviewing with personalized feedback: a brief intervention for motivating smokers with schizophrenia to seek treatment for tobacco dependence. J Consult Clin Psychol 72(4):723–728, 2004 15301657

Steinberg ML, Williams JM, Stahl NF, et al: An adaptation of motivational interviewing increases quit attempts in smokers with serious mental illness. Nicotine Tob Res 18(3):243–250, 2016 25744954

Stone WS, Faraone SV, Seidman LJ, et al: Concurrent validation of schizotaxia: a pilot study. Biol Psychiatry 50(6):434–440, 2001 11566160

Storch EA, Larson MJ, Price LH, et al: Psychometric analysis of the Yale-Brown Obsessive-Compulsive Scale Second Edition Symptom Checklist. J Anxiety Disord 24(6):650–656, 2010 20471199

Storch Jakobsen A, Speyer H, Nørgaard HCB, et al: Associations between clinical and psychosocial factors and metabolic and cardiovascular risk factors in overweight patients with schizophrenia spectrum disorders—baseline and two-years findings from the CHANGE trial. Schizophr Res 199:96–102, 2018 29501386

Strauss JL, Calhoun PS, Marx CE, et al: Comorbid posttraumatic stress disorder is associated with suicidality in male veterans with schizophrenia or schizoaffective disorder. Schizophr Res 84(1):165–169, 2006 16567080

Stroup TS, McEvoy JP, Ring KD, et al; Schizophrenia Trials Network: A randomized trial examining the effectiveness of switching from olanzapine, quetiapine, or risperidone to aripiprazole to reduce metabolic risk: Comparison of Antipsychotics for Metabolic Problems (CAMP). Am J Psychiatry 168(9):947–956, 2011 21768610

Strous RD, Patel JK, Zimmet S, et al: Clozapine and paroxetine in the treatment of schizophrenia with obsessive-compulsive features. Am J Psychiatry 156(6):973–974, 1999 10360153

Stryjer R, Dambinsky Y, Timinsky I, et al: Escitalopram in the treatment of patients with schizophrenia and obsessive-compulsive disorder: an open-label, prospective study. Int Clin Psychopharmacol 28(2):96–98, 2013 23211492

Subica AM, Claypoole KH, Wylie AM: PTSD's mediation of the relationships between trauma, depression, substance abuse, mental health, and physical health in individuals with severe mental illness: evaluating a comprehensive model. Schizophr Res 136(1–3):104–109, 2012 22104139

Subotnik KL, Nuechterlein KH, Asarnow RF, et al: Depressive symptoms in the early course of schizophrenia: relationship to familial psychiatric illness. Am J Psychiatry 154(11):1551–1556, 1997 9356563

Substance Abuse and Mental Health Services Administration: Toolkit for Integrated Dual Disorders Treatment. Integrated Treatment for Co-Occurring Disorders: How to Use the Evidence-Based Practices KITs (DHHS Publ No SMA-08-4366). Rockville, MD, Center for Mental Health Services, Substance Abuse and Mental Health Services Administration, 2009. Available at https://store.samhsa.gov/system/files/howtouseebpkits-itc.pdf. Accessed October 2019.

Swartz MS, Wagner HR, Swanson JW, et al: Substance use in persons with schizophrenia: baseline prevalence and correlates from the NIMH CATIE study. J Nerv Ment Dis 194(3):164–172, 2006 16534433

Swets M, Dekker J, van Emmerik-van Oortmerssen K, et al: The obsessive compulsive spectrum in schizophrenia, a meta-analysis and meta-regression exploring prevalence rates. Schizophr Res 152(2–3):458–468, 2014 24361303

Taipale H, Mehtala J, Tanskanen A, et al: Comparative effectiveness of antipsychotic drugs for rehospitalization in schizophrenia—a nationwide study with 20-year follow-up. Schizophr Bull 44(6):1381–1387, 2018 29272458

Takahashi H, Sugita T, Yoshida K, et al: Effect of quetiapine in the treatment of panic attacks in patients with schizophrenia: 3 case reports. J Neuropsychiatry Clin Neurosci 16(1):113–115, 2004 14990767

Taylor S: Meta-analysis of cognitive-behavioral treatments for social phobia. J Behav Ther Exp Psychiatry 27(1):1–9, 1996 8814516

Tchoukhine E, Takala P, Hakko H, et al: Orlistat in clozapine- or olanzapine-treated patients with overweight or obesity: a 16-week open-label extension phase and both phases of a randomized controlled trial. J Clin Psychiatry 72(3):326–330, 2011 20816037

Teasdale SB, Ward PB, Rosenbaum S, et al: Solving a weighty problem: systematic review and meta-analysis of nutrition interventions in severe mental illness. Br J Psychiatry 210(2):110–118, 2017 27810893

Temmingh H, Stein DJ: Anxiety in patients with schizophrenia: epidemiology and management. CNS Drugs 29(10):819–832, 2015 26482261

Tibbo P, Kroetsch M, Chue P, et al: Obsessive-compulsive disorder in schizophrenia. J Psychiatr Res 34(2):139–146, 2000 10758256

Tidey JW, Miller ME: Smoking cessation and reduction in people with chronic mental illness. BMJ 351:h4065, 2015 26391240

Tidey JW, Cassidy RN, Miller ME: Smoking topography characteristics of very low nicotine content cigarettes, with and without nicotine replacement, in smokers with schizophrenia and controls. Nicotine Tob Res 18(9):1807–1812, 2016 26995794

Tiihonen J, Mittendorfer-Rutz E, Torniainen M, et al: Mortality and cumulative exposure to antipsychotics, antidepressants, and benzodiazepines in patients with schizophrenia: an observational follow-up study. Am J Psychiatry 173(6):600–606, 2016 26651392

Tiihonen J, Mittendorfer-Rutz E, Majak M, et al: Real-world effectiveness of antipsychotic treatments in a nationwide cohort of 29,823 patients with schizophrenia. JAMA Psychiatry 74(7):686–693, 2017 28593216

Tollefson GD, Andersen SW, Tran PV: The course of depressive symptoms in predicting relapse in schizophrenia: a double-blind, randomized comparison of olanzapine and risperidone. Biol Psychiatry 46(3):365–373, 1999 10435202

Tundo A, Salvati L, Busto G, et al: Addition of cognitive-behavioral therapy for nonresponders to medication for obsessive-compulsive disorder: a naturalistic study. J Clin Psychiatry 68(10):1552–1556, 2007 17960971

Upthegrove R, Marwaha S, Birchwood M: Depression and schizophrenia: cause, consequence, or trans-diagnostic issue? Schizophr Bull 43(2):240–244, 2017 27421793

U.S. Department of Veterans Affairs: VA/DOD Clinical Practice Guideline for the Management of Posttraumatic Stress Disorder and Acute Stress Disorder. 2017. Available at: https://www.healthquality.va.gov/guidelines/MH/ptsd/VADoDPTSDCPGFinal.pdf. Accessed May 31, 2019.

van Balkom AJ, de Haan E, van Oppen P, et al: Cognitive and behavioral therapies alone versus in combination with fluvoxamine in the treatment of obsessive compulsive disorder. J Nerv Ment Dis 186(8):492–499, 1998 9717867 van den Berg DP, van der Gaag M: Treating trauma in psychosis with EMDR: a pilot study. J Behav Ther Exp Psychiatry 43(1):664–671, 2012 21963888

van den Berg DP, de Bont PA, van der Vleugel BM, et al: Prolonged exposure vs eye movement desensitization and reprocessing vs waiting list for posttraumatic stress disorder in patients with a psychotic disorder: a randomized clinical trial. JAMA Psychiatry 72(3):259–267, 2015 25607833

van den Berg DP, de Bont PA, van der Vleugel BM, et al: Trauma-focused treatment in PTSD patients with psychosis: symptom exacerbation, adverse events, and revictimization. Schizophr Bull 42:693–702, 2016 26609122

van Minnen A, Zoellner LA, Harned MS, Mills K: Changes in comorbid conditions after prolonged exposure for PTSD: a literature review. Curr Psychiatry Rep 17(3):549, 2015 25736701

van Nimwegen LJ, de Haan L, van Beveren NJ, et al: Effect of olanzapine and risperidone on subjective well-being and craving for cannabis in patients with schizophrenia or related disorders: a double-blind randomized controlled trial. Can J Psychiatry 53(6):400–405, 2008 18616861

van Rooijen G, Vermeulen JM, Ruhe HG, et al: Treating depressive episodes or symptoms in patients with schizophrenia. CNS Spectr 24(2):239–248, 2019 28927482

Vanwormer JJ, French SA, Pereira MA, Welsh EM: The impact of regular self-weighing on weight management: a systematic literature review. Int J Behav Nutr Phys Act 5:54, 2008 18983667

Varese F, Smeets F, Drukker M, et al: Childhood adversities increase the risk of psychosis: a meta-analysis of patient-control, prospective- and cross-sectional cohort studies. Schizophr Bull 38(4):661–671, 2012 22461484

Velligan DI, Sajatovic M, Hatch A, et al: Why do psychiatric patients stop antipsychotic medication? A systematic review of reasons for nonadherence to medication in patients with serious mental illness. Patient Prefer Adherence 11:449–468, 2017 28424542

Vermeulen JM, van Rooijen G, van de Kerkhof MPJ, et al: Clozapine and long-term mortality risk in patients with schizophrenia: a systematic review and meta-analysis of studies lasting 1.1–12.5 years. Schizophr Bull 45(2):315–329, 2019 29697804

Veznedaroglu B, Ercan ES, Kayahan B, et al: Reduced short-term obsessive-compulsive symptoms in schizophrenic patients treated with risperidone: a single-blind prospective study. Hum Psychopharmacol 18(8):635–640, 2003 14696023

Vickerman KA, Schauer GL, Malarcher AM, et al: Quitline use and outcomes among callers with and without mental health conditions: a 7-month follow-up evaluation in three states. Biomed Res Int 2015:817298, 2015 26273647

Vilardaga R, Rizo J, Zeng E, et al: User-centered design of Learn to Quit, a smoking cessation smartphone app for people with serious mental illness. JMIR Serious Games 6(1):e2, 2018 29339346

Walker AM, Lanza LL, Arellano F, et al: Mortality in current and former users of clozapine. Epidemiology 8(6):671–677, 1997 9345668

Weathers F, Litz B, Herman D, et al: The PTSD Checklist (PCL): reliability, validity, and diagnostic utility. Paper presented at the annual convention of the International Society for Traumatic Stress Studies, San Antonio, TX, October 1993

Weathers FW, Keane TM, Davidson JR: Clinician-Administered PTSD Scale: a review of the first ten years of research. Depress Anxiety 13(3):132–156, 2001 11387733

Weathers FW, Bovin MJ, Lee DJ, et al: The Clinician-Administered PTSD Scale for DSM-5 (CAPS-5): Development and initial psychometric evaluation in military veterans. Psychol Assess 30(3), 383–395, 2018 28493729

Williams JM, Steinberg ML, Zimmermann MH, et al: Comparison of two intensities of tobacco dependence counseling in schizophrenia and schizoaffective disorder. J Subst Abuse Treat 38(4):384–393, 2010 20363089

Williams JM, Anthenelli RM, Morris CD, et al: A randomized, double-blind, placebo-controlled study evaluating the safety and efficacy of varenicline for smoking cessation in patients with schizophrenia or schizoaffective disorder. J Clin Psychiatry 73(5):654–660, 2012 22697191

Williams JM, Steinberg ML, Griffiths KG, et al: Smokers with behavioral health comorbidity should be designated a tobacco use disparity group. Am J Public Health 103(9):1549–1555, 2013 23865661

Wing VC, Wass CE, Soh DW, et al: A review of neurobiological vulnerability factors and treatment implications for comorbid tobacco dependence in schizophrenia. Ann NY Acad Sci 1248:89–106, 2012 22129082

Wisdom JP, Manuel JI, Drake RE: Substance use disorder among people with first-episode psychosis: a systematic review of course and treatment. Psychiatr Serv 62(9):1007–1012, 2011 21885577

Zhang JP, Lencz T, Zhang RX, et al: Pharmacogenetic associations of antipsychotic drug-related weight gain: a systematic review and meta-analysis. Schizophr Bull 42(6):1418–1437, 2016 27217270

Zheng W, Xiang YT, Xiang YQ, et al: Efficacy and safety of adjunctive topiramate for schizophrenia: a meta-analysis of randomized controlled trials. Acta Psychiatr Scand 134(5):385–398, 2016 27585549

Zheng W, Zhang QE, Cai DB, et al: Combination of metformin and lifestyle intervention for antipsychotic-related weight gain: a meta-analysis of randomized controlled trials. Pharmacopsychiatry 52(1):24–31, 2019 29486513

Ziedonis D, Richardson T, Lee E, et al: Adjunctive desipramine in the treatment of cocaine abusing schizophrenics. Psychopharmacol Bull 28(3):309–314, 1992 1480735

Zimbron J, Khandaker GM, Toschi C, et al: A systematic review and meta-analysis of randomised controlled trials of treatments for clozapine-induced obesity and metabolic syndrome. Eur Neuropsychopharmacol 26(9):1353–1365, 2016 27496573

Zink M: Comorbid obsessive-compulsive symptoms in schizophrenia: insight into pathomechanisms facilitates treatment. Adv Med 2014:317980, 2014 26556409

Zink M, Knopf U, Kuwilsky A: Management of clozapine-induced obsessive-compulsive symptoms in a man with schizophrenia. Aust NZ J Psychiatry 41(3):293–294, 2007 17464712

Zisook S, McAdams LA, Kuck J, et al: Depressive symptoms in schizophrenia. Am J Psychiatry 156(11):1736–1743, 1999 10553737

Zisook S, Kasckow JW, Golshan S, et al: Citalopram augmentation for subsyndromal symptoms of depression in middle-aged and older outpatients with schizophrenia and schizoaffective disorder: a randomized controlled trial. J Clin Psychiatry 70(4):562–571, 2009 19192468

Zisook S, Kasckow JW, Lanouette NM, et al: Augmentation with citalopram for suicidal ideation in middle-aged and older outpatients with schizophrenia and schizoaffective disorder who have subthreshold depressive symptoms: a randomized controlled trial. J Clin Psychiatry 71(7):915–922, 2010 20361918

CHAPTER 11

Evidence-Based Models of Service Delivery

Michael T. Compton, M.D., M.P.H.

Marc W. Manseau, M.D., M.P.H.

Treatment for schizophrenia is effective for most individuals with the disorder. However, because there is no cure for schizophrenia, long-term engagement in comprehensive treatment and supportive interventions is necessary for individuals to have the best chance at recovery. Unfortunately, many persons with schizophrenia or other serious mental illnesses (SMIs) (e.g., other psychotic disorders, bipolar disorders, severe depressive disorders) drop out of treatment or never connect to care at all. Studies have estimated that up to half of persons with schizophrenia do not engage in care in any given year (Kreyenbuhl et al. 2009). In addition, certain circumstances may make it even more challenging for individuals to engage in treatment; these include but are not limited to first-episode psychosis (FEP), homelessness, co-occurring substance use disorders (SUDs), and a history of involvement with the criminal justice system (Dixon et al. 2016). To address this dilemma, mental health clinicians, researchers, and policy makers have increasingly developed models for *how* to effectively deliver services for the population with SMI, discovered *new* treatment modalities, and investigated *what* individual interventions are most efficacious.

In this chapter, we focus on how to deliver services to individuals with schizophrenia. Because most service delivery models focus more generally on the population with SMI rather than only on persons with schizophrenia, we will subsequently refer to SMI, unless a particular model specifies a more defined population, such as those with FEP. We describe in depth the most important and well-studied evidence-based models for organizing care and rehabilitative supports, beginning with assertive community treatment (ACT), the first intentionally designed and prospectively studied service delivery model for individuals with SMI, which still serves as a blueprint for developing and studying such models. We then review critical time intervention (CTI), a model of care coordination and support services that helps individuals avoid psychiatric relapse and other unfavorable outcomes during vulnerable transitions. Next, we discuss coordinated specialty care (CSC) for early psychosis, which is a relatively new, multipronged intervention for providing care to individuals with FEP. Finally, we describe integrated dual disorder treatment (IDDT), an approach for addressing co-occurring SMI and SUDs in a comprehensive, person-centered way within a single treatment program. Prior to the chapter's conclusion, we briefly review several other important service delivery approaches that are evidence informed and/or emerging—partial hospitalization and day treatment models; intensive case management (ICM), community support teams (CSTs), and community navigation models; and methods to collaborate with law enforcement and the criminal justice sector.

Assertive Community Treatment

ACT was one of the first mental health service delivery models to be rigorously tested, and it arguably set the foundation for the creation and study of evidence-based mental health service interventions. The model emerged in 1980 in Madison, Wisconsin, when a series of seminal papers were published in *Archives of General Psychiatry* about a novel program to treat individuals with SMI in the community rather than hospitalizing them (Stein and Test 1980; Test and Stein 1980; Weisbrod et al. 1980). The model that would eventually become ACT was called Training in Community Living (TCL) and was designed to treat individuals with SMI where they lived, rather than in a hospital setting, to better transfer, integrate, and sustain skills where they would actually be needed. The entire staff from a hospital ward was retrained to work with individuals in the community, and staff were available 24 hours a day, which may be the reason that ACT has since been commonly referred to as "a hospital without walls." Stein and Test (1980) clearly described the core concepts of the TCL model, which included requirements that the program assist clients with material resources; teach coping skills necessary for community living in vivo, where they will be used; motivate clients to "persevere and remain involved with life"; help individuals to obtain "freedom from pathologically dependent relationships" (i.e., with institutions, families, and individual treatment providers); support and educate other community members who are involved with clients; and assertively support clients by going to them and providing services where they live when necessary.

The first paper not only summarized the model but also reported striking results of a trial comparing TCL with a control group randomly assigned to inpatient state hospital admission, among a total sample of 126 individuals presenting for hospitalization (Stein and Test 1980). Compared with those assigned to the control condition, individuals assigned to TCL demonstrated a markedly reduced need for subsequent hospitalization, enhanced community tenure, and improved psychosocial functioning over the course of 14 months. Individuals in the intervention group also spent more time employed, had higher medication adherence, and had lower psychiatric symptoms. When the TCL program was discontinued, most gains among the intervention group deteriorated and hospital use rose sharply. The second paper in the series reported on a cost-benefit analysis of TCL and showed that the added benefits of the program exceeded the costs (Weisbrod et al. 1980). The third paper used local po-

TABLE 11–1.   **Core elements of assertive community treatment**

Rather than brokering services, the team directly provides treatment and support services.

Teams provide a full range of comprehensive, flexible, and individualized services.

The entire team shares responsibility for the full caseload.

Services are provided in the community where clients spend their time and live.

The team assertively engages clients in the community.

The team carefully and actively monitors medication adherence, side effects, and efficacy.

Contacts between the team and clients are regular and frequent.

The team is available for crisis management 24 hours per day, 7 days per week.

Caseloads are small (approximately 1:10 staff-to-client ratio).

There is no time-limited discharge policy; clients receive services for as long as necessary.

lice records to assess the "social cost" of TCL relative to hospitalization; the authors defined *social cost* as the additional burden that the program placed on families and communities. Finding no greater incidence of arrests, incidence of "suicidal gestures" requiring medical attention, or frequency of emergency room use, the researchers concluded that TCL placed no higher burden on families and communities than did hospitalization (Test and Stein 1980). Likely due to the clear and precise description of the model, the striking initial evidence for its efficacy and cost-effectiveness, and rapid replication of the initial results in different locations and populations (Essock et al. 1998; Hoult et al. 1984; Mueser et al. 1998; Olfson 1990; Rosenheck et al. 1995), this "home treatment" service delivery model was widely disseminated relatively quickly, and it became a mainstay of community treatment for individuals with SMI in many public mental health systems throughout the United States, and then Australia, under the "assertive community treatment" name (Burns 2010).

Table 11–1 summarizes the core elements that have come to define ACT services since the model's inception in the early 1980s (Burns 2010; Corrigan 2006). Rather than brokering services, as in traditional case management, ACT teams are designed to provide mental health treatment and support and rehabilitation services directly to the clients they serve. The teams should have available a full range of psychiatric, psychosocial, and social supportive services (e.g., medication management, psychotherapy, skills rehabilitation, case management) and should deliver them in a flexible manner, tailored to the needs of individual clients. Rather than having separate caseloads, team members are expected to share responsibility for all clients assigned to the ACT team. This feature was originally designed to align with the principle of helping clients avoid pathologically dependent relationships; however, as thinking about delivering services for individuals with SMI has evolved, this element is now justified by the need to provide comprehensive services and ensure continuity of care (Burns 2010). ACT teams are meant to keep individuals in the community (and out of institutional settings) by providing services in the communities where clients live and by assertively reaching out to individuals who may not be able or willing to independently seek out services and adhere to clinic appointments.

Because psychiatric medications are an important part of treatment for many people with SMI, a key element of ACT team services is medication monitoring. Teams are expected to make regular and frequent contact with clients and to be available for crisis management 24 hours per day, 7 days per week. To maintain such an intensive level of services, caseloads are small, with a staff-to-client ratio of around 1:10. When originally developed, TCL was supposed to be a time-limited training to permanently confer the skills necessary to maintain community tenure. However, the initial results showing that gains rapidly and significantly deteriorated led to the incorporation of a "no-discharge policy" as a core element. Not surprisingly, this policy soon led to ACT teams with full caseloads of long-term clients. Therefore, this feature has become somewhat more flexible, with the idea that clients should not be discharged after a prespecified period of time before they are ready.

These key features of ACT services are carried out by a multidisciplinary team, which at a minimum includes a psychiatrist and/or other psychiatric care provider (e.g., psychiatric nurse practitioner), a nurse, and clinicians who perform a combined case management and individual supportive psychotherapy role (e.g., social workers). In addition, many adaptations to the ACT model have been studied and implemented to include roles on the team for peer specialists (Wright-Berryman et al. 2011), addiction treatment providers, and supported employment professionals (Latimer 2005), among others. For instance, ACT teams that also provide IDDT have been created and studied (Drake et al. 1998, 2000; Essock et al. 2006; Fries and Rosen 2011; Morse et al. 2006), as discussed further in the IDDT section. Many mental health systems have implemented Forensic Assertive Community Treatment teams, with evidence supporting a decrease in arrests and detentions for clients with histories of involvement in the criminal justice system (Marquant et al. 2016). Other ACT teams have begun to experiment with integrating the ACT model with physical health care, through coordinating and/or providing medical services, to address the fact that individuals with SMI often have difficulty accessing medical care and experience much higher mortality rates than the general population (Carson Weinstein et al. 2011; Vanderlip et al. 2017).

After the seminal series of papers about the ACT model was published in 1980, the findings related to reduced hospital days were rapidly replicated numerous times in the United States (Dixon et al. 2010; Mueser et al. 1998; Olfson 1990; Scott and Dixon 1995) and Australia (Hoult et al. 1984). The cost-effectiveness of ACT was also definitively and repeatedly replicated (Essock et al. 1998; Latimer 2005), including with a randomized controlled trial (RCT) in a sample of patients with SMI in Department of Veterans Affairs (VA) settings (Rosenheck et al. 1995). In addition, multiple studies applying the ACT model to homeless individuals with SMI demonstrated that ACT not only reduced inpatient hospital use in this population but also increased the amount of time they spent in stable housing (Coldwell and Bender 2007; Essock et al. 2006; Lehman et al. 1997; Morse et al. 2006; Nelson et al. 2007). By the time two decades had passed after the initial publications, several systematic reviews and meta-analyses had confirmed the effectiveness of ACT for individuals with SMI and high inpatient hospital use, and the model was firmly established as a key evidence-based approach to delivering services in mental health systems within the United States (Bustillo et al. 2001). In fact, the Schizophrenia Patient Outcomes Research Team (PORT) recommended ACT as one of the eight evidence-based psychosocial interventions for individuals with schizophrenia (Dixon et al. 2010).

The original findings related to improved symptoms and psychosocial functioning did not hold up in subsequent research (Burns and Santos 1995; Bustillo et al. 2001), however, and even the seemingly robust effects on inpatient hospitalization were largely not replicated in the United Kingdom and then in continental Europe (Burns 2010; Dixon et al. 2010; Drukker et al. 2011, 2014; Killaspy et al. 2006; Stobbe et al. 2014; Sytema et al. 2007). Recent studies in Scandinavia have continued to show that ACT is efficacious and cost-effective, especially for individuals with high baseline inpatient service use (Aagaard and Kølbæk 2016; Aagaard and Müller-Nielsen 2011; Aagaard et al. 2017; Hastrup and Aagaard 2015). The cost-effectiveness of ACT when compared with standard case management in the United States was also questioned in a fairly large RCT (Clark et al. 1998). This led to some controversy in the field of mental health services research, as well as an international split in expert opinion.

There have been clues in the literature as to the causes of disparate findings. In the mid-1990s, a fidelity scale for ACT was developed and validated (McGrew et al. 1994), and research subsequently demonstrated that high-fidelity ACT teams were generally more effective at reducing inpatient hospitalization than low-fidelity teams (Cuddeback et al. 2013; Dixon et al. 2010; Latimer 1999; McHugo et al. 1999; Scott and Dixon 1995). However, some studies showed that fidelity to small caseloads was unnecessary for effectiveness (Burns 2010; Burns et al. 2007; Catty et al. 2002). In addition, important issues related to variation in study populations and design emerged. It seems that ACT is most effective for individuals who have a relatively high baseline use of inpatient psychiatric services (Morrissey et al. 2013; Mueser et al. 1998), and many studies in the United Kingdom and Europe included samples with low hospital use in both the control and experimental groups, making it difficult to demonstrate a difference between experimental conditions in the main outcome of interest (Burns 2010; Burns et al. 2007). Finally, interventions in the control condition varied widely (Catty et al. 2002). In U.S. studies, ACT has been consistently effective when compared with "usual treatment," which often placed a substantial and unrealistic burden on individuals with SMI to independently navigate the mental health system and adhere to treatment. However, ACT has been less consistently effective when compared with more robust and assertive control interventions, such as ICM in the United States (Latimer 1999) (a model discussed in "Other Emerging and/or Evidence-Informed Models of Service Delivery" later in this chapter) or community mental health teams in the United Kingdom and Europe (Burns 2010; Killaspy et al. 2006).

The ongoing debate about the effectiveness of ACT exemplifies the difficulty of rigorously studying models of service delivery. Studying an entire service delivery approach, unlike a medication or even a discrete psychotherapeutic intervention, inherently involves being unable to control for every aspect of a complex intervention, as well as differences in contextual factors related to the mental health system in which the model is studied (e.g., differing reliance on inpatient hospital services). However, we might consider the contingency of the model's efficacy on the system to be a feature rather than a flaw; ACT was developed to better deliver services to individuals with SMI who had failed to achieve good outcomes in a particular mental health system. It has delivered and continues to deliver results for high-service utilizers within the United States and in other settings with similar gaps in community services. Furthermore, repeated studies have shown that ACT improves outcomes related to both hospitalization and housing status for individuals who experience SMI and homelessness. While awaiting further research on how to enhance ACT and/or more effective models to deliver services to its target population, mental health policy makers and service providers can conclude that ACT is an efficacious and cost-effective option for individuals in the United States with SMI and high inpatient psychiatric hospital use and/or homelessness.

Critical Time Intervention

CTI evolved in the mid-1980s and early 1990s from the experience of mental health personnel working at two large, publicly operated men's shelters in New York City that housed up to 1,000 individuals per night, many of whom had untreated or inadequately treated SMI (Valencia et al. 1996). Mental health teams operating at these shelters developed comprehensive treatment programs providing on-site screening and outreach, psychiatric medication, rehabilitation groups, counseling about entitlements and services, and case management. In 1990, a local and state government partnership produced an unprecedented expansion of transitional and permanent housing programs for homeless persons with SMI (Lipton et al. 2000). The increased housing options made it possible for the shelter-based workers to place many of their homeless clients into housing. However, a substantial number of men provided with housing became homeless again within several months of discharge, and many returned to the shelter (Caton et al. 1993). Despite the efforts of case managers to implement carefully developed discharge plans, many men still did not have the type of help they needed to overcome the natural discontinuity in support they experienced during their transition. This dilemma led to the development of CTI.

CTI is an empirically supported service delivery model designed to reduce the risk of homelessness, psychiatric hospital recidivism, and other adverse outcomes. The model enhances continuity of support for individuals with SMI with complex psychosocial needs during transitions from institutional settings to community living. As such, it is a psychosocial support model that was developed explicitly to address a *timing-specific* need for a *time-limited* increase in support. Although the model drew from earlier approaches, such as ACT, the design of CTI was largely practical, aimed at addressing an identified service gap pertaining to critical transitions (Herman and Mandiberg 2010). Importantly, whereas ACT provides direct psychiatric treatment, CTI does not, because it is a bridging strategy meant to prevent discontinuities of care during crucial transitions.

The time following institutional release is characterized by increased risk for homelessness, hospitalization, symptom exacerbation, suicide, and violence. Having a serious psychiatric disorder and complex social needs makes garnering support, treatment, and housing in the community difficult. CTI acknowledges that transitions are inherently hazardous for a number of reasons (Herman and Mandiberg 2010). First, during the transition (e.g., after discharge from a homeless shelter, jail or prison, or inpatient care), individuals are expected to navigate a complex and fragmented system of care. Second, the transition may bring an end to personal, supportive relationships individuals developed with key people—both service providers and peers—during their institutional stay. Third, the transition period can be a difficult time in the relationship between the individual and his or her family and social network, who may not be accustomed to providing the level of support needed after discharge.

TABLE 11–2. **Key aspects of critical time intervention (CTI)**

Enhanced, time-limited, emotional and practical support is provided for individuals with serious mental illnesses with complex psychosocial needs during transitions from institutional to community settings, typically occurring over 9 months.

Help is provided with navigating an often complex and fragmented system of care.

Assistance with strengthening the individual's long-term ties to a range of supports (e.g., outpatient mental health services, family and friends) is provided.

Help is given with developing independent living skills and support networks in the community during the transition.

Postdischarge assistance is provided by a CTI worker who has already established a relationship with the individual before discharge.

CTI worker maintains a high level of contact with the client via home visits, accompanying client to appointments, and telephone calls, and mediates between client and service providers (*transition-to-the-community phase*).

CTI worker then meets with the client less frequently but maintains regular contact to observe how the plan is working and be ready to intervene when a crisis arises (*tryout phase*).

CTI worker then ensures that the most significant members of the support system come together and, along with the client, reach a consensus about the components of the ongoing system of support (*transfer-of-care phase*).

Table 11–2 lists the key aspects of CTI. The model works to strengthen an individual's long-term ties to a range of supports, including formal services, family, and friends, while also providing time-limited direct emotional and practical support during a transition (Herman and Mandiberg 2010). Importantly, postdischarge assistance is provided by a care provider who has already established a relationship with the individual before discharge. Like other care delivery models, such as ACT, CTI aims to promote the development of independent living skills and support networks in the community. However, the timing-specific and time-limited model of CTI is meant to maintain continuity of care during a critical period of transition. Then, primary responsibility gradually passes to existing community supports and other services. Thus, by providing focused support at only those points of transition known to be especially difficult for an individual's stability, CTI is an effective, relatively inexpensive patch to existing systems without requiring fundamental change to those systems (Herman and Mandiberg 2010).

CTI comprises three phases, typically occurring over 9 months (Herman and Mandiberg 2010). First, in *transition to the community*, intensive support is provided, and needs and available resources are assessed. The CTI worker maintains a high level of contact with the client via home visits, accompanying the client to appointments, and telephone calls, as well as mediating between the client and service providers. Second, in *tryout*, community providers have assumed primary responsibility for the provision of support and services, and the CTI worker meets with the client less frequently but maintains regular contact to observe how the plan is working and remains ready to intervene when a crisis arises. Third, *transfer of care* focuses on completing the transfer of responsibility to the community resources that will provide long-term support to the client. The CTI worker ensures that the most significant members of the support system meet together and, along with the client, reach a consensus about the components of the ongoing system of support.

Several quasi-experimental studies and randomized trials have been conducted. Among 96 homeless men with psychotic disorders who were placed into housing from a large municipal shelter in New York City, CTI for 9 months was associated with a statistically significant, threefold reduction in risk of postdischarge homelessness over 18 months (Susser et al. 1997). In a larger study conducted at VA medical centers, homeless psychiatric inpatients who received a 6-month version of CTI had, on average, 19% more days housed, fewer days in institutional settings, and lower alcohol and drug use and overall psychiatric symptom scores than those in a control group receiving standard case management services (Kasprow and Rosenheck 2007). In New York City, 150 men and women with schizophrenia spectrum disorders and homelessness who were being discharged from transitional residences on the grounds of state psychiatric hospitals received either usual discharge planning and follow-up services or usual services plus 9 months of CTI. The risk of homelessness at 18 months was 5 times lower in the CTI group (Herman et al. 2011), and psychiatric rehospitalization was also significantly lower for the group assigned to CTI than for the group receiving usual services (Tomita and Herman 2012).

As research evidence accumulates, CTI has been added to evidence-based practice registries in both the United States and Canada (Herman and Mandiberg 2010). Trainings, implementation support tools, and a fidelity scale have been developed and applied in a number of settings. The model's developers have created and delivered traditional classroom training curricula as well as an online curriculum that combines multimedia Web-based training modules with live person-to-person telephonic support.

Although CTI has largely focused on populations who are homeless or at risk of homelessness in the context of residential transitions, adaptations have been implemented to address other contexts involving high-risk transitions (e.g., young adults with mental illnesses aging out of residential treatment facilities, women who have been victims of domestic violence transitioning from temporary shelters). Furthermore, the tenets of CTI, or even full training in CTI with ongoing fidelity testing, have been incorporated into other service delivery models.

Coordinated Specialty Care for Early Psychosis

CSC is a multidisciplinary, recovery-oriented approach to delivering evidence-based interventions for the treatment of FEP. Table 11–3 summarizes the typical service components of CSC. The approach relies on a team of specialists who work with the client to create a personalized treatment plan using shared decision making. The team offers medication management geared toward individuals with FEP (e.g., using the lowest dose possible given that early psychosis is more responsive to medications and that individuals with FEP are more sensitive to side effects), individual psychotherapy, family psychoeducation and support, case management, and work or education support in the form of supported employment and supported education.

For several decades, a number of countries—including Australia, Canada, the United Kingdom, and several countries of Western Europe—had been providing multicomponent specialty care for early psychosis. During that time, in the United States, such services were largely confined to FEP research centers and were, as such, not widely available. As a result, most adolescents and young adults with FEP were seen in routine

TABLE 11–3. **Typical service components of coordinated specialty care for early psychosis**

Recovery-oriented principles of care

Helping young people with early psychosis achieve their goals for school, work, and social relationships

Shared decision making

Medication management using the lowest possible effective dosages

Individual psychotherapy

Family psychoeducation and support

Case management

Supported employment and supported education

Skills training

Screening, assessment, and treatment for substance use disorders

Screening, assessment, and treatment for suicidality

---

mental health services. The CSC model in the United States grew in part from the Recovery After an Initial Schizophrenia Episode (RAISE) projects funded by the National Institute of Mental Health (NIMH). Launched in 2008, RAISE aimed to develop and demonstrate effectiveness of a treatment model for FEP that could be implemented in nonresearch settings. Two RAISE studies, the RAISE Implementation and Evaluation Study (RAISE-IES; Dixon et al. 2015) and the RAISE Early Treatment Program (RAISE-ETP; Kane et al. 2016), laid the groundwork for larger-scale implementation.

The RAISE-IES feasibility study (which had no comparison condition) was carried out in Baltimore and New York City. It included 65 participants in a treatment program that provided medication management, supported employment and supported education, family psychoeducation and support, skills training, substance use treatment, and care planning for suicide prevention. Results revealed high rates of engagement, reduction of symptoms, and improvement in job and social outcomes (Dixon et al. 2015). In the RAISE-ETP trial, 34 clinics in 21 states were randomly assigned to provide CSC services called "NAVIGATE" or usual community-based care. Findings showed that those receiving NAVIGATE services had significantly better rates of engagement, improved quality of life, and reduced symptoms (Kane et al. 2016).

On the basis of, in part, the promising results from the NIMH-funded RAISE projects, in 2014, the U.S. House of Representatives bill 3547 provided an increase of 5% to the Community Mental Health Block Grant program administered by the Substance Abuse and Mental Health Services Administration (SAMHSA), requiring states to set aside 5% of their block grant allocation to support "evidence-based programs that address the needs of individuals with early serious mental illness, including psychotic disorders." The requirement was increased to 10% in 2016 and has spurred the dissemination of CSC programs across the United States. In addition to growth in funding strategies in recent years, national initiatives are now under way with regard to training, technical assistance, and developing resources for broad dissemination.

Many different programs are considered CSC in the United States; they promote recovery-oriented principles of care (e.g., shared decision making, a focus on individuals' life goals, and warm and respectful staff interactions) while aiming to minimize disability. CSC programs also strive for outreach and early detection that will hopefully reduce the *duration of untreated psychosis* (the period from onset of psychotic symptoms to engagement in specialty care); a longer duration of untreated psychosis is known to be associated with poorer outcomes (Marshall et al. 2005; Perkins et al. 2005). Examples of CSC programs include the Specialized Treatment Early in Psychosis (STEP) program (https://medicine.yale.edu/psychiatry/step/), which was established in 2006 by the Connecticut Mental Health Center; the Early Diagnosis and Preventive Treatment (EDAPT) program (https://earlypsychosis.ucdavis.edu/) at the University of California, Davis, Medical Center's Department of Psychiatry and Behavioral Sciences; and the programs of the Best Practices in Schizophrenia Treatment (BeST) Center (https://www.neomed.edu/bestcenter/) at the Department of Psychiatry at Northeast Ohio Medical University and related programs across Ohio.

In New York, OnTrackNY exemplifies the implementation and dissemination of the CSC approach across a state. OnTrackNY provides treatment to individuals ages 16–30 years with nonaffective psychosis of less than 2 years' duration (Bello et al. 2017). The program helps young people achieve their goals for school, work, and social relationships. An OnTrackNY team is composed of four full-time-equivalent staff members: two positions are staffed by licensed clinicians to fulfill the roles of the primary clinician, outreach and recruitment coordinator, and team leader (who must be full time on the team); one full-time supported education and employment specialist; a half-time peer specialist; and a part-time psychiatric care provider and nurse. Each team serves between 35 and 45 individuals, depending on staffing, and provides a range of evidence-based treatments (Bello et al. 2017). OnTrackNY emphasizes evidence-based psychopharmacology at the lowest effective doses, supported education and supported employment, health and wellness support, coordination with primary care, case management to meet concrete needs, family psychoeducation, and cognitive-behavioral–based therapy.

Integrated Dual Disorder Treatment

As described in Chapter 10, "Co-occurring Disorders and Conditions," combinations of comorbid psychiatric disorders and SUDs, also called co-occurring disorders (CODs), are common (Compton et al. 2007). SAMHSA estimated that about 3.4% of all adults in the United States experienced a COD in 2016. Among individuals with SMI, including schizophrenia, 33.8% had an addiction (Substance Abuse and Mental Health Services Administration 2017). Large, population-based, representative studies such as the Epidemiologic Catchment Area study have shown even higher rates of CODs, with around 50%–70% of those with SMI having a COD (Regier et al. 1990). The most common drugs used by individuals with SMI, in descending order of prevalence, are tobacco, alcohol, cannabis, and cocaine; use of multiple substances with multiple comorbid SUDs is common (Manseau and Bogenschutz 2016; Selzer and Lieberman 1993; Soyka et al. 1993). Tobacco use is often overlooked and is not included in the comorbidity numbers above; however, it has been estimated that almost two-thirds of individuals with schizophrenia use tobacco (Dickerson et al. 2013), and tobacco use is the leading cause of preventable death in individuals with mental illnesses (Bandiera et al. 2015). CODs are associated with worse outcomes, including more severe psychiatric symptoms, higher rates of violence and suicidality, worse overall functioning, higher rates of homelessness and legal problems, worse treatment engagement, and use of more intensive health care services (Bennett and Gjonbalaj 2007; Manseau and Bogenschutz 2016; Swofford et al. 2000; Talamo et al. 2006). In addition, comorbid SUDs place individuals with SMI at increased risk of physical health problems and death (Schulte and Hser 2014). For these reasons, CODs present significant challenges to clinicians and place substantial burdens on the health care and social services systems (Odlaug et al. 2016).

Older models of treatment for CODs include the sequential model, which posited that the SUD should be treated before the psychiatric disorder, and the parallel model, which advocated for treating both CODs simultaneously but in separate programs. Both of these models have significant drawbacks for managing CODs in individuals with mental illnesses. Because SMIs, including schizophrenia, are chronic conditions, addressing them first might lead to never treating the addiction, whereas managing SUDs first would leave the SMI untreated. Although treatment is simultaneous in the parallel model, splitting the care for the CODs can result in poor coordination, inconsistency in the treatment, and logistical burden on patients. Separating SUD and mental health care can contribute to and exacerbate difficulties engaging in and adhering to treatment that individuals with SMI already often experience (Manseau and Bogenschutz 2016; Mueser et al. 2013). Owing to such challenges, comprehensive care for CODs often did not occur at all historically. However, since the 1980s, there has been increasing recognition of the high prevalence of CODs and increasing efforts to integrate treatment for both SMIs and SUDs into single programs, commonly referred to as IDDT (Green et al. 2007; Manseau and Bogenschutz 2016).

Table 11–4 lists the key service components of IDDT. Unlike the other three main evidence-based service delivery models described in this chapter (ACT, CTI, and CSC), IDDT was not developed first for a research study; rather, it developed organically within mental health services systems, in the context of increasing recognition that nonintegrated approaches were failing to successfully serve a substantial portion of persons with SMI. Therefore, IDDT program designs tend to vary, but in general, this approach is characterized by the following (Dixon et al. 2010; Green et al. 2007; Mueser et al. 2013): SMIs and SUDs are treated in a single program by a team of clinicians with expertise in both sets of disorders; treatment plans are person centered and interventions are staged to individuals' motivation levels; motivational enhancement techniques that focus on engagement are employed; and psychotherapeutic interventions focus on coping skills, harm reduction, and relapse prevention (modified for working with individuals with SMI). Pharmacotherapy for psychiatric symptoms is guided by best practices for working with individuals with SUDs (e.g., treat psychiatric symptoms through substance use, avoid potentially addictive or unsafe medications such as benzodiazepines). Anti-addiction medications are encouraged when options are available and appropriate. Services are delivered with a long-term perspective because relapse is common and expected.

Because of an evolving model concept and wide programmatic variation, IDDT has been difficult to study systematically, which has in turn contributed to a mixed evidence base (Dixon et al. 2010). Furthermore, many studies have examined individual psychosocial components of IDDT with mixed results (Drake et al. 2008; Kirk et al. 2008), but a review of the efficacy of individual psychosocial interventions for CODs is beyond the scope of this chapter. As for the entire approach to delivering services to this population, there is some experimental evidence that an integrated approach is generally more effective than a nonintegrated (i.e., parallel) approach in terms of

TABLE 11–4.   **Key service components of integrated dual disorder treatment**

The mental illness and substance use disorder are treated in a single program by a team of clinicians with expertise in both.

Interventions are staged to individual's motivation level.

Motivational enhancement techniques are used.

Psychotherapeutic interventions focus on coping skills, harm reduction, and relapse prevention.

Pharmacotherapy for psychiatric symptoms is guided by best practices for working with individuals with substance use disorders.

Anti-addiction medications are encouraged when options are available and appropriate.

Services are delivered with a long-term perspective and expectation of relapse.

treatment engagement, substance use and addiction severity, psychiatric hospitalization rates, and likelihood of arrest (Dixon et al. 2010; Hellerstein et al. 1995; Herman et al. 1997, 2000; Mangrum et al. 2006). In addition, providing IDDT within ACT has been shown in RCTs to improve certain substance use measures (but not substance abstinence rates), quality of life, inpatient hospitalization rates, and time in stable housing for homeless individuals (Drake et al. 1998, 2000; Essock et al. 2006; Fries and Rosen 2011; Morse et al. 2006). Even with more than several positive clinical trials, many other studies have been negative, and a systematic review of IDDT and many of its component interventions that examined multiple outcomes found little consistent evidence to support one psychosocial intervention or approach to delivering services over any other (Hunt et al. 2014). Even with inconsistent and limited empirical evidence supporting IDDT, experts and mental health policy makers have recognized that CODs are common and serious problems and that integrated services are generally more engaging, person centered, and effective than older approaches. Therefore, IDDT has been recognized for over two decades in the United States as the most effective way to deliver services to individuals with CODs (Drake et al. 2000, 2001; Mueser et al. 2013) and was one of eight evidence-based psychosocial interventions for individuals with schizophrenia endorsed by the Schizophrenia PORT (Dixon et al. 2010).

Other Emerging and/or Evidence-Informed Models of Service Delivery

Partial Hospitalization Programs and Day Treatment Models

ACT is a resource-intensive service delivery model, so mental health systems must reserve this modality for the individuals who need it most. However, this leaves a relatively large group of individuals with SMI at any given time point who simultaneously do not qualify for ACT, do not meet criteria for inpatient psychiatric hospitalization, and have needs that cannot be adequately met by mental health clinics. To fill this gap, mental health systems have experimented with various (mostly Medicaid reimbursable) day treatment and rehabilitation models, including but not limited to partial hospitalization programs (PHPs), intensive outpatient programs, and continuing day treatment programs. PHPs are time-limited day treatment programs that provide active and intensive treatment for individuals with SMI. They are often used during crises to attempt to prevent inpatient hospital admission, or to shorten inpatient hospital stays and help individuals transition back to community treatment; however, they are not designed to safely care for persons who are at acute risk of self-harm/suicide or violent behavior. They tend to have staffing and provide a range of services that are similar to an inpatient unit, such as active pharmacological management, individual and group psychotherapy, skills classes, and case management/discharge planning (Khawaja and Westermeyer 2010). Two systematic reviews of PHPs found that they at least produce no worse outcomes than inpatient hospitalization among eligible patients (Horvitz-Lennon et al. 2001) and at best may lead to greater patient and family satisfaction, better symptom improvement, and fewer inpatient hospital days (Horvitz-Lennon et al. 2001; Marshall et al. 2001). It is important to note that the evidence base for PHPs remains thin, and both reviews indeed recognize limitations in the research related to widely varying definitions and components of PHPs.

Day treatment programs for individuals who are not in crisis and who need long-term care have varied widely in service content and programmatic structure, have not systematically included evidence-based interventions, and have therefore been challenging to study. However, some mental health systems have made attempts to standardize and bolster evidence-based day treatment and/or outpatient rehabilitation services for individuals with SMI. One example is the development of Personalized Recovery Oriented Services (PROS) programs in New York State in 2006. As the name suggests, the PROS model provides recovery-oriented, person-centered treatment, support, and rehabilitation services to persons with SMI. PROS programs are staffed by a combination of psychiatric care providers, community mental health nurses, individual and group therapists, and supported employment specialists; many also have peer specialists. In addition, PROS programs are required to offer a range of specific evidence-based services in an integrated manner, including IDDT, wellness self-management, family psychoeducation, evidence-based medication practices, and individual placement and support for assistance with employment- and/or education-related goals. There is some preliminary evidence that PROS might be a promising model. In a recent analysis of over 12,000 individuals discharged from PROS programs, both psychiatric and substance use–related admissions substantially decreased from the preadmission to the postdischarge periods (White et al. 2018). Although transitional treatment and rehabilitation services such as PHPs and PROS are necessary components of the services continuum for individuals with SMI, the evidence base for their effectiveness is sparse compared with the main evidence-based models described in this chapter. It will be important to continue to experiment with models of transitional services delivery and to rigorously test those that hold initial promise.

Intensive Case Management, Community Support Teams, and Community Navigation Models

Until recent decades, it was common for individuals with SMI to remain in an institution for many years, and in some cases for much of their lives; the goal now is to provide the services they need in community-based settings. Several service models have been developed to pursue this goal. ICM is one such approach. ICM consists of management of the

SMI and the rehabilitation and social supports needed, over an indefinite period of time, by a team of providers who have a fairly small group of clients. Case managers can be reached at any time, and clients are seen in nonclinical settings. A Cochrane review (Dieterich et al. 2017) evaluated evidence supporting ICM in comparison with nonintensive case management (in which individuals received the same care components but the professionals had caseloads of more than 20) and standard care (outpatient care in which support needs were less clearly defined). The review included 40 trials in Australia, Canada, China, Europe, and the United States, involving 7,524 people. Although the evidence supporting ICM was of only moderate quality, the only clear difference was that those in the ICM group were more likely to remain in care. Compared with the standard care group, those in the ICM group were more likely to stay with the service, had improved general functioning, and had shorter stays in the hospital. ICM is less intensive than ACT and thus serves outpatients in need of community-based support but not meeting the higher-level criteria for ACT.

A number of states have implemented CST services. CSTs provide community-based case management services for clients who are not making progress in office-based outpatient treatment due to psychosocial problems such as frequent crises or hospital admissions, homelessness or unstable housing, legal problems, serious psychiatric symptoms, and/or poor adherence to treatment. CST services use a team approach to assist clients in all areas of functioning so that they can reduce crisis episodes, obtain stable housing, connect with school or vocational opportunities, be more independent, improve social skills, and learn coping skills to manage their mental health and SUD symptoms (Carolina Outreach 2019). CST staff are always available in the event of a crisis.

Other related programs have been developed in specific states. For example, in Georgia, a model called Opening Doors to Recovery (ODR) was developed (Compton et al. 2011b) and preliminarily tested (Compton et al. 2016); it is now undergoing an RCT (in comparison to traditional case management and ICM). Key differences between ODR and CSTs, for example, are that 1) ODR is a *navigation* approach rather than a treatment service per se; 2) the composition of the teams differ between ODR and CST services (e.g., ODR has a novel family community navigation specialist) (Myers et al. 2015); 3) ODR has a lower caseload per team; 4) ODR is supported by a broad group of community partners; 5) ODR employs a novel police–navigation specialist linkage (Compton et al. 2017); and 6) ODR was designed specifically around recovery tenets such as creating a meaningful day (Myers et al. 2016). Similarly, New York State has created Mobile Integration Teams (MITs) across the state, funded by "preinvestment" dollars accrued as some state hospital beds are closed. The teams help clients make the transition back into the community or avoid institutional care altogether. MITs are multidisciplinary (including peer specialists, registered nurses, social workers, and others), home and community based, and flexible in their approach to providing peer support, therapy, skill building, crisis intervention, preventive care coordination, and other wrap-around services.

Collaborations With Law Enforcement and the Criminal Justice Sector

Collaboration between criminal justice/law enforcement professionals and mental health professionals is essential for diversion of individuals with SMI away from incarceration and into treatment. Guilty pleas, convictions, and incarceration histories pose challenges to successful reintegration into society after release; for example, entitlements such as Social Security benefits and Medicaid may be lost during detention, and prior convictions often limit subsidized housing and employment opportunities. Mental health services are increasingly partnering with the criminal justice sector to better address the risk of criminal justice entanglement among persons with SMI.

This entanglement is complex and can involve emergency communications, dispatch, the police encounter, arrest, transport to the station, prearraignment custody, arraignment, detention, adjudication, incarceration, release, and community corrections. The Sequential Intercept Model (Munetz and Griffin 2006) provides a framework for communities to identify specific points of intervention within the mental health and criminal justice systems to reduce fragmentation between systems and minimize the criminalization of persons with SMI. Interventions at various "intercepts" may prevent unnecessary detention of persons with SMI and more rapidly connect them to mental health services. The five intercepts within the criminal justice system are 1) law enforcement/emergency services; 2) postarrest, such as during initial bookings; 3) posthearing (e.g., specialty mental health courts); 4) reentry from jails or prisons to the community; and 5) community corrections (e.g., probation, parole). Communities can use the Sequential Intercept Model to "map" their available services and identify gaps. Although intervention at any point is better than none at all, the earlier the stage at which an individual is intercepted, the greater the effect. For example, the Crisis Intervention Team (CIT) model is a widely disseminated approach to prearrest jail diversion. Improving police responses to persons with SMI—which the CIT model aims to accomplish—is a national priority in both the criminal justice and mental health communities.

To improve police officers' responses to individuals with SMI, the CIT model was developed in 1988 in Memphis, Tennessee (Compton et al. 2011a; Dupont and Cochran 2000; Steadman et al. 2000). The now widely disseminated CIT model entails providing select officers with 40 hours of specialized training by police trainers, local mental health professionals, family advocates, and consumer groups (Cochran et al. 2000; Dupont and Cochran 2000), equipping them with the necessary knowledge, attitudes, and skills to enhance their responses to persons with SMI or those in psychiatric crisis (Deane et al. 1999; Lamb et al. 2002; Steadman et al. 2000). After training, officers are specialized first-line responders to such calls (Hails and Borum 2003; Oliva and Compton 2008). The CIT model also supports partnerships between psychiatric emergency services and police departments, encouraging treatment rather than jail when appropriate (Cochran et al. 2000; Lamb et al. 2002). In addition to being a form of pre-arrest jail diversion, the CIT model has other goals, such as improved officer and subject safety.

In addition to CIT, many other models of collaboration exist, although they have received even less research attention than CIT. Such models include mobile crisis teams that may have police collaborations, other types of psychiatric emergency response teams, community mental health officers, clinicians who ride with or consult with patrol officers, co-responder models, and various types of police officer training.

Conclusion

With regard to community-based, recovery-oriented service models for individuals with schizophrenia or other SMIs, those highlighted in this chapter—ACT, CTI, CSC, and IDDT—have substantial research support. Many other models of service delivery exist. However, research to support them as evidence-based models is limited; for many, it is nearly nonexistent. This is partly due to a paucity of funding for research on service delivery models but is also due to the complexity of such research. Studying an entire service model, as opposed to a single pharmacological agent, a device or somatic intervention, or a manualized psychotherapy, means not being able to disaggregate the multiple components, and thus the actual effective components remain unknown. The research methodologies are difficult to carry out and come with unique complexities, as exemplified by randomizing at the individual level versus cluster randomization. Finally, models are often adapted to local needs and contexts, meaning that fidelity and generalizability of earlier results are often unclear.

Because outcomes remain unsatisfactory and recovery is often unachieved for individuals with schizophrenia and other SMIs, additional service delivery models should be developed and, ideally, formally tested. Research evidence then needs to be effectively communicated to program planners, administrators, policy makers, and individuals or groups involved in funding and fiscal oversight. Input from service recipients and their family members should be included at every step. Additionally, people making decisions around implementation and dissemination should always consider culture and inclusion, while striving to reduce persistent health inequities. Services that are accessible, efficient, effective, high quality, and recovery oriented should be the gold standard. Models will undoubtedly evolve, but the goals should always be maximal recovery, community integration, and respect for dignity and human rights. The models briefly described above have this in common and provide examples for how the field must move forward.

References

Aagaard J, Kølbæk P: Predictors of clinical outcome of assertive community treatment (ACT) in a rural area in Denmark: an observational study with a two-year follow-up. Community Ment Health J 52(8):908–913, 2016 26143244

Aagaard J, Müller-Nielsen K: Clinical outcome of assertive community treatment (ACT) in a rural area in Denmark: a case-control study with a 2-year follow-up. Nord J Psychiatry 65(5):299–305, 2011 21174491

Aagaard J, Tuszewski B, Kølbæk P: Does assertive community treatment reduce the use of compulsory admissions? Arch Psychiatr Nurs 31(6):641–646, 2017 29179833

Bandiera FC, Anteneh B, Le T, et al: Tobacco-related mortality among persons with mental health and substance abuse problems. PLoS One 10(3):e0120581, 2015 25807109

Bello I, Lee R, Malinovsky I, et al: OnTrackNY: the development of a coordinated specialty care program for individuals experiencing early psychosis. Psychiatr Serv 68(4):318–320, 2017 27973999

Bennett ME, Gjonbalaj S: The problem of dual diagnosis, in Adult Psychopathology and Diagnosis, 5th Edition. Edited by Hersen M, Turner SM, Beidel DC. New York, Wiley, 2007, pp 34–77

Burns BJ, Santos AB: Assertive community treatment: an update of randomized trials. Psychiatr Serv 46(7):669–675, 1995 7552556

Burns T: The rise and fall of assertive community treatment? Int Rev Psychiatry 22(2):130–137, 2010 20504053

Burns T, Catty J, Dash M, et al: Use of intensive case management to reduce time in hospital in people with severe mental illness: systematic review and meta-regression. BMJ 335(7615):336–342, 2007 17631513

Bustillo J, Lauriello J, Horan W, Keith S: The psychosocial treatment of schizophrenia: an update. Am J Psychiatry 158(2):163–175, 2001 11156795

Carolina Outreach: Community support team. 2019. Available at: https://carolinaoutreach.com/community-support-team. Accessed May 31, 2019.

Carson Weinstein L, Henwood BF, Cody JW, et al: Transforming assertive community treatment into an integrated care system: the role of nursing and primary care partnerships. J Am Psychiatr Nurses Assoc 17(1):64–71, 2011 21659296

Caton CL, Wyatt RJ, Felix A, et al: Follow-up of chronically homeless mentally ill men. Am J Psychiatry 150(11):1639–1642, 1993 8214171

Catty J, Burns T, Knapp M, et al: Home treatment for mental health problems: a systematic review. Psychol Med 32(3):383–401, 2002 11989985

Clark RE, Teague GB, Ricketts SK, et al: Cost-effectiveness of assertive community treatment versus standard case management for persons with co-occurring severe mental illness and substance use disorders. Health Serv Res 33(5 Pt 1):1285–1308, 1998 9865221

Cochran S, Deane MW, Borum R: Improving police response to mentally ill people. Psychiatr Serv 51(10):1315–1316, 2000 11013336

Coldwell CM, Bender WS: The effectiveness of assertive community treatment for homeless populations with severe mental illness: a meta-analysis. Am J Psychiatry 164(3):393–399, 2007 17329462

Compton MT, Broussard B, Munetz M, et al: The Crisis Intervention Team (CIT) Model of Collaboration Between Law Enforcement and Mental Health. New York, Novinka/Nova Science Publishers, 2011a

Compton MT, Hankerson-Dyson D, Broussard B, et al: Opening Doors to Recovery: a novel community navigation service for people with serious mental illnesses. Psychiatr Serv 62(11):1270–1272, 2011b 22211204

Compton MT, Kelley ME, Pope A, et al: Opening Doors to Recovery: recidivism and recovery among persons with serious mental illnesses and repeated hospitalizations. Psychiatr Serv 67(2):169–175, 2016 26467907

Compton MT, Anderson S, Broussard B, et al: A potential new form of jail diversion and reconnection to mental health services, II: demonstration of feasibility. Behav Sci Law 35(5–6):492–500, 2017 29098714

Compton WM, Thomas YF, Stinson FS, et al: Prevalence, correlates, disability, and comorbidity of DSM-IV drug abuse and dependence in the United States: results from the National Epidemiologic Survey on Alcohol and Related Conditions. Arch Gen Psychiatry 64(5):566–576, 2007 17485608

Corrigan PW: Recovery from schizophrenia and the role of evidence-based psychosocial interventions. Expert Rev Neurother 6(7):993–1004, 2006 16831114

Cuddeback GS, Morrissey JP, Domino ME, et al: Fidelity to recovery-oriented ACT practices and consumer outcomes. Psychiatr Serv 64(4):318–323, 2013 23318948

Deane MW, Steadman HJ, Borum R, et al: Emerging partnerships between mental health and law enforcement. Psychiatr Serv 50(1):99–101, 1999 9890588

Dickerson F, Stallings CR, Origoni AE, et al: Cigarette smoking among persons with schizophrenia or bipolar disorder in routine clinical settings, 1999–2011. Psychiatr Serv 64(1):44–50, 2013 23280457

Dieterich M, Irving CB, Bergman H, et al: Intensive case management for severe mental illness. Cochrane Database Syst Rev 1:CD007906, 2017 28067944

Dixon LB, Dickerson F, Bellack AS, et al; Schizophrenia Patient Outcomes Research Team (PORT): The 2009 Schizophrenia PORT psychosocial treatment recommendations and summary statements. Schizophr Bull 36(1):48–70, 2010 19955389

Dixon LB, Goldman HH, Bennett ME, et al: Implementing coordinated specialty care for early psychosis: the RAISE Connection Program. Psychiatr Serv 66(7):691–698, 2015 25772764

Dixon LB, Holoshitz Y, Nossel I: Treatment engagement of individuals experiencing mental illness: review and update. World Psychiatry 15(1):13–20, 2016 26833597

Drake RE, McHugo GJ, Clark RE, et al: Assertive community treatment for patients with co-occurring severe mental illness and substance use disorder: a clinical trial. Am J Orthopsychiatry 68(2):201–215, 1998 9589759

Drake RE, Mueser KT, Torrey WC, et al: Evidence-based treatment of schizophrenia. Curr Psychiatry Rep 2(5):393–397, 2000 11122986

Drake RE, Essock SM, Shaner A, et al: Implementing dual diagnosis services for clients with severe mental illness. Psychiatr Serv 52(4):469–476, 2001 11274491

Drake RE, O'Neal EL, Wallach MA: A systematic review of psychosocial research on psychosocial interventions for people with co-occurring severe mental and substance use disorders. J Subst Abuse Treat 34(1):123–138, 2008 17574803

Drukker M, van Os J, Sytema S, et al: Function Assertive Community Treatment (FACT) and psychiatric service use in patients diagnosed with severe mental illness. Epidemiol Psychiatr Sci 20(3):273–278, 2011 21922970

Drukker M, Laan W, Dreef F, et al: Can assertive community treatment remedy patients dropping out of treatment due to fragmented services? Community Ment Health J 50(4):454–459, 2014 24178633

Dupont R, Cochran S: Police response to mental health emergencies—barriers to change. J Am Acad Psychiatry Law 28(3):338–344, 2000 11055533

Essock SM, Frisman LK, Kontos NJ: Cost-effectiveness of assertive community treatment teams. Am J Orthopsychiatry 68(2):179–190, 1998 9589757

Essock SM, Mueser KT, Drake RE, et al: Comparison of ACT and standard case management for delivering integrated treatment for co-occurring disorders. Psychiatr Serv 57(2):185–196, 2006 16452695

Fries HP, Rosen MI: The efficacy of assertive community treatment to treat substance use. J Am Psychiatr Nurses Assoc 17(1):45–50, 2011 21532920

Green AI, Drake RE, Brunette MF, et al: Schizophrenia and co-occurring substance use disorder. Am J Psychiatry 164(3):402–408, 2007 17329463

Hails J, Borum R: Police training and specialized approaches to respond to people with mental illnesses. Crime Delinq 49:52–61, 2003

Hastrup LH, Aagaard J: Costs and outcome of assertive community treatment (ACT) in a rural area in Denmark: 4-year register-based follow-up. Nord J Psychiatry 69(2):110–117, 2015 25131794

Hellerstein DJ, Rosenthal RN, Miner CR: A prospective study of integrated outpatient treatment for substance-abusing schizophrenic patients. Am J Addict 4(1):33–42, 1995

Herman DB, Mandiberg JM: Critical time intervention: model description and implications for the significance of timing in social work interventions. Res Soc Work Pract 20(5):502–508, 2010

Herman DB, Conover S, Gorroochurn P, et al: Randomized trial of critical time intervention to prevent homelessness after hospital discharge. Psychiatr Serv 62(7):713–719, 2011 21724782

Herman SE, BootsMiller B, Jordan L, et al: Immediate outcomes of substance use treatment within a state psychiatric hospital. J Ment Health Adm 24(2):126–138, 1997 9110517

Herman SE, Frank KA, Mowbray CT, et al: Longitudinal effects of integrated treatment on alcohol use for persons with serious mental illness and substance use disorders. J Behav Health Serv Res 27(3):286–302, 2000 10932442

Horvitz-Lennon M, Normand SL, Gaccione P, et al: Partial versus full hospitalization for adults in psychiatric distress: a systematic review of the published literature (1957–1997). Am J Psychiatry 158(5):676–685, 2001 11329384

Hoult J, Rosen A, Reynolds I: Community orientated treatment compared to psychiatric hospital orientated treatment. Soc Sci Med 18(11):1005–1010, 1984 6740335

Hunt GE, Siegfried N, Morley K, et al: Psychosocial interventions for people with both severe mental illness and substance misuse. Schizophr Bull 40(1):18–20, 2014 24179148

Kane JM, Robinson DG, Schooler NR, et al: Comprehensive versus usual community care for first-episode psychosis: 2-year outcomes from the NIMH RAISE Early Treatment Program. Am J Psychiatry 173(4):362–372, 2016 26481174

Kasprow WJ, Rosenheck RA: Outcomes of critical time intervention case management of homeless veterans after psychiatric hospitalization. Psychiatr Serv 58(7):929–935, 2007 17602008

Khawaja IS, Westermeyer JJ: Providing crisis-oriented and recovery-based treatment in partial hospitalization programs. Psychiatry (Edgmont Pa) 7(2):28–31, 2010 20376273

Killaspy H, Bebbington P, Blizard R, et al: The REACT study: randomised evaluation of assertive community treatment in north London. BMJ 332(7545):815–820, 2006 16543298

Kirk I, Leiknes KA, Laru L, et al: Dual Diagnoses—Severe Mental Illness and Substance Use Disorder. Part 2—Effect of Psychosocial Interventions. Report from Norwegian Knowledge Centre for the Health Services (NOKC) No 25-2008. Oslo, Knowledge Centre for the Health Services at The Norwegian Institute of Public Health, 2008

Kreyenbuhl J, Nossel IR, Dixon LB: Disengagement from mental health treatment among individuals with schizophrenia and strategies for facilitating connections to care: a review of the literature. Schizophr Bull 35(4):696–703, 2009 19491314

Lamb HR, Weinberger LE, DeCuir WJ Jr: The police and mental health. Psychiatr Serv 53(10):1266–1271, 2002 12364674

Latimer EA: Economic impacts of assertive community treatment: a review of the literature. Can J Psychiatry 44(5):443–454, 1999 10389605

Latimer E: Economic considerations associated with assertive community treatment and supported employment for people with severe mental illness. J Psychiatry Neurosci 30(5):355–359, 2005 16151541

Lehman AF, Dixon LB, Kernan E, et al: A randomized trial of assertive community treatment for homeless persons with severe mental illness. Arch Gen Psychiatry 54(11):1038–1043, 1997 9366661

Lipton FR, Siegel C, Hannigan A, et al: Tenure in supportive housing for homeless persons with severe mental illness. Psychiatr Serv 51(4):479–486, 2000 10737823

Mangrum LF, Spence RT, Lopez M: Integrated versus parallel treatment of co-occurring psychiatric and substance use disorders. J Subst Abuse Treat 30(1):79–84, 2006 16377455

Manseau M, Bogenschutz M: Substance use disorders and schizophrenia. Focus 14(3):333–342, 2016

Marquant T, Sabbe B, Van Nuffel M, et al: Forensic assertive community treatment: a review of the literature. Community Ment Health J 52(8):873–881, 2016 27422650

Marshall M, Crowther R, Almaraz-Serrano A, et al: Systematic reviews of the effectiveness of day care for people with severe mental disorders: (1) acute day hospital versus admission; (2) vocational rehabilitation; (3) day hospital versus outpatient care. Health Technol Assess 5(21):1–75, 2001 11532238

Marshall M, Lewis S, Lockwood A, et al: Association between duration of untreated psychosis and outcome in cohorts of first-episode patients: a systematic review. Arch Gen Psychiatry 62(9):975–983, 2005 16143729

McGrew JH, Bond GR, Dietzen L, et al: Measuring the fidelity of implementation of a mental health program model. J Consult Clin Psychol 62(4):670–678, 1994 7962870

McHugo GJ, Drake RE, Teague GB, et al: Fidelity to assertive community treatment and client outcomes in the New Hampshire dual disorders study. Psychiatr Serv 50(6):818–824, 1999 10375153

Morrissey JP, Domino ME, Cuddeback GS: Assessing the effectiveness of recovery-oriented ACT in reducing state psychiatric hospital use. Psychiatr Serv 64(4):303–311, 2013 23242485

Morse GA, Calsyn RJ, Dean Klinkenberg W, et al: Treating homeless clients with severe mental illness and substance use disorders: costs and outcomes. Community Ment Health J 42(4):377–404, 2006 16897413

Mueser KT, Bond GR, Drake RE, et al: Models of community care for severe mental illness: a review of research on case management. Schizophr Bull 24(1):37–74, 1998 9502546

Mueser KT, Deavers F, Penn DL, et al: Psychosocial treatments for schizophrenia. Annu Rev Clin Psychol 9:465–497, 2013 23330939

Munetz MR, Griffin PA: Use of the Sequential Intercept Model as an approach to decriminalization of people with serious mental illness. Psychiatr Serv 57(4):544–549, 2006 16603751

Myers NA, Alolayan Y, Smith K, et al: A potential role for family members in mental health care delivery: the family community navigation specialist. Psychiatr Serv 66(6):653–655, 2015 25828874

Myers NA, Smith K, Pope A, et al: A mixed-methods study of the recovery concept, "a meaningful day," in community mental health services for individuals with serious mental illnesses. Community Ment Health J 52(7):747–756, 2016 26659600

Nelson G, Aubry T, Lafrance A: A review of the literature on the effectiveness of housing and support, assertive community treatment, and intensive case management interventions for persons with mental illness who have been homeless. Am J Orthopsychiatry 77(3):350–361, 2007 17696663

Odlaug BL, Gual A, DeCourcy J, et al: Alcohol dependence, co-occurring conditions and attributable burden. Alcohol Alcohol 51(2):201–209, 2016 26246514

Olfson M: Assertive community treatment: an evaluation of the experimental evidence. Hosp Community Psychiatry 41(6):634–641, discussion 649–651, 1990 2193868

Oliva JR, Compton MT: A statewide Crisis Intervention Team (CIT) initiative: evolution of the Georgia CIT program. J Am Acad Psychiatry Law 36(1):38–46, 2008 18354122

Perkins DO, Gu H, Boteva K, et al: Relationship between duration of untreated psychosis and outcome in first-episode schizophrenia: a critical review and meta-analysis. Am J Psychiatry 162(10):1785–1804, 2005 16199825

Regier DA, Farmer ME, Rae DS, et al: Comorbidity of mental disorders with alcohol and other drug abuse: results from the Epidemiologic Catchment Area (ECA) study. JAMA 264(19):2511–2518, 1990 2232018

Rosenheck R, Neale M, Leaf P, et al: Multisite experimental cost study of intensive psychiatric community care. Schizophr Bull 21(1):129–140, 1995 7770734

Schulte MT, Hser YI: Substance use and associated health conditions throughout the lifespan. Public Health Rev 35(2), 2014 28366975

Scott JE, Dixon LB: Assertive community treatment and case management for schizophrenia. Schizophr Bull 21(4):657–668, 1995 8749892

Selzer JA, Lieberman JA: Schizophrenia and substance abuse. Psychiatr Clin North Am 16(2):401–412, 1993 8332568

Soyka M, Albus M, Kathmann N, et al: Prevalence of alcohol and drug abuse in schizophrenic inpatients. Eur Arch Psychiatry Clin Neurosci 242(6):362–372, 1993 8323987

Steadman HJ, Deane MW, Borum R, et al: Comparing outcomes of major models of police responses to mental health emergencies. Psychiatr Serv 51(5):645–649, 2000 10783184

Stein LI, Test MA: Alternative to mental hospital treatment, I: conceptual model, treatment program, and clinical evaluation. Arch Gen Psychiatry 37(4):392–397, 1980 7362425

Stobbe J, Wierdsma AI, Kok RM, et al: The effectiveness of assertive community treatment for elderly patients with severe mental illness: a randomized controlled trial. BMC Psychiatry 14:42, 2014 24528604

Substance Abuse and Mental Health Services Administration: Key Substance Use and Mental Health Indicators in the United States: Results From the 2016 National Survey on Drug Use and Health (HHS Publ No SMA 17-5044, NSDUH Series H-52). Center for Behavioral Health Statistics and Quality, 2017. Available at: https://www.samhsa.gov/data/sites/default/files/NSDUH-FFR1-2016/NSDUH-FFR1-2016.htm. Accessed May 31, 2019.

Susser E, Valencia E, Conover S, et al: Preventing recurrent homelessness among mentally ill men: a "critical time" intervention after discharge from a shelter. Am J Public Health 87(2):256–262, 1997 9103106

Swofford CD, Scheller-Gilkey G, Miller AH, et al: Double jeopardy: schizophrenia and substance use. Am J Drug Alcohol Abuse 26(3):343–353, 2000 10976661

Sytema S, Wunderink L, Bloemers W, et al: Assertive community treatment in the Netherlands: a randomized controlled trial. Acta Psychiatr Scand 116(2):105–112, 2007 17650271

Talamo A, Centorrino F, Tondo L, et al: Comorbid substance-use in schizophrenia: relation to positive and negative symptoms. Schizophr Res 86(1–3):251–255, 2006 16750347

Test MA, Stein LI: Alternative to mental hospital treatment, III: social cost. Arch Gen Psychiatry 37(4):409–412, 1980 7362426

Tomita A, Herman DB: The impact of critical time intervention in reducing psychiatric rehospitalization after hospital discharge. Psychiatr Serv 63(9):935–937, 2012 22810163

Valencia E, Susser E, McQuiston H: Critical time points in the clinical care of homeless mentally ill individuals, in Practicing Psychiatry in the Community: A Manual. Edited by Vaccaro J, Clark G. Washington, DC, American Psychiatric Press, 1996, pp 259–276

Vanderlip ER, Henwood BF, Hrouda DR, et al: Systematic literature review of general health care interventions within programs of assertive community treatment. Psychiatr Serv 68(3):218–224, 2017 27903142

Weisbrod BA, Test MA, Stein LI: Alternative to mental hospital treatment, II: economic benefit-cost analysis. Arch Gen Psychiatry 37(4):400–405, 1980 6767462

White C, Frimpong E, Huz S, et al: Effects of the Personalized Recovery Oriented Services (PROS) program on hospitalizations. Psychiatr Q 89(2):261–271, 2018 28971347

Wright-Berryman JL, McGuire AB, Salyers MP: A review of consumer-provided services on assertive community treatment and intensive case management teams: implications for future research and practice. J Am Psychiatr Nurses Assoc 17(1):37–44, 2011 21659293

CHAPTER 12

Person- and Family-Centered Care

Nev Jones, Ph.D.
Lisa B. Dixon, M.D., M.P.H.

Patient- and *family-centered care* is one of a handful of aspirational service constructs that have entered the psychiatry lexicon over the past few decades. Unfortunately, as with other trendy buzzwords, it is not always clear what this term actually means in the context of real-world psychiatric services. Rather than getting stuck on high-level or abstract principles and values, our goal in this chapter is to draw attention to important nuances and distinctions, explore tensions and areas of controversy, and concretize patient- and family-centered practices. Throughout, we emphasize the importance of ongoing critical reflection on the provider's personal interactions and practices and their effects and implications with respect to service users and family members—a process for which no amount of knowledge or education can substitute.

Principles, Values, and Best Practices

The Institute of Medicine (now part of the National Academies of Sciences, Engineering, and Medicine) defined *patient-centered care* (PCC) as "care that is respectful of, and responsive to, individual patient preferences, needs and values, and ensur[es] that patient values guide all clinical decisions" (Institute of Medicine 2001, p. 40). In a complementary way, Gerteis et al. (1993), early health architects of patient-centered practice, defined PCC as "an approach that consciously adopts the patient's perspective as to what matters" (p. 5). *Family-centered care* (FCC) is simply the family analogue of PCC and is arguably particularly important—and also challenging—in the context of schizophrenia. In place of the more traditional emphasis on top-down decision making, with the provider positioned as the expert and the patient as the beneficiary of that expertise, PCC seeks to promote meaningful dialogue and discussion

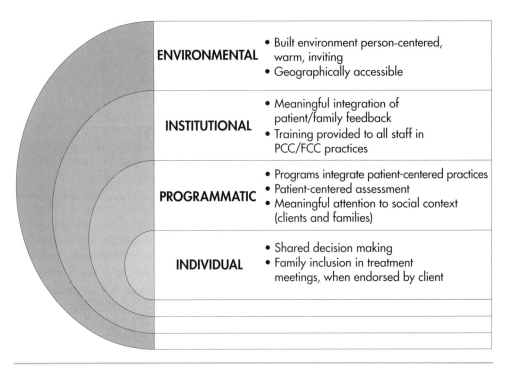

FIGURE 12–1. Levels of patient- and family-centered care.

FCC=family-centered care; PCC=patient-centered care.

and to recenter patient values, perspectives, and preferences, including views that may clash with those of a given provider (Barry and Edgman-Levitan 2012; Rudnick and Roe 2011). Listening to individual patient and family views is a critical component of PCC, as is the cultivation of greater sensitivity to, attunement to, and empathy for the patient's or family's experience of behavioral health challenges, services, and broader impacts on quality of life.

Although individual or interpersonal skills serve as the foundation for PCC/FCC in most settings, similar principles hold at the level of programs, institutions, and environments (Figure 12–1). At these more macro levels, key considerations extend beyond clinical interactions to patient-centered infrastructure, the systemic integration of specific patient- and family-centered practices, and careful integration of stakeholders' views within ongoing processes and outcomes measurement, quality improvement, and performance monitoring (Epstein et al. 2010).

With PCC and FCC, as is true in many other values-driven areas of psychiatry and medicine, a risk is that abstract or high-level claims—for example, slogans or mission statements claiming patient centeredness—substitute for practices that actually include patients and families (Davidson et al. 2005). The influential Public Participation Spectrum schema of the International Association for Public Participation (IAP2) (International Association for Public Participation 2014; Nabatchi 2012) is one example of a framework that can be helpful in gauging both current and potential stakeholder involvement (Figure 12–2). Across the IAP2 spectrum, key distinctions include level of accountability to stakeholders and the extent to which stakeholders are able to exercise direct power or influence over decision-making processes.

INCREASING IMPACT ON THE DECISION

	INFORM	CONSULT	INVOLVE	COLLABORATE	EMPOWER
PUBLIC PARTICIPATION GOAL	To provide the public with balanced and objective information to assist them in understanding the problem, alternatives, opportunities and/or solutions.	To obtain public feedback on analysis, alternatives and/or decisions.	To work directly with the public throughout the process to ensure that public concerns and aspirations are consistently understood and considered.	To partner with the public in each aspect of the decision including the development of alternatives and the identification of the preferred solution.	To place final decision making in the hands of the public.
PROMISE TO THE PUBLIC	We will keep you informed.	We will keep you informed, listen to and acknowledge concerns and aspirations, and provide feedback on how public input influenced the decision.	We will work with you to ensure that your concerns and aspirations are directly reflected in the alternatives developed and provide feedback on how public input influenced the decision.	We will look to you for advice and innovation in formulating solutions and incorporate your advice and recommendations into the decisions to the maximum extent possible.	We will implement what you decide.

FIGURE 12–2. International Association for Public Participation's (IAP2) Public Participation Spectrum.

Source. Reprinted with permission from International Association for Public Participation: IAP2's Public Participation Spectrum. 2018. © International Association for Public Participation www.iap2.org.

Although the fundamental principles of PCC apply equally across diagnoses, schizophrenia and other psychotic disorders pose some additional challenges. By definition, many psychotic symptoms involve a "break" from reality, and many providers and family members struggle with what they perceive to be a more fundamental "lack of insight" into the nature and impact of symptoms. Empirically, a diagnosis of schizophrenia has been found to significantly heighten the risk of involuntary interventions (Hustoft et al. 2013). Engaging people actively struggling with psychosis in PCC may require providers to grapple even more carefully with assumptions regarding reason and irrationality; patient autonomy and mental capacity and their implications with respect to a patient's sense of self; relationships and dignity; and human rights (see Jones and Shattell 2014). For similar reasons, families can easily find themselves entangled in complex and difficult decisions regarding the treatment of their family member, including when to intervene and how to interact with clinicians with respect to the care of an adult child. There are numerous challenges and no easy answers.

In the following sections, we discuss five specific areas of central concern to PCC: implementing PCC against a historical backdrop of segregation, stigma, and family blame; balancing patient and family needs and goals; shared decision making (SDM); patient-centered design (PCD); and values-based measurement, quality improvement, and performance monitoring. Later in this chapter, we describe specific evidence-based and evidence-informed practices built on the principles of PCC.

Understanding the Historical and Sociopolitical Context of Contemporary Care

The history of psychiatry is fraught with examples of the poor treatment of persons with schizophrenia and their families. For substantial portions of the twentieth century, practices such as frontal lobotomy, hydrotherapy, forced sterilization, and extended institutionalization were common (Braslow 1997). On the family side, the psychoanalytic construct of the "schizophrenogenic mother" held mothers responsible for the onset of schizophrenia in a child, leading to clinical recommendations that required the forcible separation of the minor or adult child from his or her mother and in extreme cases focused treatment not on the affected child but on the mother, who was construed as the true "source" of the problem (Hartwell 1996). Both the consumer/ex-patient movement, on the one hand, and the family advocacy movement, on the other, arose in large part in reaction to these practices, and that legacy continues to color relationships between patients, families, and providers, as well as public discourse (Adame et al. 2017; McLean 1995; Sommer 1990).

More specifically, power relations, as they might manifest in a provider-patient relationship, are also influenced by history and societal context. Effective PCC requires that practitioners remain cognizant of the possibility that not only an individual patient's personal experiences but also larger legacies and contexts have shaped the patient's responses or reactions to a provider. For example, consumers from minority groups with a long historical legacy of discrimination (e.g., African Americans, American Indians in the United States; Dovidio et al. 2008) and those who experienced interventions (e.g., forced sterilization) or conditions of treatment in state institutions that would now be considered a violation of basic human rights may be more likely to bring these legacies to bear on current relationships with providers. Considerable efforts may be required to establish trust and rapport and to validate and acknowledge underlying personal, historical, and sociological contexts and experiences that may be driving a given patient's or family's views of providers, particular treatments, or the mental health system more broadly.

Balancing Patient and Family Needs and Goals

Although "patient- and family-centered care" is often used as a single phrase, the reality is that, depending on circumstances, a patient's and his or her family's needs or views may be at odds with one another (or the trio of provider, patient, and family member might all disagree on key decisions or ways forward; Rowe 2012). Specific evidence-informed interventions related to patient-directed family involvement are discussed in the later section "Evidence-Based and Evidence-Informed Interventions." At this point in the chapter, we want to underscore the cross-cutting importance of attention to sometimes fraught family and patient relationships, as well as both the importance of and challenges in weighing needs and concerns from different perspectives and points of view. In most U.S. states, families can petition the court for guardianship of a seriously disabled family member and/or initiate an involuntary inpatient hold or assisted outpatient treatment order (Testa and West 2010). In other cases, family members may serve as representative payees for the more limited purpose of administering Supplemental Security Income (SSI) or Social Security Disability Insurance (SSDI) (Luchins et al. 2003). In all cases, legal arrangements in which "normative" relationships and adult autonomy are compromised require clinicians to exercise care and sensitivity as they work with both families and patients. In this context, it is also important to keep in the mind the singular challenges that family members often face in navigating treatment decisions for an otherwise independent adult child (or family member) and the importance of providing as much support as possible; see inset that follows for a more extended discussion.

Shared Decision Making

SDM is generally framed as an alternative to older and more paternalistic models of clinical decision making in which providers, on the basis of their expertise, made decisions "for" patients. SDM, in contrast, aspires to be a far more collaborative and dialogic process in which providers contribute information, clinical experience, and knowledge; lay out treatment options; and support and encourage patients to weigh pros and cons and identify preferences that align with their personal values and priorities (Drake et al. 2010; Slade 2017). SDM aligns strongly with the principles of informed consent—namely, that patients be made fully aware of the range of potential risks and benefits associated with a particular treatment and that patients provide explicit, active consent only once these risks are known and considered.

To date, a variety of SDM interventions have been tested for adults with schizophrenia, including interventions that use paper or electronic decision aids and interven-

---

Issues for Consideration

Families confronted with involuntary treatment decisions

Unfortunately, many family members who have a loved one with schizophrenia are likely at some point to find themselves confronted by the perceived need to initiate an involuntary examination (or enlist police support). Although clinicians will inevitably become involved at some stage, family members are often the ones forced to "make the call." For many people, such decisions are heart-wrenching and may lead to significant rifts and tensions, as well as guilt and regret, even when involuntary treatment initiation was or is unavoidable.

Validating and supporting all parties through involuntary treatment decisions and their aftermath are critical for providers. At a minimum, clinicians should validate the ethical uncertainties, conflicted feelings, and sense of guilt that may arise for families and provide as much support as possible in reestablishing a relationship of trust and mutual respect between a family and the loved one.

---

tions aimed at increasing SDM skills among providers and empowerment and activation among service users. Although the quality of trials has varied, with some inconsistent findings, a recent meta-analysis focused on SDM and psychosis found small but significant improvements in patient empowerment and a trend in the direction of reduced longer-term compulsory treatment (Stovell et al. 2016), while a Web-based quasi-experimental study of medication-related SDM found significant increases in adherence for the 12-month period following the intervention (Finnerty et al. 2018). Both inconsistency in SDM strategies and implementation and psychometric limitations of existing measures are hypothesized to have contributed to the variability of SDM trials in mental illness thus far (Perestelo-Perez et al. 2017). In the future, comparative effectiveness research focused on establishing best practices in SDM training, and implementation of these practices will be key to the development of well-operationalized clinical guidelines.

Three major challenges associated with SDM in schizophrenia, unlike in many other areas of physical medicine, are the following: 1) widespread lack of access to evidence-based interventions; 2) the need to adapt SDM approaches for team-based services and nonpharmacological/nonmedical interventions; and 3) the realities of decision making as they play out in the context of involuntary treatment, court-mandated treatment, and assisted outpatient treatment. Beginning with access, the inability to exercise choice due to lack of availability or access to evidence-based interventions can render SDM a hollow exercise (Drake 2017). For team-based service models such as assertive community treatment and coordinated specialty care (both discussed in Chapter 11, "Evidence-Based Models of Service Delivery"), the operationalization of SDM is not always clear. Finally, SDM almost by definition begins to break down when a patient's decision-making capacity or insight is seriously compromised (Meadows 2017), arguably requiring deeper investigation into best practices for the navigation of involuntary treatment and the development of postdischarge interventions explicitly designed to reestablish trust and process the sequelae of the patient's loss of autonomy and associated threats to self-concept and identity. The use of psychiatric advance directives—essentially treatment plans created by patients to guide future treatment in situations in which their capacity becomes impaired—is one potentially promising approach to maximizing patient self-direction and autonomy even during acute crises or episodes when SDM would otherwise break down (Zelle et al. 2015).

Patient-Centered Design

PCD draws on and extends the user-centered design movement as it has developed within the areas of product design, architecture, and urban planning (Douglas and Douglas 2005; Schnall et al. 2016). The core principle of PCD is the development of practices and interventions as well as treatment spaces that, from their inception, integrate and reflect the needs and preferences of end users (patients and families) rather than administrators or providers (Lyon and Koerner 2016). For example, when a new social network or smartphone application is developed on the open market, when user-centered design is standard, the new product undergoes extensive user testing, including the development of "user profiles" intended to maximize designers' engagement with the types of individuals expected to use the product, and ongoing pilot testing and focus groups to improve and refine the product, including its appeal and usability.

In the areas of mHealth and eHealth (i.e., the use of mobile and electronic technologies for health), which have tended to maintain much stronger ties non-technology-related mental health research to conventional tech sector research and development practices, user-centered design (or PCD) is far more common. The principles of PCD, however, can—and likely will—be used in more areas, including inpatient and outpatient clinic architecture and interior design, as well as development of new behavioral health interventions.

Measurement, Quality Improvement, and Performance Monitoring

Across fields, performance monitoring and evaluation are increasingly recognized as essential to quality assurance as well as quality improvement. To strengthen a program, program leaders and staff must understand, as objectively as possible, what is actually going on—for example, the extent to which patients and families are actually engaging with a given service, the program's impact on key outcomes, and patient satisfaction (Boswell et al. 2015). One key component of more patient-centered evaluation and quality improvement is the integration of patient-centered and/or patient-selected outcomes (Reininghaus and Priebe 2012). Whereas clinicians and administrators might prioritize change in symptomatology, patients might find the measure of functional recovery or community involvement a more important metric for adjudicating the relative success of a service program (Crawford et al. 2011; Thornicroft and Slade 2014).

Evidence-Based and Evidence-Informed Interventions

Peer Support and Peer-Led Interventions

Peer Support

In a seminal early paper, Solomon (2004) defined *peer support* as "social emotional support, frequently coupled with instrumental support, that is mutually offered or provided by persons having a mental health condition to others sharing a similar mental health condition to bring about a desired social or personal change" (p. 393). Peer support may occur between two individuals or within a group, but regardless of setting, the peer practice community has overwhelmingly endorsed the core operating principles of mutuality and reciprocity, the minimization or (ideally) elimination of the tacit power hierarchies conventionally found in provider-recipient relationships, free choice (freedom from coercion), and a commitment to "meeting people where they are" in terms of their needs, preferences, or ways of understanding or navigating behavioral health–related challenges (International Association for Public Participation 2014; Mead et al. 2001). Peer support nurtures a sense of belonging and/or community through shared experiences, but it also facilitates the exchange of experiential knowledge regarding such issues as treatment, systems navigation, and emotional healing. Peer specialists or group facilitators may also serve as role models for patients in their recovery journeys and serve as "living proof" that recovery is possible (Swarbrick and Brice 2006).

Peer Specialists

In the contemporary service landscape, "peer support roles" need to be distinguished from "peer support" in a strict sense. The Substance Abuse and Mental Health Services Administration (2019) defines *peer specialist* (or *peer provider*) as a person "who uses his or her lived experience of recovery from mental illness and/or addiction, plus skills learned in formal training, to deliver services in behavioral health settings." In practice, peer specialists may be responsible for a wide variety of activities and functions, including community outreach, case management, vocational support, organizational planning, and quality improvement, provider training, and evaluation (Salzer et al. 2010). The hope or expectation is that peer staff, across these diverse roles, will serve more instrumental functions and contribute to the "normalization" of mental health challenges between and among agency staff, as well as help introduce perspectives grounded in lived experience that might otherwise drop out of conversations regarding policy and practice. Peer specialists may be individuals with experience of mental illness, more narrowly, or persons with a specific set of intersectional experiences and identities (e.g., a member of a sexual minority community who has sought services for self-harm, a survivor of childhood sexual abuse with PTSD). Peer support in the strict sense, in contrast, refers to a mutual and nonhierarchical support *relationship* in which both parties share challenges and receive advice and support from the other (Mead et al. 2001, 2013). In real-world services, peer specialist roles may or may not include explicit provision of peer support, for example, a given position might instead revolve around case management or vocational support.

Early empirical research on peer workers found no decrement in quality or impact for case management performed by peer providers versus traditional case managers (Davidson et al. 2012; Pitt et al. 2013). Positive effects over and above those of non-peer providers have proven more elusive, and although a handful of studies have demonstrated significant additive benefits, both a recent Cochrane review and two independent meta-analyses found overall study quality to be low with significant risk of bias and selective reporting (Fuhr et al. 2014; Lloyd-Evans et al. 2014; Pitt et al. 2013). As the authors of these meta-analyses and other commentators (King and Simmons 2018) have noted, inconsistencies in the roles, responsibilities, and training of peer specialists across research trials, as well as in outcome metrics, limit the generalizability of this body of literature and underscore the importance of careful empirical investigations, including studies aimed at teasing out mechanisms of action.

Semistructured Peer-Led Group Interventions

In addition to peer support and peer specialist interventions, there are also a growing number of semistructured peer-led (or family-led) interventions, including Wellness Recovery Action Planning (WRAP; Cook et al. 2012a; Jonikas et al. 2013), Building Recovery of Individual Dreams and Goals through Education and Support (BRIDGES; Cook et al. 2012b), and Peer to Peer (Lucksted et al. 2009). Unlike completely open topic groups, in which participants can choose their own focus, semi-structured interventions tend to have specific training protocols and in some cases certification pathways for facilitators; a set number of meetings; and ready-to-use materials or a specified curriculum that covers particular topics, such as wellness planning, identifying triggers, or physical health issues. In under-resourced public mental health settings, structured and semistructured interventions therefore offer advantages in terms of ease of implementation, as well as quality assurance. Examples of emerging, peer-led group interventions include economic empowerment (Jiménez-Solomon et al. 2016) and hearing voices groups, in which the explicit focus of the group is on exploring the experience, content, and possible meanings behind the experience of voices or auditory hallucinations (Corstens et al. 2014).

In part because it is easier to study discrete, structured group interventions as opposed to generalist, full-time provider roles spanning different functions, the evidence base for semistructured groups is more robust. RCTs have found significant effects on such outcomes as physical health (Druss et al. 2018), internalized stigma (Mulfinger et al. 2018), personal recovery (Cook et al. 2012a), and quality of life (Cook et al. 2012b).

Focus on the Family

Over the past few decades, a number of family-focused interventions have been developed and tested, including family psychoeducation, multifamily and family-to-family groups, and family partners/navigators as integrated members of treatment programs.

Family Psychoeducation

The majority of family members involved in caring for a loved one with schizophrenia are likely to have never had formal academic or clinical training in serious mental illness, and many will not have basic mental health literacy. Major goals of psychoeducation interventions therefore typically span content regarding symptoms and diagnosis, medications and side effects, psychosocial treatment options, prognosis and recovery, and the links between family and patient well-being. In addition, many psychoeducational interventions provide structured skill building, including problem solving, crisis planning, and systems navigation (for a systematic review, see Lucksted et al. 2012). Group (multifamily) psychoeducational intervention provides the added benefit of mutual support and emotional validation from others with similar experiences.

Although models vary to some degree, overarching empirical support for family psychoeducation is extremely strong (Eassom et al. 2014; Lucksted et al. 2012; Sin and Norman 2013). The 2009 Schizophrenia Patient Outcomes Research Team (PORT) clinical guidelines for schizophrenia recommend that psychoeducational interventions be provided for a minimum duration of 6–9 months and include education, crisis intervention and planning, support, and skills training (Kreyenbuhl et al. 2010). McFarlane's (2002) multifamily groups model, specifically, has been adopted as a core evidence-based practice, and a federally funded toolkit was developed to aid its implementation and dissemination (Substance Abuse and Mental Health Services Administration 2010). Although these existing tools are invaluable, it is worth keeping in mind that as the scientific literature on the epidemiology and underlying mechanisms of psychotic disorders continues to evolve, public-facing educational materials must be regularly updated. The following inset also explores some of the potential complications suggested by a series of recent stigma reviews and meta-analyses; the upshot of which is that, at least when it comes to stigma reduction, a strong emphasis on biogenetic mechanisms may actually have unexpected negative effects on public attitudes, including the perceived dangerousness and permanence of schizophrenia.

Issues for Consideration

Turning to the stigma reduction literature for insights into effective psychoeducation?

Although stigma reduction and family psychoeducation are orthogonal to some extent, the stigma literature may offer important insights into the attitudinal impact of different explanatory frameworks, particularly for psychotic disorders. Stigma-focused systematic reviews and meta-analyses, for example, have consistently found that strongly biogenetic explanations of schizophrenia, but not depression, predict greater desired social distance, perceived permanence, and perceived dangerousness, while nevertheless decreasing blame (Angermeyer et al. 2015; Kvaale et al. 2013; Schomerus et al. 2012). Similarly, categorical models of schizophrenia appear to exacerbate stigma more than continuum models (i.e., models in which mental illness and mental health are described on a continuum; Thibodeau et al. 2018). Conversely, although both educational anti-stigma programs and programs involving contact with patients have been found to weaken negative stereotypes and increase positive attitudes, effect sizes indicate that contact with actual patients has significantly more impact than education alone (Corrigan et al. 2012; Griffiths et al. 2014).

Family-Led Groups

Similar to semistructured peer-led groups, family-led groups significantly improve a variety of outcomes, including caregiver-related coping, empowerment, knowledge, and distress (Dixon et al. 2011; Lucksted et al. 2013; Pickett-Schenk et al. 2008). The most prominent example in the United States is the Family-to-Family program of the National Alliance on Mental Illness (available at www.nami.org/find-support/nami-programs/nami-family-to-family). Family-to-Family is a free, 12-session group psychoeducation program, widely available throughout the United States, that helps bring together family members struggling with similar challenges, to share, find mutual validation, and access information and build skills in such areas as self-care, family advocacy, and local systems navigation. Unlike some professionally led family psychoeducation models (which require the consent of the patient on behalf of a family member), programs like Family-to-Family can be freely accessed without explicit patient consent, and they create avenues for greater family member involvement as Family-to-Family facilitators.

Family Involvement Planning

Given the need to respect the individual autonomy of adults, the potential for tensions between patients and family members, and possible estrangement over time, provider navigation of the involvement of families of adults can be challenging. Many family-focused psychotherapeutic models include strategies for facilitation, mediation, and strengthened communication (e.g., Lobban and Barrowclough 2016); however, family therapy involving adult consumers is often not accessible within real-world mental health systems in the United States. The Recovery-Oriented Decisions for Relatives' Support (or REORDER) intervention is a brief, manualized intervention designed to structure and support patient-led consideration of family involvement in care (Dixon et al. 2014). REORDER involves two phases: the first focuses on structured conversations with patients regarding their goals and preferences for family involvement, and the second focuses on bringing in family members for those patients who have opted for this. A pilot RCT found that the intervention led to 59% of the patient participants scheduling at least one family session, significantly decreased patients' levels of paranoia, and bolstered recovery.

Conclusion

The goal of patient- and family-centered care is to move away from paternalistic, top-down models of services provision and to reorient to the perspectives, goals, and needs of those receiving services and their caregivers. As the implementation science and systems change literature has underscored, meaningful shifts to PCC/FCC must span changes in practice across levels, including individual-focused clinical practices, organizational climate, institutional policies, and the built environment. Likewise, PCC/FCC frameworks stress the integration of patient and family feedback—in policy, planning, and evaluation—as well as direct involvement in the form of paraprofessional family and peer worker roles, as consultants and advisors, and ideally also leaders in practice, program development, and research. An array of patient- and family-centered interventions have been rigorously evaluated and found to be effective. Emerging, innovative practices promise to further bolster the potential transformative impact of work in this area.

References

Adame AL, Bassman R, Morsey M, et al: A brief history of the psychiatric survivor movement, in Exploring Identities of Psychiatric Survivor Therapists: Beyond Us and Them. London, Palgrave Macmillan, 2017, pp 33–53

Angermeyer MC, Daubmann A, Wegscheider K, et al: The relationship between biogenetic attributions and desire for social distance from persons with schizophrenia and major depression revisited. Epidemiol Psychiatr Sci 24(4):335–341, 2015 24786227

Barry MJ, Edgman-Levitan S: Shared decision making—pinnacle of patient-centered care. N Engl J Med 366(9):780–781, 2012 22375967

Boswell JF, Kraus DR, Miller SD, et al: Implementing routine outcome monitoring in clinical practice: benefits, challenges, and solutions. Psychother Res 25(1):6–19, 2015 23885809

Braslow J: Mental Ills and Bodily Cures: Psychiatric Treatment in the First Half of the Twentieth Century. Berkeley, University of California Press, 1997

Cook JA, Copeland ME, Floyd CB, et al: A randomized controlled trial of effects of Wellness Recovery Action Planning on depression, anxiety, and recovery. Psychiatr Serv 63(6):541–547, 2012a 22508435

Cook JA, Steigman P, Pickett S, et al: Randomized controlled trial of peer-led recovery education using Building Recovery of Individual Dreams and Goals through Education and Support (BRIDGES). Schizophr Res 136(1–3):36–42, 2012b 22130108

Corrigan PW, Morris SB, Michaels PJ, et al: Challenging the public stigma of mental illness: a meta-analysis of outcome studies. Psychiatr Serv 63(10):963–973, 2012 23032675

Corstens D, Longden E, McCarthy-Jones S, et al: Emerging perspectives from the hearing voices movement: implications for research and practice. Schizophr Bull 40 (suppl 4):S285–S294, 2014 24936088

Crawford MJ, Robotham D, Thana L, et al: Selecting outcome measures in mental health: the views of service users. J Ment Health 20(4):336–346, 2011 21770782

Davidson L, O'Connell MJ, Tondora J, et al: Recovery in serious mental illness: a new wine or just a new bottle? Prof Psychol Res Pr 6:480–486, 2005

Davidson L, Bellamy C, Guy K, et al: Peer support among persons with severe mental illnesses: a review of evidence and experience. World Psychiatry 11(2):123–128, 2012 22654945

Dixon LB, Lucksted A, Medoff DR, et al: Outcomes of a randomized study of a peer-taught Family to-Family Education Program for mental illness. Psychiatr Serv 62(6):591–597, 2011 21632725

Dixon LB, Glynn SM, Cohen AN, et al: Outcomes of a brief program, REORDER, to promote consumer recovery and family involvement in care. Psychiatr Serv 65(1):116–120, 2014 24177229

Douglas CH, Douglas MR: Patient-centred improvements in health care-built environments: perspectives and design indicators. Health Expect 8(3):264–276, 2005 16098156

Dovidio JF, Penner LA, Albrecht TL, et al: Disparities and distrust: the implications of psychological processes for understanding racial disparities in health and health care. Soc Sci Med 67(3):478–486, 2008 18508171

Drake RE: Mental health shared decision making in the U.S. World Psychiatry 16(2):161–162, 2017 28498589

Drake RE, Deegan PE, Rapp C: The promise of shared decision making in mental health. Psychiatr Rehabil J 34(1):7–13, 2010 20615839

Druss BG, Singh M, von Esenwein SA, et al: Peer-led self-management of general medical conditions for patients with serious mental illnesses: a randomized trial. Psychiatr Serv 69(5):529–535, 2018 29385952

Eassom E, Giacco D, Dirik A, et al: Implementing family involvement in the treatment of patients with psychosis: a systematic review of facilitating and hindering factors. BMJ Open 4(10):e006108, 2014 25280809

Epstein RM, Fiscella K, Lesser CS, et al: Why the nation needs a policy push on patient-centered health care. Health Aff (Millwood) 29(8):1489–1495, 2010 20679652

Finnerty MT, Layman DM, Chen Q, et al: Use of a Web-based shared decision-making program: impact on ongoing treatment engagement and antipsychotic adherence. Psychiatr Serv 69(12):1215–1221, 2018 30286709

Fuhr DC, Salisbury TT, De Silva MJ, et al: Effectiveness of peer-delivered interventions for severe mental illness and depression on clinical and psychosocial outcomes: a systematic review and meta-analysis. Soc Psychiatry Psychiatr Epidemiol 49(11):1691–1702, 2014 24632847

Gerteis M, Edgman-Levitan S, Daley J, et al (eds): Through the Patient's Eyes: Understanding and Promoting Patient-Centered Care. San Francisco, CA, Jossey-Bass, 1993

Griffiths KM, Carron-Arthur B, Parsons A, et al: Effectiveness of programs for reducing the stigma associated with mental disorders: a meta-analysis of randomized controlled trials. World Psychiatry 13(2):161–175, 2014 24890069

Hartwell CE: The schizophrenogenic mother concept in American psychiatry. Psychiatry 59(3):274–297, 1996 8912946

Hustoft K, Larsen TK, Auestad B, et al: Predictors of involuntary hospitalizations to acute psychiatry. Int J Law Psychiatry 36(2):136–143, 2013 23395506

Institute of Medicine, Committee on Quality of Health Care in America: Crossing the Quality Chasm: A New Health System for the 21st Century. Washington, DC, National Academy Press, 2001

International Association for Public Participation: IAP2 Public Participation Spectrum. International Association for Public Participation, 2014. Available at: https://cdn.ymaws.com/www.iap2.org/resource/resmgr/pillars/Spectrum_8.5x11_Print.pdf. Accessed October 2019.

Jiménez-Solomon OG, Méndez-Bustos P, Swarbrick, M, et al: Peer-supported economic empowerment: A financial wellness intervention framework for people with psychiatric disabilities. Psychiatr Rehabil J 39(3), 222–233, 2016 27618459

Jones N, Shattell M: Beyond easy answers: facing the entanglements of violence and psychosis. Issues Ment Health Nurs 35(10):809–811, 2014 25259645

Jonikas JA, Grey DD, Copeland ME, et al: Improving propensity for patient self-advocacy through wellness recovery action planning: results of a randomized controlled trial. Community Ment Health J 49(3):260–269, 2013 22167660

King AJ, Simmons MB: A systematic review of the attributes and outcomes of peer work and guidelines for reporting studies of peer interventions. Psychiatr Serv 69(9):961–977, 2018 29962310

Kreyenbuhl J, Buchanan RW, Dickerson FB, et al; Schizophrenia Patient Outcomes Research Team (PORT): The Schizophrenia Patient Outcomes Research Team (PORT): updated treatment recommendations 2009. Schizophr Bull 36(1):94–103, 2010 19955388

Kvaale EP, Gottdiener WH, Haslam N: Biogenetic explanations and stigma: a meta-analytic review of associations among laypeople. Soc Sci Med 96:95–103, 2013 24034956

Lloyd-Evans B, Mayo-Wilson E, Harrison B, et al: A systematic review and meta-analysis of randomised controlled trials of peer support for people with severe mental illness. BMC Psychiatry 14:39–45, 2014 24528545

Lobban F, Barrowclough C: An interpersonal CBT framework for involving relatives in interventions for psychosis: evidence base and clinical implications. Cognit Ther Res 40:198–215, 2016 27069287

Luchins DJ, Roberts DL, Hanrahan P: Representative payeeship and mental illness: a review. Adm Policy Ment Health 30(4):341–353, 2003 12870559

Lucksted A, McNulty K, Brayboy L, et al: Initial evaluation of the Peer-to-Peer program. Psychiatr Serv 60(2):250–253, 2009 19176421

Lucksted A, McFarlane W, Downing D, et al: Recent developments in family psychoeducation as an evidence-based practice. J Marital Fam Ther 38(1):101–121, 2012 22283383

Lucksted A, Medoff D, Burland J, et al: Sustained outcomes of a peer-taught family education program on mental illness. Acta Psychiatr Scand 127(4):279–286, 2013 22804103

Lyon AR, Koerner K: User-centered design for psychosocial intervention development and implementation. Clin Psychol (New York) 23(2):180–200, 2016 29456295

McFarlane WR: Multifamily Groups in the Treatment of Severe Psychiatric Disorders. New York, Guilford Press, 2002

McLean A: Empowerment and the psychiatric consumer/ex-patient movement in the United States: contradictions, crisis and change. Soc Sci Med 40(8):1053–1071, 1995 7597459

Mead S, Hilton D, Curtis L: Peer support: a theoretical perspective. Psychiatr Rehabil J 25(2):134–141, 2001 11769979

Mead S, Kuno E, Knutson S: Intentional peer support [in Spanish]. Vertex 24(112):426–433, 2013 24511559

Meadows G: Shared decision making: a consideration of historical and political contexts. World Psychiatry 16(2):154–155, 2017 28498601

Mulfinger N, Müller S, Böge I, et al: Honest, Open, Proud for adolescents with mental illness: pilot randomized controlled trial. J Child Psychol Psychiatry 59(6):684–691, 2018 29205343

Nabatchi T: Putting the "public" back in public values research: designing participation to identify and respond to values. Public Adm Rev 72(5):699–708, 2012

Perestelo-Perez L, Rivero-Santana A, Alvarez-Perez Y, et al: Measurement issues of shared decision making in mental health: challenges and opportunities. Mental Health Review Journal 22(1):214–232, 2017

Pickett-Schenk SA, Lippincott RC, Bennett C, et al: Improving knowledge about mental illness through family led education: the Journey of Hope. Psychiatr Serv 59(1):49–56, 2008 18182539

Pitt V, Lowe D, Hill S, et al: Consumer-providers of care for adult clients of statutory mental health services. Cochrane Database Syst Rev (3):CD004807, 2013 23543537

Reininghaus U, Priebe S: Measuring patient-reported outcomes in psychosis: conceptual and methodological review. Br J Psychiatry 201(4):262–267, 2012 23028084

Rowe J: Great expectations: a systematic review of the literature on the role of family carers in severe mental illness, and their relationships and engagement with professionals. J Psychiatr Ment Health Nurs 19(1):70–82, 2012 22070436

Rudnick AE, Roe DE: Serious Mental Illness: Person-Centered Approaches. London, Radcliffe Press, 2011

Salzer MS, Schwenk E, Brusilovskiy E: Certified peer specialist roles and activities: results from a national survey. Psychiatr Serv 61(5):520–523, 2010 20439376

Schnall R, Rojas M, Bakken S, et al: A user-centered model for designing consumer mobile health (mHealth) applications (apps). J Biomed Inform 60:243–251, 2016 26903153

Schomerus G, Schwahn C, Holzinger A, et al: Evolution of public attitudes about mental illness: a systematic review and meta-analysis. Acta Psychiatr Scand 125(6):440–452, 2012 22242976

Sin J, Norman I: Psychoeducational interventions for family members of people with schizophrenia: a mixed-method systematic review. J Clin Psychiatry 74(12):e1145–e1162, 2013 24434103

Slade M: Implementing shared decision making in routine mental health care. World Psychiatry 16(2):146–153, 2017 28498575

Solomon P: Peer support/peer provided services underlying processes, benefits, and critical ingredients. Psychiatr Rehabil J 27(4):392–401, 2004 15222150

Sommer R: Family advocacy and the mental health system: the recent rise of the alliance for the mentally ill. Psychiatr Q 61(3):205–221, 1990 2075224

Stovell D, Morrison AP, Panayiotou M, Hutton P: Shared treatment decision-making and empowerment-related outcomes in psychosis: systematic review and meta-analysis. B J Psychiatry 209(1):23–28., 2016 27198483

Substance Abuse and Mental Health Services Administration: Family Psychoeducation Evidence-Based Practices (EBP) Kit (Publ No SMA09-4423). Rockville, MD, Substance Abuse and Mental Health Services Administration, March 2010. Available at: https://store.samhsa.gov/product/Family-Psychoeducation-Evidence-Based-Practices-EBP-KIT/sma09-4423. Accessed September 2019.

Substance Abuse and Mental Health Services Administration: Making Integrated Care Work. Rockville, MD, Substance Abuse and Mental Health Services Administration and Health Resources and Services Administration. Available at: www.integration.samhsa.gov/workforce/team-members/peer-providers#who are peer providers. Accessed September 2019.

Swarbrick M, Brice GH Jr: Sharing the message of hope, wellness, and recovery with consumers psychiatric hospitals. Am J Psychiatr Rehabil 9:101–109, 2006

Testa M, West SG: Civil commitment in the United States. Psychiatry (Edgmont Pa) 7(10):30–40, 2010 22778709

Thibodeau R, Shanks LN, Smith BP: Do continuum beliefs reduce schizophrenia stigma? Effects of a laboratory intervention on behavioral and self-reported stigma. J Behav Ther Exp Psychiatry 58:29-35, 2018 28803131

Thornicroft G, Slade M: New trends in assessing the outcomes of mental health interventions. World Psychiatry 13(2):118–124, 2014 24890055

Zelle H, Kemp K, Bonnie RJ: Advance directives in mental health care: evidence, challenges and promise. World Psychiatry 14(3):278–280, 2015 26407773

Index

Page numbers printed in **boldface type** refer to tables or figures.

Abnormal Involuntary Movement Scale (AIMS), 161
Acamprosate, 211
ACC. *See* Anterior cingulate cortex
Acculturative stress, 56, 114
N-acetylcysteine (NAC), 170–171
ACT (assertive community treatment), 251, 252–256, **253**, 262
Active-phase syndrome, 44–45
Adherence to treatment, 27, 48, 166, 217
Adolescents
    age at onset, 4, 13–14, 35
    cannabis use by, 27, **89**, 91, 118
    cognitive impairment and, 13, 118–119
    diagnostic criteria for, 35
    pathophysiology of schizophrenia in, 86, 94–95, 118–119, 131–132
    psychosocial stressors as risk factor for, 6–7, 117, **119**
Adoption studies, 81
Affective flattening (diminished emotional expression), 40, 42, 149, 218
African Americans
    depressive symptoms among, 217
    quality of mental health care for, 63, 276–277
    schizophrenia prevalence, 62–63
    symptom manifestation, 61
Age. *See* Adolescents; Children; Geriatric patients; Onset; Paternal age
Aggressive behavior (hostility), 149, 153, 158, 168–169, 170
Agitation, 48, 211
Agranulocytosis, 150–151, 153, 167, 170
AIMS (Abnormal Involuntary Movement Scale), 161
Akathisia, 158–159
    antipsychotics with risk of, 156, 157, 161
    defined, 150, 158

differential diagnosis, 220
    management of, 158–159
    monitoring for, 158
    suicidal behavior and, 158
Akinesia, 218
AKT1 (AKT serine/threonine kinase 1 gene), **89**, 91
Alcohol use. *See* Substance use disorders
Alogia, 40, 42, 149, 218
α-Amino-3-hydroxy-5-methyl-4-isoxazolepropionic acid (AMPA) receptors, 92
American Psychiatric Association, 67, 164
Amisulpride, 160, 163, 164–165
Amotivation, 41, 42, 218
Anandamide, 112–113
Anergia, 218
Anhedonia, 40–41, 47, 149, 218
Anterior cingulate cortex (ACC)
    dopamine system and, 135
    neuronal distribution in, 129
    neuronal somal size in, 131
    pathophysiology of, 42, **115**, 116
Antiadrenergic side effects
    antipsychotics with high risk of, 151, **152**, 153, 155, 156, 157
    antipsychotics with low risk of, **152**, 156
Anticholinergic agents, 158–159
Anticholinergic side effects, 151, **152**, 153, 157
Antidepressants, 169
    as adjunctive treatment, 149, 169
    for cocaine use disorder, 210
    for depressive disorders, **206**, 218–219
    for panic disorder, 221
    for posttraumatic stress disorder management, **206**, 224
    for social phobia, **206**
    for tobacco use disorder, 213
Antiepileptic drugs, 149, 169–170

Anti-inflammatory drugs, 172–173
Antipsychotic medications, 150–168. *See also specific drugs*
  adherence to treatment, 27, 48, 166, 217
  adverse effects of, 47, 151, **152**, 153, 158–163. *See also* Antiadrenergic side effects; Anticholinergic side effects; Cardiovascular effects; Diabetes; Extrapyramidal side effects; Prolactin elevation; Weight gain
  for attenuated psychosis, 14
  breast-feeding precautions, 168
  choice of, 96, 164–165
  for co-occurring disorder management, 209–210, 220, 221, 222–223, 226
  course of schizophrenia with, 20–21
  course of schizophrenia without, 15–17, **19**
  cultural variations in prescribing, 63
  development of, 20–23, 150–151, 157–158
  dosage of, **152**, **154**, 165–166
  end state of schizophrenia with, 21–23, **22**, 24
  end state of schizophrenia without, 15, 17–20, **19**, 23, 24
  for first-episode psychosis, 165, 166, 167
  genetic counseling and, 96
  maintenance treatment and relapse prevention with, 28–29, 163–164, 253–254, 258–260
  mechanism of action, 150, 151
  monitoring of, 161, **161**, 253–254
  overview, 149, 150–151, **152**, **154**
  patient education on, 28–29
  polypharmacy, 165, 218
  potency classification, 151–153
  pregnancy precautions, 168
  prognosis of schizophrenia with, 25–26
  response factors, 167
  route of administration, **154**, 166, 210
  targeted, intermittent therapy with, 164
  for treatment-resistant schizophrenia, 153, 167–168, 218
  treatment targets, 166–167
Anxiety symptoms and disorders, **206**, 220–223
  detection and management of, 221
  management of, 149, 171
  overview, 220–221
  panic attacks and disorders, 221
  prevalence of, 47–48, 220
  in prodromal phase, 14
  psychopathology of, 47–48
  social anxiety disorder, 222–223
Anxiolytics, 149
Apathy, 41, 42, 218
Aripiprazole, **152**, **154**, 156–157
  for cocaine use disorder, 210
  for OCD and OCS management, 226
  prolactin levels and, 163
  weight-gain liability of, 216
Arsenic, 94
Asenapine, **152**, 157
Asians, 56, 62
Asociality, 40, 218
Asphyxia, 88
Assertive community treatment (ACT), 251, 252–256, **253**, 262
Association studies (genetic), 82
Astrocyte-related genes, **107**, 108
Attentional bias, 40
Attenuated psychosis, 14, 36
Auditory hallucinations, 38, 39, 56–57, 173–174
Autoimmune disorders
  depressive symptoms and, 47
  as environmental risk factor, 38, **89–90**, 91–92
Avolition, 40, 149, 218

Basket cells, 132
BDNF (brain-derived neurotrophic factor), 135–136
Beads task, 39–40
Benzodiazepines, 168–169
  for akathisia management, 158–159
  catatonia and, 173
  for neuroleptic malignant syndrome management, 160
  for panic disorder management, 221
  precautions with schizophrenia, 159, 169, 174, 211
Benztropine, 159
ß-Blockers
  for akathisia management, 158–159
  for cardiovascular side effects, 163
Biases
  of clinicians, 60, 62, 70
  delusions and, 39–40
Bipolar depression, 46–47
Bipolar disorder, 45
Birth risk factors, 6–7, 88, **89–90**, 92
Birth weight, 88
Black Caribbeans, 59, 62, 80

Blacks. *See* African Americans; Black Caribbeans

Bleuler, Eugen, 15–16, 20, 21, 28

Bleuler, Manfred, 17–18, 23

Bleuler's scale, 21

Blunted affect, 40, 47

Body/mind control delusions, 37

Bradykinesia, 41, 150

Brain-derived neurotrophic factor (BDNF), 135–136

Breast-feeding, 168

Brexpiprazole, **152**, 157

Brief Social Phobia Scale, 222

Bromocriptine, 159–160

Building Recovery of Individual Dreams and Goals through Education and Support (BRIDGES), 281

Bupropion, 169, 210, 212, 213–214

C4A and *C4B* (complement component 4 genes), 86

Calcium channel genes, **85**, 96, 107, **107**

Calgary Depression Scale for Schizophrenia, 218

Canadian Psychiatric Association, 188

Cannabidiol (CBD), 113

Cannabis use
adolescents and, 27, **89**, 91, 118
as co-occurring substance use disorder, 206, 207, 260. *See also* Substance use disorders
disorganization symptom and, 44
endocannabinoid models on, 113
management of, 209, 211
prevalence of, 49
prognosis and, 27, 49, 113
as risk factor, 8–9, 27, 49, **89**, 91

CAPS (Clinician-Administered PTSD Scale), 223

Carbamazepine, 169–170

Cardiovascular effects, **152**, 162–163
antipsychotics with high risk of, 153, 155, 156, 157
antipsychotics with low risk of, 153, 157
hypotension, 151, 153, 155, 157
management of, 163
monitoring, **161**, 162–163
QT prolongation, 156, 157

Cariprazine, **152**, 157, 210

CASPR2 (contactin-associated protein-like 2) receptors, 92

Catatonia, 45, 160, 173

CATIE (Clinical Antipsychotic Trials of Intervention Effectiveness) study, 50, 151–152

Causes. *See* Etiology

CBD (cannabidiol), 113

CBT. *See* Cognitive-behavioral therapy

CBTp. *See* Cognitive-behavioral therapy for psychosis

CDC42 effector protein (CDC42EP), 130

Celiac disease, 91

Cesarean section (emergency), 88

CFI. *See* DSM-5 Cultural Formulation Interview

Chandelier cells, 132, 133

Children
adoption studies, 81
age at onset, 35–36
birth and place of residence as risk factor, 6–7, 92–93
cognitive symptoms for, 13, 46
conduct problems during childhood, as risk factor, 50
diagnostic criteria for, 35–36
infection and inflammation during childhood, as risk factor, 6, **89–90**, 90–91, **119**
migration status as risk factor, 117, **119**
nutrition as risk factor, 117
pathophysiology of schizophrenia in, 94–95, 111, 117
premorbid phase of schizophrenia and, 13
socioeconomic status as risk factor, 59, 92, **119**
trauma during childhood, as risk factor, 3, 7, **90**, 92, 117, **119**, 223
twin studies, 81

Chlorpromazine, 20, 150, 151, **152**

Chondroitin sulfate proteoglycans (CSPGs), 131

Choreoathetoid movements. *See* Tardive dyskinesia

Circuit models, **106**, 113–117, **115**
for cognitive deficits, 116–117
for negative symptoms, 116
for psychosis, 114–116

CIT (Crisis Intervention Team) mode, 265

Citalopram, 218

Clinical Antipsychotic Trials of Intervention Effectiveness (CATIE) study, 50, 151–152

Clinician-Administered PTSD Scale (CAPS), 223

Clinician bias, 60, 62, 70

Clomipramine, 226

Clonazepam, 160

Clozapine, **152**, 153–155
adverse effects of, 150–151, 153–155, 163, 164, 165, 214
agranulocytosis risk and, 150–151, 153, 167, 170
antidepressants and, 169
contraindications, 165, 167
ECT and, 173
efficacy of, 150–151, 153, 164–165
neuroleptic malignant syndrome incidents and, 160
for OCD and OCS management, 226
for social anxiety disorder management, 222
substance use disorder management, 209–210
suicidal behavior management with, 153, 220
for tardive dyskinesia treatment, 160
for treatment-resistant schizophrenia, 153, 167–168, 218

Clozapine-refractory schizophrenia, 173

Clozapine Risk Evaluation and Mitigation Strategy (REMS) Program, 153

CNS viral infections, 6

Cocaine use disorder, 48–49, 207, 210. *See also* Substance use disorders

Coercion, 61–62

Cognitive-behavioral therapy (CBT), 218–219
for OCS or OCD, 226
for panic disorder management, 221
for posttraumatic stress disorder management, 224
for social anxiety disorder management, 222

Cognitive-behavioral therapy for psychosis (CBTp)
ABC model of, 186
description, 186
goals and treatment principles, 185, 186–187, **187**
illness management and recovery (IMR) and, 196
implications for clinical practice, 188
intervention rationale, 186
research support, 187–188

Cognitive remediation (CR), 188–191
description, 188–189
goals and treatment principles, 185, 187, 189, **190**
implications for clinical practice, 190–191
intervention rationale, 188
research support, 189–190
for social-cognitive deficits, 190

Cognitive Remediation Expert Working Group (CREW), 188–189

Cognitive symptoms
during adolescents, 13, 118–119
dopamine system and, 134
employment and, 193–195
functional outcomes for, 46
OCS and OCD correlations, 225
pathophysiological theories on, 113–114, **115**, 116
pharmacological management of, 149, 167
posttraumatic stress disorder and, 48
in prodromal phase, 14
psychopathology of, 45–46
psychosocial therapies for, 188–190, 191–193
social skills and, 191–193
suicide risk and, 48

Community navigation models, 252, 264

Community support teams (CSTs), 252, 264

Comorbidity. *See* Co-occurring disorders and conditions

Complexin I, 130

Complexin II, 130

COMT (catechol O-methyltransferase), 91

Congenital malformations, 88

Contactin-associated protein-like 2 (CASPR2) receptors, 92

Co-occurring disorders (CODs) and conditions, 46–50, 205–249, **206**
anxiety symptoms and disorders, 46–48, 220–223. *See also* Anxiety symptoms and disorders
depressive symptoms and disorders, 46–47, 217–220. *See also* Depressive symptoms and disorders
management of, 168–173, 209, **209**, 260–262, **262**
obesity, 8, 214–217
obsessive-compulsive disorder, 48, 205, **206**
obsessive-compulsive symptoms and disorder, 224–226

overview, 7–8, 205, **206**, 260–261
posttraumatic stress disorder, 47–48,
    223–224
substance use disorders, 8–9, 49, 206–214.
    See also Substance use disorders
suicidal behavior, 8, 48–49, 219–220. *See
    also* Suicidal behavior
tobacco use disorder, 207, 211–214, 260
violence, 9, 49–50
Coordinated specialty care (CSC), 26, 252,
    258–260, **259**
Copy number variations (CNVs), 83, **84**, 86,
    87, 107
Core symptoms, 37–44
    after first episode, 15, 113, 114, 118
    disorganization, 42–44, 45, 149–150
    negative symptoms, 40–42, 45. *See also*
        Negative symptoms
    positive symptoms, 37–40. *See also*
        Positive symptoms
Cortical gene expression, 107–108, **107**
Cortical interneurons, 86
Course. *See* Natural history
Coxsackie B5, 6
CpG islands, 94–95
CR. *See* Cognitive remediation
Creatine kinase, 159
CREW (Cognitive Remediation Expert
    Working Group), 188–189
Criminal justice collaborations, 252, 264–265
Crisis Intervention Team (CIT) mode, 265
Critical time intervention (CTI), 251–252,
    256–258, **257**
Cross-cultural variations. *See* Cultural
    assessments; Cultural variations
Cross-national variations, 57–58, 60–61
CTI (critical time intervention), 251–252,
    256–258, **257**
Cultural assessments
    about, 63–64
    DSM-5 Cultural Formulation Interview
        (CFI), 63–71, **64–67**, **69**
    importance of, 53–54
    methodological concerns, 57
    patient-centered approaches to, 55
    symptom evaluation, 55–58
Cultural Formulation Interview (CFI). *See*
    DSM-5 Cultural Formulation Interview
Cultural psychiatry, 54–55, 61
Cultural variations, 53–75
    about, 53–54

assessment of, 53–58. *See also* Cultural
    assessments
diagnosis considerations, 57, 60, 61, 62–63
epidemiological estimates and, 57–58
further recommendations, 55, 71
illness manifestations attributed to, 54–55
mental health care delivery and, 61–62, 63
outcomes and, 55–56, 58
as risk factor, 4–5, 59–63. *See also*
        Migration status; Race and ethnicity
symptom evaluation and, 55–58
Culture, defined, 53, 55
Culture, Medicine, and Psychiatry (journal), 55
D-cycloserine, 170
Cytochrome P450 enzymes, 156, 211
Cytomegalovirus, 6, 219

Dantrolene, 160
Day treatment models, 252, 262–263
Deficit syndrome, 40–41
Delusions. *See also specific delusions*
    as active-phase symptom, 45
    as antipsychotic response factor, 167
    defined, 225
    differential diagnosis for, 38
    epidemiology, 37–38
    etiology, 39–40
    management of, 149, 150
    obsessions versus, 225
    pathophysiological theories on, 40, 115
    suicidal behavior and, 219
Dendritic spine density, 86, 91, 129–131
De novo mutations, 86
Dentate gyrus, 115
Depot antipsychotics (LAI antipsychotics),
    154, 166, 210
Depressive symptoms and disorders, **206**,
    217–220
    as antipsychotic side effect, 47
    as co-occurring disorder, 41, 46–47, **206**,
        217–220
    cross-cultural presentation of, 54–55
    detection of, 217–218
    diagnosis criteria for, 46–47
    differential diagnosis, 41, 47, 218
    management of, 169, 173, **206**, 217–220
    OCS and OCD correlations, 224, 225
    overview, 217
    pathophysiological theories on, 217
    prevalence of, 46, 217
    in prodromal phase, 14

Depressive symptoms and disorders
    (*continued*)
    psychopathology of, 46–47
    suicidal behavior and, 47, 48, 217–218,
        219–220
Desipramine, 210
Determinants of Outcome Study, 58
Deutetrabenazine, 160
Developmental risk factors, 117–119
Diabetes
    as antipsychotic medication side effect, 162
    as environmental risk factor, 91–92
    gestational, 88
    management of, 162, 168
    monitoring for, 162, 168
Diagnosis
    for adolescents, 35
    for children, 35–36
    clinician bias and, 60, 62, 70. *See also*
        DSM-5 Cultural Formulation
        Interview
    cultural considerations for, 57, 60, 61,
        62–63
    disorganization symptom and, 44
    DSM-5 criteria for, 35–36, 44–45, 173
    prior to antipsychotic medication era,
        15–16, 18–20
*Diagnostic and Statistical Manual of Mental
    Disorders. See* DSM-IV; DSM-5
Digit Symbol Coding test, 46
Diminished emotional expression (affective
    flattening), 40, 42, 149, 218
Dipeptidyl peptidase-like protein 6 (DPPX)
    receptors, 92
Diphenhydramine, 159
Disorganization, 42–44
    as active-phase symptom, 45
    description, 40, 42–43
    epidemiology, 43–44
    etiology, 43
    functional outcomes, 44
    management of, 149, 150
Disorganized speech, 45
Disorganized thinking (formal thought
    disorder), 43
Disulfiram, 210
Dizziness, 157. *See also* Orthostatic
    hypotension
DNA methylation, 94–95, 108
DNA sequencing studies, 82–83, 94
DOPA decarboxylase, 110

Dopamine D$_2$ receptors
    antipsychotics and, 151, 156, 157, 210
    autoimmune disorders and, 92
    DRD2, 83, **85**, 96, 106, **107**
    obesity and, 215
    pathophysiology of, 108–110, **109**, 134–135
Dopamine D$_3$ receptors, 82, 109–110, 157
Dopamine system
    antipsychotics and, 150, 151
    depressive symptoms and, 47
    negative symptoms and, 42, 116, 134
    neurobiology of, 134–135
    pathophysiological theories on, 114,
        115–116
    positive symptoms and, 40, 115, 134
    risk genes and, 82
    substance use disorders and, 208
Dorsal prefrontal cortex (DPFC), 129, 130,
    131, 134–136
DPPX (dipeptidyl peptidase-like protein 6)
    receptors, 92
Drug-induced parkinsonism, 159
Drugs. *See* Antipsychotic medications;
    specific drugs
Drug use. *See* Cannabis use; Substance use
    disorders
DSM-IV, 54
DSM-5
    on active-phase symptoms, 44–45
    catatonia diagnostic criteria, 173
    on cultural influence, 53
    on cultural risk factors, 5
    on culture, definition of, 53
    on disorganization as symptom, 42–43
    on negative symptoms, 40
    schizophrenia diagnostic criteria, 35–36,
        44–45, 173
    tardive dyskinesia (TD) diagnostic
        criteria, 160
DSM-5 Cultural Formulation Interview
    (CFI), **64–67**, 67–71
    about, 63–64
    design of, 67–68
    domains of, 68–70
    supplementary modules, 68, **69**
    versions of, 68, 70–71
DSM-5 Gender and Cross-Cultural Issues
    Study Group, 67
Dyslipidemia, 151, 162
Dystonias, 158, 159, 161. *See also* Tardive
    dystonia

Early-onset (acute) schizophrenia, 14–15, 44

Early Psychosis Prevention and Intervention Centre (EPPIC) study, **22**, 23

Economic risk factors, 7, 58, 59–61, 68, **90**, 92, **119**

Efference copy system, 39

eHealth, 279

Elderly patients, 128, 160, 161

Electroconvulsive therapy (ECT), 160, 168, 173, 218

Emergency cesarean section, 88

Employment. *See* Supported employment

Endophenotypes, 82

Entorhinal cortex, 114, 129, 133–134, 135

Environmental risk factors, 87–93, **89–90**
  autoimmune disorders, 38, 91–92
  childhood trauma, 3, 7, 92, 117, 223
  epigenetics *versus*, 94
  genetic factors *versus*, 80–82, 87–88, 91, 93, 97
  infections and, 5–6, 88, 90–91, **119**
  malnutrition (maternal), 88, 91
  migration status, 5, 59–61, 93, 117
  obstetric complications, 88, 94, 167
  paternal age, 5, 93
  pathophysiological theories for, **106**, 117–119
  posttraumatic stress disorder and, 47–48, 223
  prenatal stress and exposures, 5–6, 88–90
  prognosis and, 27
  race and ethnicity, 4–5, 59–61, 93
  socioeconomic status and disparities, 7, 58, 59–61, 68, 92
  substance use, 8–9, 27, 91
  urban birth and residence, 6–7, 92

Epidemiology, 3–11
  cross-cultural variations, 56–57
  cross-national variations, 57–58
  descriptive epidemiology, 3–4
  of disorganization, 43–44
  further recommendations, 9
  of negative symptoms, 41
  outcomes, 7–9, 79
  overview, 3, 79–80
  of positive symptoms, 37–38
  risk factors, 4–7. *See also specific risk factors*
  risk factors *versus* risk indicators, 80

Epigenetics, 81, 93–96, 107–108, **107**

EPPIC (Early Psychosis Prevention and Intervention Centre) study, **22**, 23

Errorless learning, 194

Estrogen, 163

Ethnicity. *See* Race and ethnicity

Etiology, 79–104. *See also* Neurobiology; Pathophysiological theories
  cross-cultural variations, 53–75. *See also* Cultural variations
  delusions, 39–40
  disorganization, 43
  environmental risk factors, 87–93, **89–90**. *See also* Environmental risk factors
  epigenetics and, 81, 93–96, 107–108, **107**
  future promises and challenges, 96–97
  future research, 97
  genetic factors, 80–87, 96–97
  hallucinations, 38–39
  for negative symptoms, 42
  for positive symptoms, 38–40

Evidence-based models of service delivery, 251–271, 280–283
  approaches to, 251–252
  assertive community treatment, 252–256, **253**, 262
  community navigation models, 264
  community support teams, 264
  coordinated specialty care, 26, 258–260, **259**
  critical time intervention, 256–258, **257**
  cultural considerations, 61–62, 63
  day treatment models, 262–263
  family-centered, 281–283. *See also* Family-centered care
  further recommendations, 265–266
  integrated dual disorder treatment, 209, **209**, 254, 260–262, **262**
  intensive case management, 263–264
  law enforcement/criminal justice collaborations, 264–265
  partial hospitalization programs, 262–263
  patient-centered, 280–281. *See also* Patient-centered care

Exome sequencing, 82–83

Extrapyramidal side effects (EPS), **152**, 158–161. *See also* Akathisia; Dystonias; Neuroleptic malignant syndrome; Parkinsonism; Tardive dyskinesia; Tardive dystonia
  as antipsychotic response factor, 167
  antipsychotics with high risk of, 151, 153, 157
  antipsychotics with low risk of, 150–151, 155, 156, 157

Extrapyrmidal side effects (EPS) (*continued*)
　depression differential, 218
　monitoring for, 161
　negative symptom resemblance of, 41
　onset of, 158

Familial studies, 80–82, **81**, 207
Family-centered care (FCC), 273–287
　balancing patient and family needs, 277
　defined, 273
　family involvement planning, 283
　family-led groups, 283
　family psychoeducation, 199–200, 281–282
　historical and sociopolitical context of,
　　276–277
　involuntary treatment decisions, 278
　levels of, **274**
　peer support and peer-led interventions,
　　254, 280–283
　performance monitoring and evaluation,
　　279
　principles, values, and best practices for,
　　273–276, **274–275**
　shared decision making (SDM), 277–279
Family psychoeducation, 199–200, 281–282
Family-to-Family program, 283
Famines, 88, **89**, 91
First-episode psychosis (FEP)
　depression and, 217
　mortality risk, 15, 24
　neuropathology of, 128, 134, 136
　obesity and, 214
　overview, 14
　pathophysiological theories on, 15, 113,
　　114, 118
　pharmacological therapies, 165, 166, 167
　prognosis for, 15–20, **19**, 21–23, 25–26, 164
　psychosocial therapies, 187
　service delivery for, 61–62, 63, 251–252,
　　258–260, **259**
　substance use and, 49, 207–208, 209
　symptoms of, 15, 41, 46, 217
First-rank symptoms, 37
Fluoxetine, 226
Fluphenazine, 150, **152**, **154**, 221
Fluvoxamine, 169, 226
Folate, **89**, 91, **119**, 171
Forensic Assertive Community Treatment
　teams, 254
Formal thought disorder (disorganized
　thinking), 43

Fragile X mental retardation protein
　(FMRP), 107
Frontal cortex, 114, 129
Functional candidate genes, 82
Functional recovery, 23–24

GABA (γ-Aminobutyric acid) system
　autoantibodies and, 92
　dysregulation of, **106**, **109**, 111–112, 114
　neuropathology of, 129, 130, 132–133,
　　135–136
　NMDA and, 133
GABA$_A$ (type A), 92, 132
GABA membrane transporter (GAT-1), 130,
　132
GAF (Global Assessment of Functioning)
　Scale, 21
Gender differences
　age at onset, 4, 15
　as antipsychotic response factor, 167
　anxiety symptoms and, 220
　genetic epidemiology, 5
　prevalence of schizophrenia and, 3, 4
　suicide risk and, 48, 219
　tardive dyskinesia and, 160
　violent behavior and, 9
Gene annotation, 88
Genetic counseling, 96
Genetic factors, 80–87, 93–97
　adoption studies, 81
　endophenotypes, 82
　environmental risk factors *versus*, 80–82,
　　87–88, 91, 93, 97
　epigenetics, 81, 93–96, 107–108, **107**
　familial studies, 80–82, **81**, 207
　genome-wide association studies, 82,
　　83–88, **85**, 94–97, 106–107
　for obesity, 215
　paternal age, 5, 93
　pathophysiological theories on, 83–87,
　　84–85, 106–108, **107**
　postmortem studies of, 107–108, **107**
　risk genes, 82–83, 96–97, 118
　of substance use disorders, 207
　twin studies, 80–82, **81**, 106–107, 207
Genetic loci, 82, 83–84, 94–95, 106–107
Genome-wide association studies (GWAS),
　82, 83–88, **85**, 94–97, 106–107
Geriatric patients, 128, 160, 161
Gestational diabetes, 88, 168
Glia and glial markers, 127–128

Glial fibrillary acidic protein (GFAP), 127–128
Global Assessment of Functioning (GAF) Scale, 21
Glucose abnormalities (side effect), 155, 156, 157, **161**
Glutamate system
circuit models and, 106, 111–112
dendritic spine density and, 130
drugs targeting, 14, 170–171
environmental risk factors for, 92, 117–118
genetic models and, **106**, **107**
molecular models and, 111–112
neuropathology of, 133–134
risk genes of, 83, **85**, 96
Glutamic acid decarboxylase 67 (GAD$_{67}$), 132, 136
Glutathione, 170–171
Glycine, 170
Grandiose delusions, 37
GRIN2A (glutamate ionotropic receptor NMDA type subunit 2A gene), 96
Grooved Pegboard test, 46
Guanine, 94–95
Guilt, delusions of, 37
Gustatory hallucinations, 37
GWAS (genome-wide association studies), 82, 83–88, **85**, 94–97, 106–107

Hallucinations
acculturative stress and, 56
as active-phase symptom, 45
as antipsychotic response factor, 167
differential diagnosis for, 38
epidemiology of, 37–38
etiology for, 38–39
management of, 149, 173–174
pathophysiological theories on, 115
suicidal behavior and, 219
treatment of, 150
Haloperidol, 150, **152**, **154**
adverse effects of, 153, 167
dopamine system and, 134–135
for dystonia management, 159
neurobiological effects of, 134–135
for women of reproductive age, 168
HCN1 (hyperpolarization activated cyclic nucleotide gated potassium channel 1 gene), 96
Headaches, 157

Head circumference, 88
Hepatic impairment, 155
Herpes simplex virus (HSV), 5, **89**, 91, 219
High-potency antipsychotics, 153, 159
Hippocampus, 114, 115–116, 129, 130, 131
Histone modification, 94, 95, 107, **107**
Histopathology, 127–132
glia and glial markers, 127–128
neuronal somal size, 131
neurons and neuronal distribution, 128–129
neuropil markers, 129–131
perineuronal nets (PNNs), 131–132
synaptic markers, 129–131. *See also* Synaptic transmission
HLA (human leukocyte antigen) locus, 82, **85**, 86
Homelessness, 251, 254, 255–258, 264
Homocysteine, **89**, 91, 171
Homovanillic acid, 42
Hopelessness, feelings of, 48
Hormone replacement therapy, 163
Hospitalization
alternatives to, 252–255, 262–263
clozapine efficacy and reduction of, 153
posttraumatic stress disorder and, 48
substance use and, 27
for suicidal behavior, 220
as suicide risk factor, 48
symptoms related to, 44
transitioning from, 256–258
Hostility, 149, 153, 158, 168–169, 170
HSV (herpes simplex virus), 5, **89**, 91, 219
Human leukocyte antigen (HLA) locus, 82, **85**, 86
Hyaluronan, 131
Hyperdopaminergia, 134–135
Hyperprolactinemia. *See* Prolactin elevation
Hyperthermia, 159–160
Hypodopaminergia, 134–135
Hypoglutamatergia, 134
Hypotension (side effect), 151, **152**, 153, 155, 157

IAP2 (International Association for Public Participation), 274, **275**
Iatrogenic negative symptoms, 41
ICM (intensive case management), 252, 263–264
IDDT (integrated dual disorder treatment), 209, **209**, 252, 254, 260–262, **262**

Illness management and recovery (IMR), 195–197
  description, 195–196
  goals and treatment principles, 185, 196
  implications for clinical practice, 197
  intervention rationale, 195
  research support, 196–197
Iloperidone, **152**, 157, 210, 214
Imipramine, 42, 210, 221, 226
Immigrants. *See* Migration status
Indigenous populations, 55
Individual placement support, 193–195
Infections, 5–6, 88, **89**, 90–91, **119**
Inflammation
  as environmental risk factor, 5–6, **90**, **119**
  management of, 172–173
  negative symptoms and, 42
  pathophysiological theories on, 111–113
Influenza virus, 5, 90–91
Insomnia, 156, 157
Institutionalization, 256–258
Integrated dual disorder treatment (IDDT), 209, **209**, 252, 254, 260–262, **262**
Intensive case management (ICM), 252, 263–264
Interleukin 6, 118
International Association for Public Participation (IAP2), 274, **275**
Interviews, 63–71, **64–67**, **69**
Involuntary treatment decisions, 278
IQ, 13, 46
IREB2 (iron-responsive element–binding protein 2 gene), 85
Iron, 6, 85, **89**, 91

"Jumping-to-conclusions" bias, 39–40

Ketamine, 111
Kraepelin, Emil
  on course of schizophrenia, 16, 28
  on cross-cultural variation, 54–55
  on diagnosis of schizophrenia, 15, 17, 20
  on end state of schizophrenia, 17
  on full recovery, 24
  on prognosis of schizophrenia, 18, 20
  "Vergleichende Psychiatrie" "Comparative Psychiatry," 54
Kynurenic acid, 111–112, 118

LAI (long-acting injectable) antipsychotic medications, **154**, 166, 210

Lamotrigine, 226
Late-onset schizophrenia, 4, 44
Latinos
  acculturative stress and, 56–57
  diagnosis rates and, 62–63
  quality of care and, 63
  symptom manifestation and, 61
Latitude of birth, as risk factor, 6, **89**
Law enforcement collaborations, 252, 264–265
Lecticans, 131
Leucine-rich, glioma inactivated 1 (LGI1) receptor, 92
Life expectancy, 8
Linkage studies, 82
Link proteins, 131
Lipid abnormalities (side effect), 155, 156, 157, **161**, 162
Liraglutide, 216
Lithium, 149, 169
Liver disease, 155
Living arrangements, 48, 50, 192, 252, 256–257
Locus coeruleus, 115–116
Long-acting injectable (LAI) antipsychotic medications, **154**, 166, 210
Lorazepam, 160
Low birth weight, 88
Low-potency antipsychotics, 151
Loxapine (oral), **152**
Lurasidone, **152**, 156

Major depressive disorder
  as co-occurring disorder, 217–218
  differential diagnosis, 36, 38, 45
Malnutrition (maternal), 88, **89**, 91, 94
Manic-depressive insanity, 15
MAPK3 (mitogen-activated protein kinase 3 gene), 85
Marijuana. *See* Cannabis use
Maternal risk factors
  infections during pregnancy, 5–6, 88, **89**, 90–91, **119**
  inflammation, 5–6, **119**
  malnutrition, 88, **89**, 91, 94
Medium-potency antipsychotics, 151–153
Medium spiny neurons (MSNs), 85–86
Men. *See* Gender differences
Metabolic side effects, 161–162, **161**. *See also* Diabetes; Lipid abnormalities; Weight gain
Metabolic syndrome, 156

Metabotropic glutamate receptor 5 (mGluR5), 92
Metformin, 162, **206**, 216–217
Methadone, 210
3-methoxy-4-hydroxy-phenylglycol, 42
Methylazoxymethanol acetate, 117
N-methyl-D-aspartate (NMDA) system
    cognitive deficits and, 116
    drugs targeting, 170–171
    environmental risk factors and, 92, 117–118
    GABA system and, 114, 133
    glutamate system and, 96, **109**, 111–112, 118, 133–134
    negative symptoms and, 42, 43
    pyramidal cells and, 133
    risk genes and, 107
Mexican Americans, 61
MFPT (multifactorial polygenic threshold) model, 87
mGluR5 (metabotropic glutamate receptor 5), 92
mHealth, 279
Microglia, 128
microRNA-137 (miR-137), 131
microRNAs (miRNAs), 94, 95–96, 107, 131
Midbrain, 109–110, 111, 114, 115–116
Migration status
    acculturative stress and, 56
    Cultural Formulation Interview, 63–71
    outcomes and, 53–54
    as risk factor, 5, 59–61, **90**, 93, 117
Minorities. *See* Migration status; Race and ethnicity
Mitogen-activated protein kinase 3 gene (*MAPK3*), 85
Mobile Integration Teams (MITs), 264
Molecular models, 108–113, **109**
    dopamine models, 108–110
    endocannabinoid models, **109**, 112–113
    GABA (γ-Aminobutyric acid) models, **109**, 112
    glutamate models, **109**, 111–112
Mood stabilizers, 149
Mood symptoms. *See* Anxiety symptoms and disorders; Depressive symptoms and disorders
Mortality risk
    after first episode, 15, 24
    clozapine efficacy for reduction of, 153
    suicidal behavior and, 8, 48, 219

tobacco use disorder and, 211
    unnatural death rates, 8, 24
mRNA, 130
MSNs (medium spiny neurons), 85–86
Multifactorial polygenic threshold (MFPT) model, 87
Mumps, 6

NAC (N-acetylcysteine), 170–171
NADPH-d (nicotinamide adenine dinucleotide phosphate–diaphorase), 129
Naltrexone, 210–211, 216
National Alliance on Mental Illness, 283
National Institute for Health and Care Excellence (NICE), 188
National Institute of Mental Health (NIMH), 40, 97, 150, 151–152, 195, 259
National Institute of Mental Health Measurement and Treatment Research to Improve Cognition in Schizophrenia (NIMH MATRICS), 40, 45–46
National Latino and Asian American Study (NLAAS), 56
Natural history, 13–34
    chronic, symptomatic course, 16–17, 21
    course, after first episode, 15–23
    course, with antipsychotics, 20–21
    course, without antipsychotics, 15–17, **19**
    end state, with antipsychotics, 21–23, **22**, 24
    end state, without antipsychotics, 15, 17–20, **19**, 23, 24
    mortality risk, 8, 15, 24, 48, 153, 219
    outcome ratings, 21–23, **22**
    prognostic factors, 25–27
    psychoeducation on, 28–29
    recovery from schizophrenia, 18–20, **19**, 23–24
    stages of schizophrenia, 13–15, 44–45, 47, 217
Nausea, 156, 157
NAVIGATE services, 259
NCAM (neural cell adhesion molecule), 130
Negative symptoms, 40–42
    as active-phase symptom, 45
    descriptions, 40–41, 43
    differential diagnosis, 41, 47, 218
    dopamine system and, 42, 116, 134
    epidemiology of, 41
    etiology for, 42
    functional outcomes, 42

Negative symptoms (*continued*)
　management of, 149, 157, 166, 169
　pathophysiological theories on, 113–114,
　　115, 116
　in prodromal phase, 14
　psychosocial therapies for, 186–188
　treatment of, 156
　violent behavior and, 50
Negative thought disorder, 43
Neural cell adhesion molecule (NCAM), 130
Neuregulin 1 gene (*NRG1*), 82
Neurobiology, 127–145
　dopamine system, 134–135
　further recommendations, 136–137
　GABA system, 129, 130, 132–133,
　　135–136
　glia and glial markers, 127–128
　glutamate system, 133–134
　histopathology, 127–132
　neurochemistry, 132–136
　neuronal somal size, 131
　neurons and neuronal distribution, **107**,
　　108, 128–129, 131
　neuropil and synaptic markers, 129–131
　neurotrophins, 135–136
　perineuronal nets (PNNs), 131–132
　of substance use disorders, 208
Neurocognitive deficits. *See* Cognitive
　symptoms
Neuroleptic malignant syndrome (NMS),
　159–160
Neuromodulation, 173–174
Neuronal somal size, 131
Neurons and neuronal distribution, **107**, 108,
　128–129, 131
Neuropil markers, 129–131
Neuroplasticity, 106, 110, 116, 118, 189
Neurotrophins, 135–136
Niacin, 171
NICE (National Institute for Health and
　Care Excellence), 188
Nicotinamide adenine dinucleotide
　phosphate–diaphorase (NADPH-d),
　129
Nicotine dependence. *See* Tobacco use
　disorder
Nicotine replacement therapy (NRT), 212,
　213–214
NIDA-Modified ASSIST, 208
NIMH (National Institute of Mental Health),
　40, 97, 150, 151–152, 195, 259

NIMH MATRICS (National Institute of
　Mental Health Measurement and
　Treatment Research to Improve
　Cognition in Schizophrenia), 40
NLAAS (National Latino and Asian
　American Study), 56
NMDA receptor coagonists, 170
NMDA system. *See* N-methyl-D-aspartate
　system
NMS (neuroleptic malignant syndrome),
　159–160
Noradrenaline, 42
NOTCH4 (Notch receptor 4 gene), 82
NRG1 (neuregulin 1 gene), 82
NRT (nicotine replacement therapy), 212,
　213–214
Nucleus accumbens, 111, 114, 129
Nutrition (maternal), 88, **89**, 91, 94

Obesity, 214–217
　detection of, 215
　management of, **206**, 215–217
　overview, **206**, 214–215
　prevalence of, 8, 214
　risk factors for. *See* Weight gain
Obsessive-compulsive disorder (OCD), 48,
　205, **206**
Obsessive-compulsive symptoms (OCS) and
　disorder (OCD), 224–226
Obstetric complications, 88, **89**, 94, 167
Occupational functioning, 46
ODR (Opening Doors to Recovery), 264
Olanzapine, 155–156
　adverse effects of, **152**, 155, 160, 165, 167,
　　214
　dosage, **152**, **154**
　efficacy of, 164–165
　OCD and OCS management with, 226
　route of administration, **154**, 155–156
　substance use disorder management and,
　　210
　suicidal behavior management with,
　　220
Olfactory hallucinations, 37
Omega-3 fatty acids, 14, 172
Onset, 14–15
　age ranges, 4, 13–14, 35–36
　gender differences, 4, 15
　neuronal pruning and, 86
　OCS and OCD correlations, 224–225
　stages, 13–15

OnTrackNY, 260
Opening Doors to Recovery (ODR), 264
Opioid agonists and antagonists, 211
Opioid use, 206–207, 210. *See also* Substance
   use disorders
Oral hypoesthesia, 157
Orlistat, 216
Orthodenticle homeobox 2 (OTX2), 131–132
Orthostatic hypotension, 151, **152**, 153, 155,
   157
Over-the-counter adjunctive
   pharmaceuticals, 170–173. *See also*
   specific products by name

Paliperidone, **152**, **154**, 155, 163, 210
Panic attacks and disorders, 47, **206**, 221
Panic Disorder Severity Scale (PDSS), 221
PANSS (Positive and Negative Syndrome
   Scale), 221
Parahippocampal gyrus, 43
Paranoia, 41, 48
Parkinsonism, 41, 158, 159, 161
Parkinson's disease, 157
Partial hospitalization programs (PHPs),
   252, 262–263
Parvalbumin (PV) neurons
   density of, 112, 117, 130
   GABA system neuropathology and,
      132–133
   glutamate system neuropathology and,
      133–134
   perineuronal nets and, 131–132
Paternal age, 5, **90**, 93
Pathophysiological theories, 105–126
   approaches, 105–106, **106**
   circuit models, **106**, 113–117, **115**
   for developmental risk factors, **106**,
      117–119
   for environmental risk factors, **106**,
      117–119, **119**
   further recommendations, 119–120
   genetic factors, 83–87, **84–85**
   genetic models, 106–108, **106–107**
   molecular models, **106**, 108–113, **109**
Patient-centered care (PCC), 273–287
   balancing patient and family needs, 277
   defined, 273
   historical and sociopolitical context of,
      276–277
   levels of, **274**
   patient-centered design (PCD), 279

peer support and peer-led interventions,
   280–283
performance monitoring and evaluation,
   279
principles, values, and best practices for,
   273–276, **274–275**
shared decision making (SDM), 277–279
Patient-centered design (PCD), 279
PCL (PTSD Checklist), 223–224
PDSS (Panic Disorder Severity Scale), 221
Peer support and peer-led interventions,
   254, 280–283
Peer to Peer (intervention), 281
Pellagra, 171
Perineuronal nets (PNNs), 131–132
Perphenazine, 150, **152**
   adverse effects of, 151–152
   efficacy of, 150
   lower weight gain liability of, 216
Persecutory delusions, 37, 40
Personalized Recovery Oriented Services
   (PROS) programs, 263
PFC. *See* Prefrontal cortex
PGRS (polygenic risk score), 88
Pharmacological therapies, 149–183. *See also*
   specific drugs
   antidepressants, 169. *See also*
      Antidepressants
   antiepileptic drugs, 149, 169–170
   antipsychotic medications, 150–168. *See*
      also Antipsychotic medications
   benzodiazepines, 168–169. *See also*
      Benzodiazepines
   further recommendations, 174
   lithium, 149, 169
   over-the-count adjunctives, 170–173
Phencyclidine, 111
PHPs (partial hospitalization programs),
   252, 262–263
Pimavanserin, 157
Placental abruption, 88
PNNs (perineuronal nets), 131–132
"Polyenviromic" score, 93
Polygenic risk score (PGRS), 88
Polypharmacy, 165, 218
Positional candidate genes, 82
Positive and Negative Syndrome
   Scale (PANSS), 221
Positive symptoms, 37–40. *See also*
   Delusions; Hallucinations
   differential diagnosis for, 38

Positive symptoms (*continued*)
dopamine system and, 40, 115, 134
epidemiology of, 37–38
etiology for, 39–40
as first-rank symptom, 37
management of, 149, 166
negative symptom resemblance, 41
pathophysiological theories on, 113–116, **115**
psychosocial therapies for, 186–188
suicide risk and, 48
treatment of, 150, 156
Positive thought disorder, 43
Postmortem studies, 107–108, **107**
Posttraumatic stress disorder, 47–48, **206**, 223–224
Precentral gyrus, 43
Preeclampsia, 88
Prefrontal cortex (PFC). *See also* Dorsal prefrontal cortex
developmental risk factors and, 118–119
environmental risk factors and, 117
GABA system and, 132–133
GFAP-reactive astroglia, 128
glutamate system and, 111, 134
perineuronal nets and, 132
positive symptoms and, 115–116
Pregnancy precautions, 168
Premorbid phase, 13
Prenatal Determinants of Schizophrenia study, 5
Prenatal exposures and stress, as risk factor, 5–6, 88–90, **89–90**
Presentation. *See* Cultural variations; Natural history; Psychopathology
Pressured speech, 43
Primary negative symptoms, 40–41
Prodromal phase, 14, 44–45, 47, 217
Progestogen, 163
Prognosis
disorganization symptom and, 44
other factors affecting, 26–27
substance use's effect on, 27
with treatment, 25–26
Prolactin elevation
antipsychotics with high risk of, 155, 156, 168
antipsychotics with low risk of, 156, 157
diagnosis of, 163
management of, 163
monitoring for, 163
overview, **152**
pathophysiology of, 163
pregnancy precautions and, 168
Prolonged exposure and cognitive processing therapy, 224
Promethazine, 159
PROS (Personalized Recovery Oriented Services) programs, 263
Pruning
complement activity, 107, **107**
synaptic, 86, 119
PsychENCODE initiative, 97
Psychoeducation, 197–200
coordinated specialty care and, 258
description, 197–198
for families, 28–29, 199, 281–282
goals and treatment principles, 196, 198–199, **198**
implications for clinical practice, 199–200
intervention rationale, 197
for patients, 28–29, 198–199
prognosis and, 26
research support, 199
for suicidal behavior, 220
Psychopathology, 35–52. *See also* Diagnosis; Symptoms
anxiety symptoms, 47–48
cognitive symptoms, 45–46
complications of schizophrenia, 48–50. *See also* Substance use disorders; Suicidal behavior; Violence and violent behavior
core symptoms, 37–44. *See also* Core symptoms
depression, 46–47
diagnostic criteria, 35–36, 44–45
further recommendations, 50
Psychosis. *See* Positive symptoms
Psychosocial and rehabilitative therapies, 185–204
approaches to, 185
cognitive-behavioral therapy, 186–188
cognitive remediation, 188–191
for depression management, 218–219
further recommendations, 200
illness management and recovery, 195–197
psychoeducation, 197–200
social skills training (SST), 191–193
supported employment, 193–195
for tobacco use disorder management, 212–213

Psychotherapy, 14
Psychotic agitation, 158
Psychotic disorder due to medical conditions, 45
Psychotic-like symptom evaluation, 55–58
PTSD Checklist (PCL), 223–224
Public Participation Spectrum schema, 274, **275**
PV neurons. *See* Parvalbumin neurons
Pyramidal cells, 86, 130–131, 132–133

Quetiapine, **152**, 156, 210, 218, 221

Race and ethnicity
    diagnosis rates and, 62–63
    illness manifestations and, 54–55
    outcomes and, 53–54
    quality of care and, 63, 276–277
    as risk factor, 4–5, 59–61, **90**, 93
    routes of entry into mental health care and, 61–62
    symptom manifestation and, 61
RAISE (Recovery After an Initial Schizophrenia Episode) projects, 259
Recovery-Oriented Decisions for Relatives' Support (REORDER) intervention, 283
Rehabilitative therapies. *See* Psychosocial and rehabilitative therapies
Relapses
    depressive symptoms and, 217
    illness management and recovery (IMR) and, 196
    prevention with antipsychotic medications, 28–29, 163–164, 253–254, 258–260
    prevention with psychosocial therapies, 196
    prior to antipsychotic medications, 16–17
    route of antipsychotic administration and, 166
Religious delusions, 37
Renal failure, 159
REORDER (Recovery-Oriented Decisions for Relatives' Support) intervention, 283
Repetitive transcranial magnetic stimulation (rTMS), 173–174, 214, 226
Residual symptoms, 44, 45
Rey Total Recall test, 46
Rhabdomyolysis, 159
Rheumatoid arthritis, 92
Rh incompatibility, 88

Rigidity, 41, 150
Risk factors, 4–7. *See also* Developmental risk factors; Environmental risk factors; Genetic factors
Risk genes, 82–83, 96–97, 118
Risperidone, **154**, 155
    adverse effects of, **152**, 163
    depression management with, 218
    efficacy of, 164–165
    for OCD and OCS management, 226
    substance use disorder management and, 210
RNA (noncoding), 95–96
rTMS (repetitive transcranial magnetic stimulation), 173–174, 214, 226
Rubella, 91
Rural birth and residence, 6–7, 92

SAMHSA (Substance Abuse and Mental Health Services Administration), 259, 280
Sarcosine, 170
Schizoaffective disorder
    antipsychotic response factors, 167
    depressive symptoms and, 46–47
    as differential diagnosis, 45
    negative symptoms and, 41
Schizophrenia. *See also* Co-occurring disorders and conditions
    causes. *See* Etiology
    definition, 15–16
    diagnostic criteria. *See* Diagnosis
    differential diagnosis, 45
    pathophysiology. *See* Neurobiology; Pathophysiological theories
    presentation. *See* Cultural variations; Epidemiology; Natural history; Psychopathology
    risk factors, 4–7. *See also* Developmental risk factors; Environmental risk factors; Genetic factors
    treatment and rehabilitative therapies. *See* Antipsychotic medications; Family-centered care; Patient-centered care; Pharmacological therapies; Psychosocial and rehabilitative therapies; Service delivery; Somatic therapies
Schizophrenia Patient Outcomes Research Team (PORT), 155, 164, 165, 170, 188, 254, 282

Schizophrenogenic mother, 276
SDM (shared decision making), 200, 211, 217, 258–260, **259**, **274**, 277–279
SE. *See* Supported employment
Season of birth, as risk factor, 6, **89**
Secondary negative symptoms, 40–41
Second-generation antipsychotic medications, 151, 209–210
Sedation (side effect)
　antipsychotics with low risk of, 156
　antipsychotics with risk of, 151, **152**, 153, 155, 156, 157
　depression differential, 218
Seizures, 163
Selective serotonin reuptake inhibitors (SSRIs), 169
Selfhood, cultural identity and, 53
Self-medication hypothesis, 207–208
Semistructured peer-led (or family-led) interventions, 281
Sequential Intercept Model, 265
D-serine, 170
Serotonin 5-HT$_{1A}$ receptors, 157, 225
Serotonin receptors, 42, 82, 151, 157, 225
Serotonin reuptake inhibitors (SRIs), 222–223, 226
Service delivery, 251–271. *See also* Family-centered care; Patient-centered care
　approaches to, 251–252
　assertive community treatment, 252–256, **253**, 262
　community navigation models, 264
　community support teams, 264
　coordinated specialty care, 26, 258–260, **259**
　critical time intervention, 256–258, **257**
　cultural considerations, 61–62, 63
　day treatment models, 262–263
　further recommendations, 265–266
　integrated dual disorder treatment, 209, **209**, 254, 260–262, **262**
　intensive case management, 263–264
　law enforcement/criminal justice collaborations, 264–265
　partial hospitalization programs, 262–263
Shared decision making (SDM), 200, 211, 217, 258–260, **259**, **274**, 277–279
Shock therapy, 18, 25
Single nucleotide polymorphisms (SNPs), 82, 87–88, 94, 106
Sleep spindles, 114

Smoking. *See* Tobacco use disorder
SNAP-25 (synaptosomal nerve-associated protein 25), 130
Social anxiety disorder (social phobia), **206**, 222–223
Social cost, 253
Social Interaction Anxiety Scale, 222
Socialization impairments. *See* Cognitive symptoms
Social phobia (social anxiety disorder), **206**, 222–223
Social Phobia Scale, 222
Social skills training (SST), 185, 191–193, 196, 222
Social withdrawal, 149
Socioeconomic status, 7, 58, 59–61, 68, **90**, 92, **119**
Sodium benzoate, 170
Somatic delusions, 37
Somatic hallucinations, 37
Somatic therapies, 173–174
Somnolence, 157
Specialized Treatment Early in Psychosis (STEP) program, 260
Spontaneous improvement or recovery, 15, 17, 20, 28
SRIs (serotonin reuptake inhibitors), 222–223, 226
SSRIs (selective serotonin reuptake inhibitors), 169
SST (social skills training), 185, 191–193, 196, 222
Stages, of schizophrenia, 13–15, 44–45, 47, 217
STAT6 (signal transducer and activator of transcription 6 gene), 85
Statistical Manual for the Use of Institutions for the Insane, 18
Stem cells, 97
STEP (Specialized Treatment Early in Psychosis) program, 260
Stigmatization, 63, 70, 186, 197–200, 282
Stress
　DNA methylation and, 94
　endocannabinoid models on, 112–113
　prenatal, as risk factor, 88–90, **90**
　urban residence and, 6–7, **90**, 92
Stress-vulnerability model, 196, 207
Striatum, 114, 116, 134
Substance Abuse and Mental Health Services Administration (SAMHSA), 259, 280

Substance-induced psychotic disorders, 45
Substance use disorders (SUDs)
    as co-occurring disorder, 8–9, 206–214,
        206
    detection of, 208
    management of, **206**, 208–211, **209**, 212–
        214, 252. *See also* Integrated dual
        disorder treatment
    overview, 206–208
    prevalence of, 49
    prognosis affected by, 27
    prognosis and, 27, 49
    as risk factor, 8–9, 27, **89**, 91
    suicidal behavior and, 48–49, 219
    violent behavior and, 9, 50
Substantia nigra, 114, 134–135
Suffolk County Mental Health Project study,
    23
Suicidal behavior
    akathisia and, 158
    anxiety symptoms and, 221
    clozapine efficacy for reduction of, 153
    as comorbid condition, 8, 48–49, 219–220
    depression and, 47, 217, 219–220
    detection of, 219–220
    management of, 149, 218, 219–220
    OCS and OCD correlations, 224
    overview, 219
    posttraumatic stress disorder and, 48
    prevalence of, 219
    risk of, 48–49
Sulpiride, 163
Supported employment (SE)
    description, 193
    goals and treatment principles, 185, 193
    implications for clinical practice, 195
    intervention rationale, 193
    research support, 194–195
Symptomatic recovery, 24
Symptoms
    acculturative stress, 56
    active-phase syndrome pattern, 44–45
    anxiety symptoms, 47–48
    cognitive symptoms, 14, 45–46. *See also*
        Cognitive symptoms
    core symptoms, 37–44. *See also*
        Disorganization; Negative
        symptoms; Positive symptoms
    cross-cultural variations, 56–57, 60–61
    depression, 46–47
    further recommendations, 50

Synaptic transmission
    pathophysiology of, 107–108, **107**,
        109–110, **109**
    studies on, 83, **85**
    synaptic markers, 129–131
    synaptic pruning, 86, 119
Synaptophysin, 130
Synaptosomal nerve-associated protein 25
    (SNAP-25), 130
Systemic lupus erythematosus, 91

Tachycardia (side effect), 153, 163
Tardive dyskinesia (TD)
    after antipsychotic withdrawal, 160
    antipsychotics with high risk of, 150, 153,
        157
    antipsychotics with low risk of, 150, 155,
        160
    diagnosis, 160
    incidence of, 160
    management of, 160
    monitoring for, 161
    onset of, 158, 160
    overview, **152**
Tardive dystonia, 158, 160
Tardive syndromes, 160
Targeted, intermittent therapy with, 164
TCL (Training in Community Living), 252–253
Telephone tobacco quit lines, 212–213
Temporal lobe, 113–114
tES (transcranial electrical stimulation), 174
Testosterone replacement therapy, 163
Tetrabenazine, 160
Tetrahydrocannabinol (THC), 211
Thalamic reticular nucleus (TRN), 114
Thalamus, 114, 129
L-theanine, 171
Therapies. *See* Pharmacological therapies;
    Psychosocial and rehabilitative
    therapies; Service delivery; Somatic
    therapies
Thioridazine, 150
Thought broadcasting, 37
Thought disorder (disorganized thinking),
    43
Thyroid disease, 91
Tiagabine, 112
TLEQ (Traumatic Life Events
    Questionnaire), 223
TMS (transcranial magnetic stimulation),
    173–174, 214

Tobacco use disorder, 49, 94, **206**, 207, 211–214, 260

Topiramate, 216

Toxoplasma gondii, 91

Toxoplasmosis, 5

Trails A & B tests (neurocognitive tests), 46

Training in Community Living (TCL), 252–253

Transcranial electrical stimulation (tES), 174

Transcranial magnetic stimulation (TMS), 173–174, 214

Transcultural Psychiatry (journal), 55

Transitions, to community, 256–257

Transtheoretical model of IMR, 196

Trauma
  during childhood, 7, **90**, 92, 223
  DNA methylation and, 94
  posttraumatic stress disorder, 47–48, **206**, 223–224

Traumatic Life Events Questionnaire (TLEQ), 223

Treatment-resistant schizophrenia, 167–168
  antipsychotic recommendations for, 167–168, 218
  depression and, 218
  drug of choice for, 153, 155
  ECT for, 168
  trial treatment duration recommendation, 155

Treatments. *See* Pharmacological therapies; Psychosocial and rehabilitative therapies; Service delivery

Tremor, Parkinsonian, 150

Tricyclic antidepressants, 210

Trihexyphenidyl, 159

TRN (thalamic reticular nucleus), 114

Tropomyosin receptor kinase B (TrkB), 136

Twin studies, 80–82, **81**, 106–107, 207

Tyrosine hydroxylase (TH), 109, 135

Ultrahigh-risk status, 80, 114, 128, 134

Unipolar depression, 46–47

Urban birth and residence, 6–7, **90**, 92

Uterine atony, 88

Valbenazine, 160

Valproate, 170

Varenicline, 211, 212, 213–214

Ventral striatal dysfunction, 42

Ventral tegmental area (VTA), 110, 114

Veterans Affairs (VA), 195, 197, 258

Veterans Affairs/Department of Defense Clinical Practice Guideline for PTSD, 224

Violence and violent behavior, 9, 49–50

Viruses, maternal exposure to, 5–6

Visual hallucinations, 37, 39, 56–57

Vitamin B_6, 158–159

Vitamin B_{12}, 162, 171

Vitamin D, 172

Vocational rehabilitation. *See* Coordinated specialty care; Supported employment

VTA (ventral tegmental area), 110, 114

Weight gain (side effect), **152**, 161–162
  antipsychotics with high risk of, 151, 153, 155, 156, 157, 214
  antipsychotics with low risk of, 151, 153, 156, 157
  management of, 161–162, 215–217
  monitoring for, 161, 215
  pathophysiological theories on, 214–215

Wellness Recovery Action Planning (WRAP), 281

Whites, 61–63

WHO. *See* World Health Organization

Whole-genome sequencing, 82–83

Withdrawal dyskinesias, 160

Women. *See* Gender differences

Women of reproductive age, 168

Work skills. *See* Coordinated specialty care; Supported employment

World Health Organization (WHO)
  cross-national studies by, 58
  incidence cohort study, 21, **22**, 24
  long-term observation studies, 25
  on prevalence, 3

WRAP (Wellness Recovery Action Planning), 281

Ziprasidone, **152**, 156, 160, 216